W9-BTZ-919

Complex Coronary Lesions in Acute Coronary Syndromes

edited by

John A. Ambrose, MD

Professor of Medicine
Director
Cardiac Catheterization Laboratory
Mount Sinai Medical Center
New York, New York

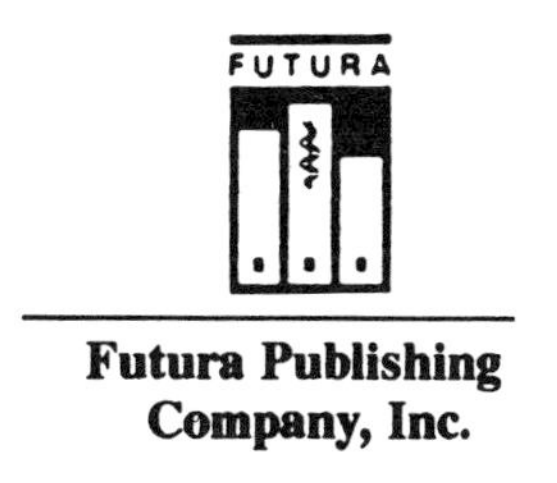

Futura Publishing Company, Inc.

Library of Congress Cataloging-in-Publication Data
Complex coronary lesions in acute coronary syndromes
/ edited by Ambrose, John A.
p. cm.
Includes bibliographical references and index.
ISBN 0-87993-6304
1. Coronary Angiography. 2. Coronary Arteriosclerosis.
3. Coronary Thrombosis.
[WG 300 C7365 1996]: OXNLM
(P): 02NLM 95-33648

Published by
Futura Publishing Company, Inc.
135 Bedford Road
Armonk, NY 10504

LC#: 95-33648
ISBN#: 0-87993-630-4

Printed in the United States of America
This book is printed on acid-free paper.

This book is dedicated
to the memory of
my father and mother,
Victor J. and Adrienne Ambrose,
who taught me at an early age
the value of intellectual pursuits.

Contributors

Philip C. Adams, MD
Consultant Cardiologist, The Royal Victoria Infirmary and the Freeman Hospital, Newcastle-upon-Tyne, United Kingdom

John A. Ambrose, MD
Professor of Medicine, Director, Cardiac Catheterization Laboratory, Mount Sinai Medical Center, New York, New York

Juan J. Badimon, PhD
Associate Professor, Department of Medicine, The Cardiovascular Institute, Mount Sinai Medical Center, New York, New York

Alberico Borghi, MD
Institute of Patologia Medica, University of Bologna, Italy

Raffaele Bugiardini MD, FACC, FESC
Chief of Hemodynamics-CCU, Institute of Patologia Medica, University of Bologna, Italy

Raymond E. Carnes, MD
Director of Pathology, Department of Cardiology, Saint Michael's Medical Center, Newark, New Jersey

James H. Chesebro, MD
Professor of Medicine, Department of Medicine, The Cardiovascular Institute, Mount Sinai Medical Center, New York, New York

Christos P. Christou, MD
Department of Cardiology, Saint Michael's Medical Center, Newark, New Jersey

Marc Cohen, MD
Chief of Cardiology, Likoff Cardiovascular Institute, Department of Medicine, Hahnemann University Hospital, Philadelphia, Pennsylvania

Srinivas Duvvuri, MD
Instructor of Medicine, Mount Sinai Medical Center, New York, New York

Ari Ezratty, MD
Cardiology Associate, Saint Francis Hospital, Roslyn, New York

Erling Falk, MD, PhD
Institute of Forensic Medicine, Odense University, Odense, Denmark
John T. Fallon, MD, PhD
Professor of Pathology, Department of Pathology, Mount Sinai Medical Center and the Cardiovascular Institute, New York, New York
Richard Gallo, MD
Research Associate, Department of Medicine, The Cardiovascular Institute, Mount Sinai Medical Center, New York, New York
Jonathan E. Goldstein, MD
Director, Cardiac Catheterization Laboratory, Department of Cardiology, Saint Michael's Medical Center, Newark, New Jersey
Jacob I. Haft, MD
Chief of Cardiology, Department of Cardiology, Saint Michael's Medical Center, Newark, New Jersey
Craig E. Hjemdahl-Monsen, MD
Assistant Professor of Medicine, New York Medical College, Westchester County Medical Center, Valhalla, New York
Douglas Israel, MD
Cardiology Associate, New Haven, Connecticut
Jonathan D. Marmur, MD
Assistant Professor of Medicine, Mount Sinai Medical Center, New York, New York
Stephen R. Ramee, MD
Director, Cardiac Catheterization Laboratory, Ochsner Hospital, New Orleans, Louisiana
Samin Sharma, MD
Assistant Professor of Medicine; Associate Director, Cardiac Catheterization Laboratory, Mount Sinai Medical Center, New York, New York
Sabino Torre, MD
Morristown Medical Hospital, Morristown, New Jersey
John Venditto, MD
Cardiology Associate, Saint Francis Hospital, Roslyn, New York
Christopher J. White, MD
Director of Invasive Cardiology, Cardiac Catheterization Laboratory, Health Care International, Glasgow, Scotland

Foreword

The acute coronary syndrome is the major contributor to death in the Western world. The understanding and management of this critical cardiovascular condition has evolved since the beginning of this century. That is, in 1910, Dr. V. Obrastzow, a Russian physician, was the first to describe the clinical presentation of acute myocardial infarction. In 1912, Dr. J. B. Herrick associated the clinical presentation of acute infarction with a thrombotic coronary occlusion. In 1959, Drs. A. P. Fletcher and S. Sherry were the first to use intravenous thrombolytic therapy. That same year, the development of selective coronary angiography by Dr. M. Sones not only served to outline the importance of coronary occlusion in myocardial infarction, but eventually led to the systematic development of coronary artery bypass graft surgery by Dr. R. Favaloro in 1970 and percutaneous transluminal coronary angioplasty by Dr. A. Gruntzig in 1979. In 1980, Dr. M. DeWood clearly demonstrated the importance of thrombotic occlusion in the early stages of myocardial infarction. In 1985, Drs. M. Davies and E. Falk described plaque disruption in a large population of patients with the acute coronary syndromes, including myocardial infarction and unstable angina. That same year, Dr. J. A. Ambrose, editor of this book, described the angiographic morphology of the complex coronary lesions in unstable angina, and in 1989, Dr. E. Braunwald developed the clinical/prognostic classification of unstable angina. Such historical landmarks have rapidly accelerated over the last 5 years during which contributions to the understanding and management of acute coronary syndromes have been seminal.

The first question, in regard to a new book, is "Is it really necessary?" A recent editorial in the *New England Journal of Medicine* by its editors, Drs. J. P. Kassirer and M. Angel, calls for caution regarding redundant publications, while a simultaneous editorial in *Nature* by the editor Dr. J. Maddox points out that each new book or journal may offer something with a special focus that can be of wide general interest. Indeed, Dr. John A. Ambrose and his collaborators at The Mount Sinai Cardiovascular Institute, together with other national and international experts, have put together an outstanding book written from the perspective of the cardiac catheterization diagnostic laboratory and the interventional cardiologist, which has special focus: the so-called complex, thrombus-containing lesions seen in a majority of patients with acute coronary syndromes.

Despite multiple authors, this is one of the few books that appears to have been written by a single author: indeed, over the years, most of the expert contributors to the book have interacted with Dr. Ambrose on a clinical or research basis; this integration of effort results in such consistency from chapter to chapter that is rewarding to the reader. The book's illustrations elucidate many concepts in the text and great care has been invested in such a didactic approach. Finally, this book even includes a chapter that integrates the most recent data through the summer of 1995.

Dr. John A. Ambrose and his collaborators have to be congratulated for what will become a "standard book" on the understanding and management of acute coronary syndromes. Such a well-integrated, didactic, and practical book will be invaluable to clinical and interventional cardiologists, investigators, and students who wish to be informed about this number-one killer in the Western world. I am proud, as a member of the team of collaborators and a friend of Dr. John A. Ambrose, to have had the opportunity to write this foreword for an outstanding contribution.

Valentin Fuster, M.D., Ph.D.
Arthur M. & Hilda A. Master
Professor of Medicine
Director Cardiovascular Institute
Vice Chairman, Department of Medicine
Mount Sinai Medical Center
New York, New York

Preface

The therapy for coronary artery disease is changing rapidly. Over the past 10 to 15 years, significant strides have been made that reduced the morbidity and mortality of coronary disease. Techniques or therapies such as thrombolytic therapy in acute myocardial infarction, antithrombotic and anticoagulant therapy in unstable angina and acute myocardial infarction and coronary bypass surgery have all been shown in randomized trials to improve survival. Central to many of these techniques and therapies has been the role and importance of coronary arteriography in defining the presence and extent of coronary artery disease. Angiography has also been essential in understanding the pathogenesis of coronary disease. The appreciation of the central importance of coronary thrombus superimposed on a disrupted atherosclerotic plaque in the pathogenesis of myocardial infarction as well as unstable angina has been made possible largely in the living patient by analysis of coronary arteriography.

The main subject of this book is the patient with an acute coronary syndrome. However, unlike many books on unstable angina or acute myocardial infarction, the book attempts to focus on the so-called complex, thrombus-containing lesions seen in a majority of these patients. Therefore, the pathology, physiology, angiographic and angioscopic findings of these lesions are discussed in the first section of the book. In the second section the medical and interventional approaches to these lesions are outlined. As the lesion separated from the patient has little practical or clinical importance, the relationship of such therapy to the clinical presentation is intertwined with the angiographic or lesional response. When the data relating complex lesions or intracoronary thrombi (vida infra) to such therapy are scant or absent, the authors have focused their comments on the clinical presentation of the patient, e.g., unstable angina, postinfarct angina, and acute myocardial infarction.

To avoid confusion, it is necessary to define the word *complex* as it is used in this book. *Complex* refers to the "acute" lesions representing plaque fissuring/disruption and thrombus found in a large number of patients with unstable angina and acute myocardial infarction. This definition should not be confused with the interventional cardiology literature definition of complex. Often, the word *complex* in interventional cardiology refers to various anatomic characteristics of a lesion or its location that may complicate the procedure. According to the American Heart Association/American College of Cardiology classification of lesions, this would be a type B_2 or a C lesion.

Finally, the distinction between a complex lesion and intracoronary thrombus should be mentioned. Due to a lack of standardization in the literature, there is no clear separation between the angiographic definitions of complex lesion and intracoronary thrombus particularly when the "culprit" lesion is <100% occluded. While these terms are not completely interchangeable (a more detailed discussion is contained in Chapter 3), several chapters refer to the presence of an intracoronary thrombus in their discussions of the subject matter. The reader should for all practical purposes consider intracoronary thrombus and complex as similiar. Therefore, angiographic lesions that possess one or more of the following characteristics are considered complex: overhanging edges, irregular borders, ulcerations, or filling defects proximal or distal to a lesion. Some of these same characteristics are utilized for a definition of intracoronary thrombus. In totally occluded vessels, when dye staining or a convex cut-off of the vessel is present, one usually refers to this as a thrombotic occlusion and not a complex lesion. However, in reality, all of the above are complex and all likely contain some amount of intracoronary thrombus formation.

In approaching a book such as this one, one may not necesarily need to read the entire book to understand the subject. Certain sections may be more appealing to some individuals than others. This is often my approach in reading medical text books. Because of this, I have maintained a little redundancy to some chapters. Sections of Chapters 3 and 4 overlap as well as Chapters 8 and 11. This redundancy gives the reader a sense of completeness in reviewing a given section.

Finally, I am indebted to the authors of the different chapters for providing their manuscripts in timely fashion. I also greatly appreciate the invaluable work of my staff, including Sonia Castro and Ram Bongu for their help in preparation of the book.

John A. Ambrose, MD

Contents

I

Pathophysiology and Dianosis

1

Pathological Considerations of Coronary Lesions in Acute Coronary Syndromes

Erling Falk, MD, PhD,
John T. Fallon, MD, PhD

Introduction

The occurrence and course of coronary atherosclerosis and ischemic heart disease (IHD) are largely unpredictable. For individuals with the same number and degree of stenoses evaluated angiographically, some live for years without any symptoms while others are severely handicapped by angina pectoris, experience life-threatening heart attacks, or die suddenly and unexpectedly. Disease severity is often equated with "number and degree of stenoses," but recent observations indicate that it is not the severity of stenosis (plaque volume) that determines the outcome, but the type of stenosis (plaque composition) and the extent of collateral development. Patients with IHD have many plaques in their coronary arteries, probably tenfold more than judged from a coronary angiogram, and survival depends much more on the common but clinically silent nonstenotic plaques than on the few stenotic ones. Stable angina is usually due to stenotic but stable or very slowly progressing lesions, while acute coronary syndromes and sudden death are usually due to sudden and rapid progression of nonstenotic lesions

From: Ambrose JA (ed): *Complex Coronary Lesions in Acute Coronary Syndromes.* © Futura Publishing Co., Inc., Armonk, NY, 1996.

due to plaque disruption, often complicated by thrombosis, with or without concomitant vasospasm.[1] Postmortem studies performed in the early 1980s revealed that unstable and dangerous plaques/stenoses could be identified angiographically due to irregular borders and/or intraluminal lucencies giving rise to a "complex" angiographic morphology.[2] A few years later, this was confirmed in vivo and culprit lesions responsible for acute coronary syndromes are now often identified on angiography.[3–5] This chapter will review and discuss the pathoanatomic features of unstable atherosclerotic plaques—the ones underlying acute coronary syndromes that often give rise to angiographically complex coronary lesions.

Atherosclerosis

The type of plaque determined by composition, consistency, vulnerability, and thrombogenicity varies considerably from patient to patient, even from plaque to plaque in the same coronary artery. There is no simple relation among plaque type, plaque volume, or stenosis severity.

Plaque Composition

Atherosclerosis is an intimal disease characterized by two main components: atheromatous material (the "gruel") and sclerotic tissue (Figure 1). The former is lipid-rich and soft, while the latter is collagen-rich and "hard," i.e., noncompliant. Lipid accumulation and monocyte/macrophage infiltration with foam cell formation are key events in the atherosclerotic process, preceded, accompanied, or followed by smooth muscle cell proliferation and matrix synthesis, causing slowly progressive luminal narrowing over years, frequently associated with dystrophic calcification. In patients with ischemic heart disease, the coronary arteries are often diffusely involved with confluent "plaquing."[6] The composition of coronary plaques varies greatly without any obvious relation to risk factors for IHD or types of ischemic syndrome.[7,8] The most voluminous plaque component is the sclerotic one, but a significant atheromatous component is usually present in culprit lesions responsible for acute coronary syndromes.[9] The sclerotic plaque component may, of course, limit coronary flow and give rise to chronic angina

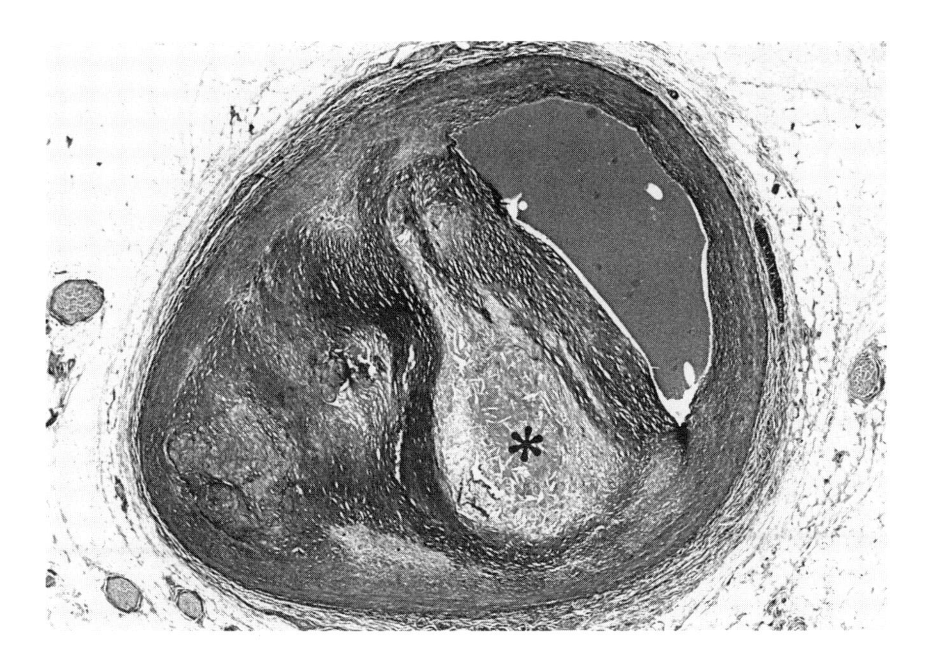

Figure 1: By definition, atherosclerosis is characterized by two main components: atheromatous "gruel" and sclerotic tissue. The atheromatous component (asterisk) is lipid-rich and dangerous because it softens plaques, making them vulnerable to rupture with subsequent thrombosis. The sclerotic collagen-rich component is, like here, usually the most voluminous plaque component. Sclerosis is, however, rather innocuous; it may, in fact, be good because it conveys stability to the lesion.

pectoris, but it may, in fact, stabilize the plaque by hardening and is, therefore, rather innocuous. On the contrary, the atheromatous component is dangerous, because it softens and destabilizes plaques making them vulnerable, i.e., prone to rupture, a process that frequently is complicated by thrombosis and responsible for the great majority of acute coronary syndromes.[10]

Plaque Vulnerability

The atheromatous gruel is separated from the vascular lumen by a fibrous cap which may be very thin and is often heavily infiltrated with foam cells of macrophage origin. The fibrous cap is often thinnest and macrophage-richest and, therefore, probably weakest at the junction between the cap and the adjacent more normal intima, also called the shoulders of the lesion.[11] Macrophages may degrade the cap matrix by phagocytosis or by secreting proteolytic enzymes, in particular plasminogen activators and matrix metalloproteinases such as stromelysin and collagenase,[12,13] which weaken the fibrous component of the cap, predisposing it to rupture. Compared with intact caps, ruptured ones contain less collagen and their tensile strength is reduced.[14] The size of the atheromatous core, the thickness of the cap, and macrophage density are possibly major determinants of plaque vulnerability.[14–16]

Plaque Rupture

Rupture of the plaque surface occurs frequently during plaque growth.[14] It is probably the most important mechanism underlying the unpredictable rapid progression of coronary lesions.[17] Most importantly, rupture and rapid plaque progression are clinically silent in the great majority of instances. Only if a major luminal thrombus evolves at the rupture site causing acute flow obstruction will a person experience new or changing symptoms. As mentioned, rupture of the plaque surface occurs most frequently where the cap is thinnest and most heavily infiltrated by macrophages and therefore probably weakest, namely at the cap's shoulders. The shoulder regions are not only weak points, they are also points where the circumferential tensile stress is probably maximal during systole.[11,18] Therefore, the propensity for plaque rupture is both a function of internal plaque changes (vulnerability) and external stresses (triggers). As the presence of a vulnerable plaque is a prerequisite for plaque rupture, vulnerability is probably more important than triggers in determining the risk of a future heart attack. If no vulnerable plaques are present in the coronary arteries, there is no rupture-prone substrate for a potential trigger to work on. This may explain why rupture/thrombus-related acute heart attacks rarely occur during exercise stress testing (thought to be a potent trigger activity) of patients with advanced coronary artery disease. A high fraction of acute coronary syndromes may be triggered by normal daily activities,[19] but only about 5% of all acute myocardial infarctions (AMI) seem to be related, or triggered by heavy physical exertion such as shoveling snow.[20–22] On the other hand, people who do not exercise regularly may have a 100-fold increased risk of an AMI during physical activity,[22] although it is unknown whether refraining from heavy physical activities reduces or only postpones heart attacks in such individuals.[20]

Plaque Thrombogenicity

The atheromatous "gruel" is not only the most vulnerable plaque component, it is also the most thrombogenic component. In vitro studies reveal that the "gruel" is up to sixfold more thrombogenic than other plaque components.[23] The substance(s) responsible for this high thrombogenicity is still unknown, but tissue factor is one candidate.[24]

Thrombosis

About ¾ of thrombi responsible for acute heart attacks are precipitated by plaque rupture whereby thrombogenic material is exposed to the flowing blood (Figure 2).[10] Minor and superficial intimal irregularities without frank rupture, i.e., no deep injury, are found beneath the rest of the thrombi, usually in combination with a severe atherosclerotic stenosis. After plaque rupture, there are three major determinants for the thrombotic response: (1) the character and extent of exposed thrombogenic plaque material (the thrombogenic substrate); (2) the degree of stenosis causing shear-induced platelet activation (local flow disturbances); and (3) the actual thrombotic-thrombolytic equilibrium (the thrombotic propensity). The latter may be modified therapeutically, substantially improving the outcome.

Platelet-Rich Thrombus

Platelets are responsible for the initial flow limitation at the rupture site, but early platelet-rich thrombus is very unstable and is easily swept away unless fibrin subsequently stabilizes the aggregated platelets. Therefore, both platelets and fibrin play a role in the evolution of a persistently occlusive coronary thrombus.

Dynamic Thrombosis

The thrombotic response to plaque rupture is dynamic: thrombosis/rethrombosis and thrombolysis/embolization occur simultaneously, with or without concomitant vasospasm, causing intermittent flow ob-

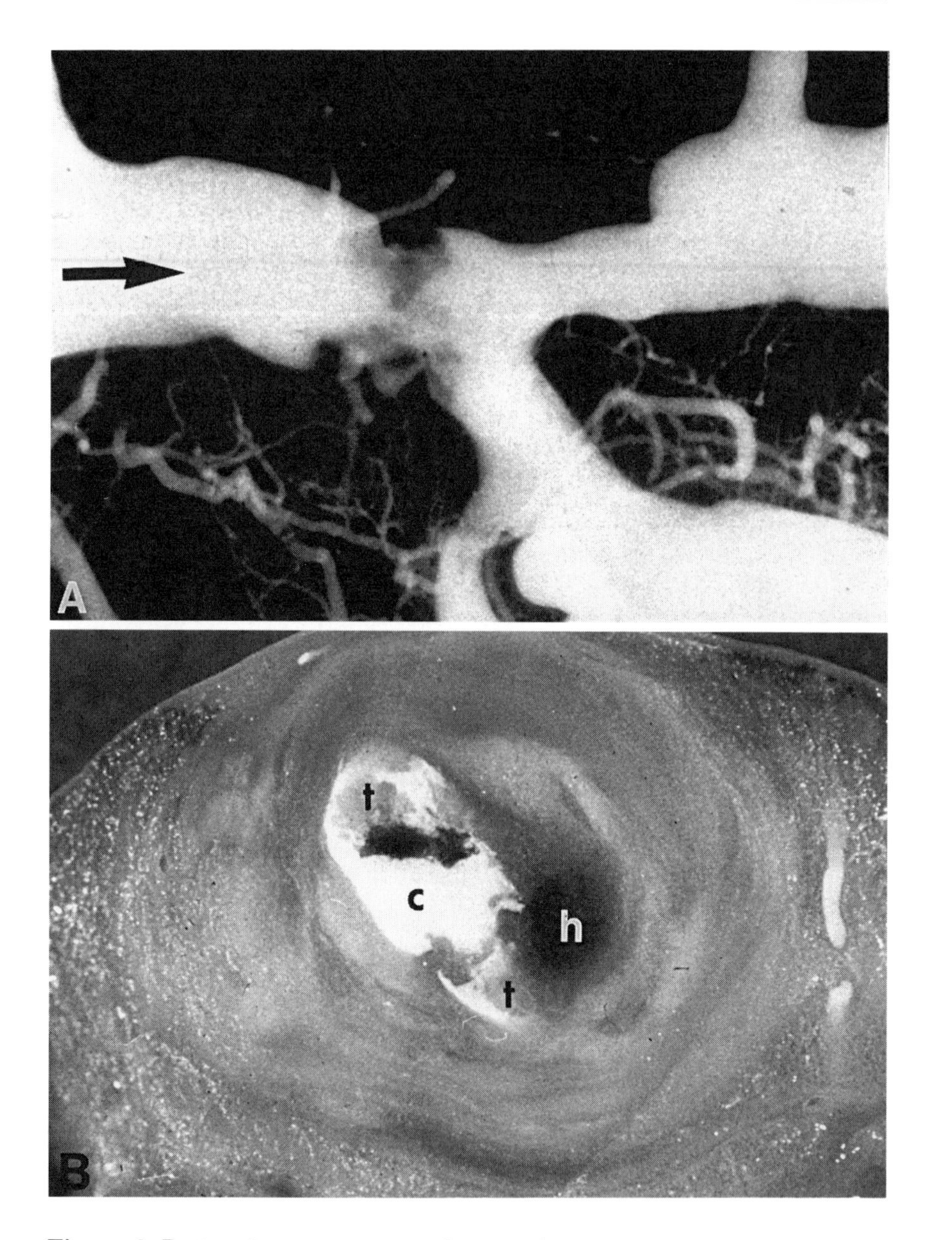

Figure 2: Postmortem coronary angiogram showing a complex lesion in the circumflex branch with irregular borders and intraluminal lucencies (**A**), and the corresponding cross-section (**B**) revealing plaque rupture with hemorrhage into the plaque (h) and nonoccluding thrombi (t) projecting into the narrowed lumen. Arrow in **A** = flow direction; c = contrast medium injected postmortem.

struction.[10,25,26] Therefore, depending on the relative amount of thrombus (labile) and plaque (fixed) in luminal obstruction, coronary morphology may change dramatically or not at all within a short period of time.

Stagnation Thrombosis

Secondary to the reduced flow caused by the white platelet-rich thrombus at the rupture site, a red, erythrocyte and fibrin-rich, low-flow thrombus may form and propagate proximally and distally, contributing to the overall thrombotic burden. This phenomenon tends to regularly occur in coronary vein bypass grafts which, compared to the native coronary arteries, are of larger caliber without side branches.[27]

Clinical Correlations

The culprit lesion responsible for stable angina is probably most often collagenous and lipid-poor (i.e., hard and stable), while ruptured lipid-rich atheromatous (i.e., soft and vulnerable) plaques with or without superimposed thrombus underlie the great majority of acute coronary syndromes.[1] As fibrous tissue, atheromatous gruel, and thrombus have different mechanical as well as thrombogenic properties, and therefore different risk profiles, these features should be taken into account when interventional procedures are considered.

Stable Angina

Davies et al. categorized the plaque type in 54 men with stable angina and found that 60% of the plaques were fibrous and 40% were lipid-rich.[28] More interestingly, all the plaques were fibrous in 15% of the patients and not a single plaque with a large lipid pool was found in as many as 1/3 of the patients. Apparently, many patients with stable angina lack the appropriate pathoanatomic substrate for plaque rupture and may, consequently, be at low risk of an acute coronary syndrome. It should be noted, however, that in the same patient individual plaques may differ significantly, and the composition of one plaque does not predict the composition of a nearby plaque in the same artery.

Acute Coronary Syndromes

Rapid plaque progression due to plaque rupture with variable degrees of plaque hemorrhage and luminal thrombosis, with or without additional vasospasm, may occur silently, or may give rise to an acute coronary syndrome in the form of primary unstable angina, non-Q-wave infarction (often but not always subendocardial), Q-wave infarction (often but not always transmural), or sudden death. The culprit lesion is frequently "dynamic" causing intermittent flow obstruction, and the clinical presentation and the outcome depend on the severity and duration of myocardial ischemia. In addition to the size of the myocardial risk area, the degree and duration of thrombotic obstruction and the available collateral flow are the chief determinants of the extent of infarction. Necrosis following coronary occlusion progresses from the subendocardium to the epicardium in a time-dependent fashion (the wavefront phenomenon), and timely reperfusion by recanalization and/or via collaterals may prevent or interrupt the process, thereby limiting infarction to the subendocardial zone and sparing myocardium at risk. Furthermore, collaterals may extend the time window for achieving myocardial salvage by reperfusion therapy.[29–31] Clinical trials have clearly shown that antithrombotic therapy reduces infarction rate and mortality in primary unstable angina with pain at rest and in non-Q-wave infarction, probably by reducing the thombotic response and preventing the progression from mural to occlusive thrombosis.[32] In Q-wave infarction, thrombolysis may open occluded arteries and conjunctive antithrombotic therapy may prevent reocclusion, improving the prognosis further. An open artery may convey benefit beyond that achieved by myocardial salvage alone.[33]

Coronary Angiography

Evaluated angiographically, coronary atherosclerosis appears to be a focal disease, and it is so in the sense that it gives rise to intimal plaques that involve the coronary tree unevenly, longitudinally as well as circumferentially. However, in many patients with IHD, the extent of "plaquing" is usually so widespread ("diffuse") that virtually no vascular segment is left entirely unaffected.[6] Coronary arteries undergo compensatory enlargement during early plaque growth and may thus preserve a normal lumen despite rather severe vessel wall disease.[34,35] Therefore, angiography usually underestimates the extent of disease as well as the degree and length of stenoses, and vascular segments judged normal (because the lumen appears normal) are frequently severely diseased.

The extent of circumferential vessel wall involvement differs from plaque to plaque and along the course of a stenotic lesion, giving rise to quite variable shapes and position of the residual lumen. On cross-section, the shape of the narrowed lumen may be round, oval, or D-shaped, but it is virtually never crescentic or slit-like in pressure-fixed specimens, unless the underlying plaque is rapidly progressing due to ruptured surface, plaque hemorrhage, and/or luminal thrombosis. Irrespective of luminal shape, the residual lumen may be positioned centrally encircled entirely by plaque or eccentrically, with or without an adjacent plaque-free arc of normal vessel wall. As plaques enlarge, more of the arterial circumference is involved, so the proportion of plaques with a normal wall segment becomes lower with increasing severity of stenosis. Eccentric plaques (asymmetric stenoses) with a plaque-free wall segment seem to have a greater vasospastic potential than that of concentric stenoses encircled entirely by rigid plaque tissue.[36]

Ruptured plaques with or without superimposed nonocclusive thrombus may be identified angiographically due to irregular luminal borders and/or intraluminal lucencies: the complex lesion (Figure 3).[2–5] Acute vasospasm frequently accompanies such lesions and may contribute to the dynamic flow obstruction. A nonocclusive thrombus formed within a stenosis is usually platelet-rich, relatively resistant to pharmacological thrombolysis (may constitute a persisting thrombogenic surface) and is easily missed angiographically because it rarely projects into the lumen (Figure 4). A free-floating tail of thrombus extending downstream poststenotically may be much more voluminous, much more labile (embolizes frequently and disappears spontaneously or rapidly with thrombolytic therapy) and is readily visualized angiographically as an intraluminal filling defect (Figure 4). Although the final and critical flow obstruction responsible for primary unstable angina usually is thrombotic in nature, on a volume basis, thrombus may constitute only a small fraction of the entire lesion—the main component being atherosclerotic in nature—giving no great potential for improvement with thrombolytic therapy (Figure 4). On the other hand, there may be a critical amount of myocardium at risk that may be salvaged if the progression of an atherothrombotic lesion to total occlusion is prevented or rapidly reversed.

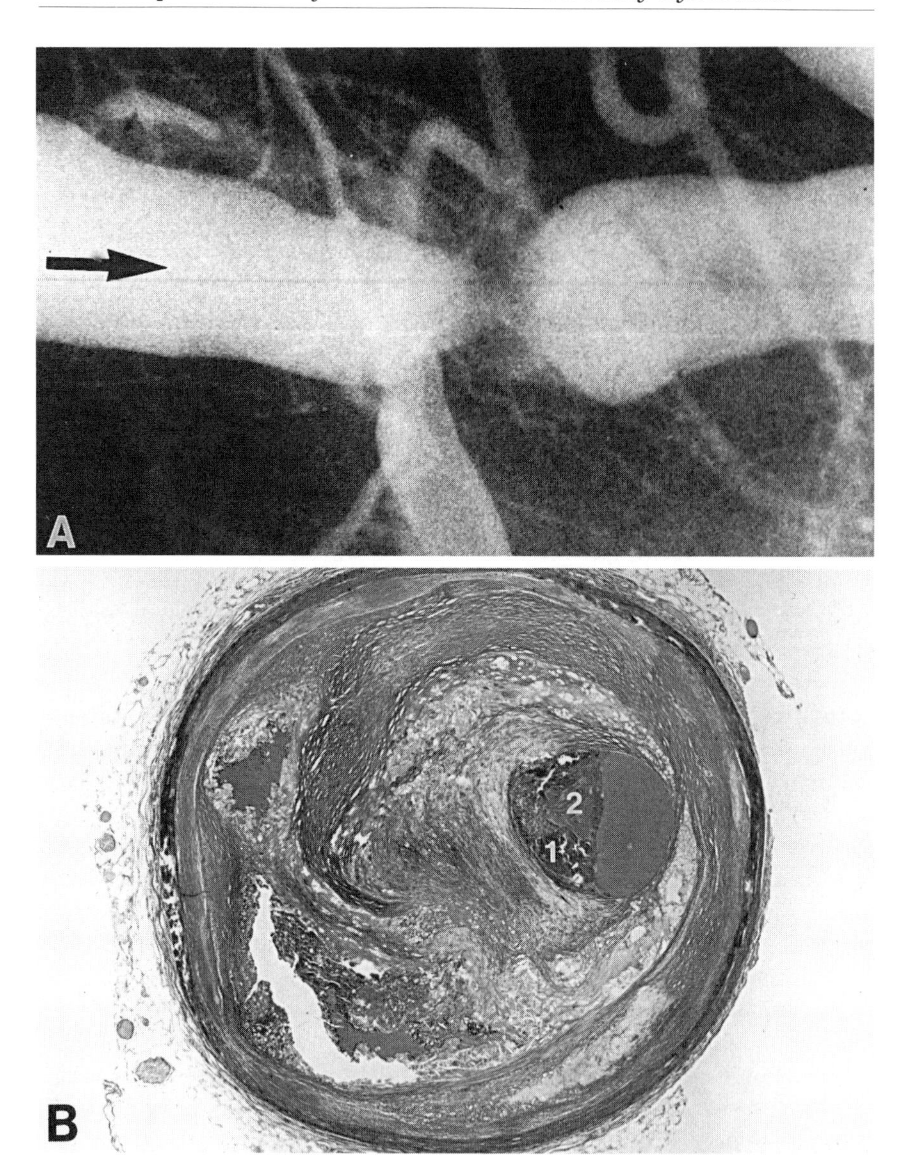

Figure 3: Postmortem coronary angiogram showing a severe stenosis in the right coronary artery **(A)**, and the corresponding cross-section **(B)**. This case illustrates that (1) a small nonoccluding thrombus may be hard to see angiographically, (2) although the final and critical flow obstruction is thrombotic in nature, the bulk of the obstruction may be atherosclerotic and, consequently, thrombolytic therapy will cause no significant angiographic improvement, and (3) the nonoccluding thrombus has a layered structure (1 and 2, in **B**), indicating episodic growth. Arrow in **A**: flow direction.

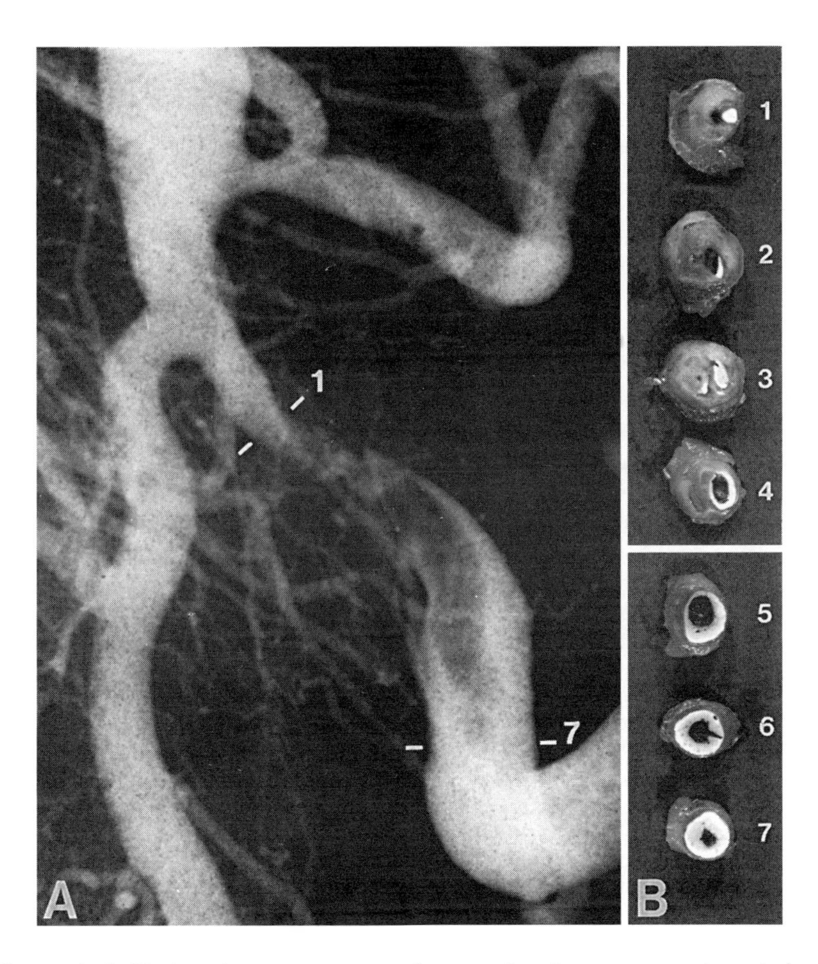

Figure 4: A. Postmortem coronary angiogram showing a severe stenosis in a circumflex sidebranch, with a prominent filling defect extending downstream. **B.** Consecutive cross-sections cut at 2-mm intervals through the lesion, revealing a severe atherosclerotic stenosis with ruptured surface and plaque hemorrhage (section #1), an adjacent nonoccluding thrombus within the stenosis (section #2), and a much more impressive free-floating tail of thrombus extending downstream poststenotically (sections #3–7). Such a thrombus tail is probably very labile and prone to embolize, explaining why poststenotic filling defects may disappear rapidly, either spontaneously or during brief lytic therapy.

Conclusions

The composition, consistency, vulnerability, and thrombogenicity of atherosclerotic plaques differ markedly, even for plaques that have been exposed to the same systemic risk factors (lipids, "smoke," blood pressure, glucose, insulin, etc.). Unfortunately, very little is known about the initiation and progressive growth of the soft lipid-rich atheromatous core—the most dangerous plaque component, being mainly responsible for vulnerability, rupture, and thrombogenicity and, therefore, underlying most acute coronary syndromes. Although the degree of stenosis determined angiographically is a risk marker for thrombotic occlusion, it is a poor predictor of acute coronary syndromes because: (1) the most severe stenoses are often "protected" by collateral vessels, and (2) vulnerability and rupture risk are not a simple function of stenosis severity.[14,37] Stenotic plaques are not necessarily vulnerable and vulnerable plaques are not necessarily stenotic. This is why rupture-prone plaques are easily missed on coronary angiograms. As soon as rupture occurs, it may give rise to a "complex" lesion that may be identified angiographically and which is associated with an increased risk of an acute clinical event.[1,3–5] In patients with stable angina, therapies directed against stenotic lesions only (angioplasty and bypass surgery) may relieve pain but do not improve prognosis to any extent, if at all, because infarction and mortality depend more on coexisting nonstenotic vulnerable plaques than on angina-producing stenotic lesions.[38] Therefore, the challenge of today is to identify and treat the vulnerable plaques—to find and treat only stenotic lesions is no longer enough. The focus of research is now shifting from the visualization of the lumen (angiography) to imaging of the vessel wall and the plaque itself (intravascular ultrasound[39]) and angioscopy,[40] for example) to get a better understanding of the biology of the disease. For effective prevention and treatment, a systemic approach that addresses all coronary plaques may prove to be most rewarding.[41]

References

1. Fuster V, Badimon L, Badimon JJ, Chesebro JH. The pathogenesis of coronary artery disease and the acute coronary syndromes: Parts 1 and 2. N Engl J Med 1992; 326:242–250, 310–318.
2. Levin D, Fallon JT. Significance of the angiographic morphology of localized coronary stenoses: histopathologic correlations. Circulation 1982; 66: 316–320.
3. Ambrose JA, Winters SL, Stern A, Eng A, Teicholz LE, Gorlin R, Fuster

V. Angiographic morphology and the pathogenesis of unstable angina pectoris. J Am Coll Cardiol 1985; 5:609–614.
4. Ambrose JA, Winters SL, Arora RR, Eng A, Riccio A, Gorlin R, Fuster V. Angiographic evolution of coronary artery morphology in unstable angina. J Am Coll Cardiol 1986; 7:472–478.
5. Gorlin R, Fuster V, Ambrose JA. Anatomic-physiologic links between acute coronary syndromes. Circulation 1986; 74:6–9.
6. Roberts WC. Diffuse extent of coronary atherosclerosis in fatal coronary artery disease. Am J Cardiol 1990; 65: 2F-6F.
7. Kragel AH, Reddy SG, Wittes JT, Roberts WC. Morphometric analysis of the composition of atherosclerotic plaques in the four major epicardial coronary arteries in acute myocardial infarction and in sudden coronary death. Circulation 1989; 80:1747–1756.
8. Kragel AH, Reddy SG, Wittes JT, Roberts WC. Morphometric analysis of the composition of coronary arterial plaques in isolated unstable angina pectoris with pain at rest. Am J Cardiol 1990; 66:562–567.
9. Gertz SD, Roberts WC. Hemodynamic shear force in rupture of coronary arterial atherosclerotic plaques. Am J Cardiol 1990; 66:1368–1372.
10. Falk E. Coronary thrombosis: pathogenesis and clinical manifestations. Am J Cardiol 1991; 68:28B-35B.
11. Richardson PD, Davies MJ, Born GVR. Influence of plaque configuration and stress distribution on fissuring of coronary atherosclerotic plaques. Lancet 1989; 2:941–944.
12. Henney AM, Wakeley PR, Davies MJ, Foster K, Hembry R, Murphy G, Humphries S. Localization of stromelysin gene expression in atherosclerotic plaques by in situ hybridization. Proc Natl Acad Sci 1991; 88: 8154–8158.
13. Shah PK, Falk E, Badimon JJ, Levy G, Fernandez-Ortiz A, Fallon J, Fuster V. Human monocyte-derived macrophages express collagenase and induce collagen breakdown in atherosclerotic fibrous caps: implications for plaque rupture (abstract). Circulation 1993; 88:I-254.
14. Falk E. Why do plaques rupture? Circulation 1992; 86(suppl III):III-30-III-42.
15. Davies MJ, Richardson PD, Woolf N, Katz DR, Mann J. Risk of thrombosis in human atherosclerotic plaques: role of extracellular lipid, macrophage, and smooth muscle cell content. Br Heart J 1993; 69:377–381.
16. Moreno PR, Falk E, Palacios IF, Newell JB, Fuster V, Fallon JT. Macrophage infiltration in acute coronary syndromes: implications for plaque rupture. Circulation (submitted for publication).
17. Haft JI, Al-Zarka AM. The origin and fate of complex coronary lesions. Am Heart J 1991; 121:1050–1061.
18. Cheng GC, Loree HM, Kamm RD, Fishbein MC, Lee RT. Distribution of circumferential stress in ruptured and stable atherosclerotic lesions: a structural analysis with histopathological correlation. Circulation 1993; 87:1179–1187.
19. Willich SN, Maclure M, Mittleman M, Arntz H-R, Muller JE. Sudden cardiac death: support for a role of triggering in causation. Circulation 1993; 87:1442–1450.
20. Mittleman MA, Maclure M, Tofler GH, Sherwood JB, Goldberg RJ, Muller

JE. Triggering of acute myocardial infarction by heavy physical exertion: protection against triggering by regular exertion. N Engl J Med 1993; 329: 1677–1683.

21. Willich SN, Lewis M, Lowel H, Arntz H-R, Schubert F, Schroder R. Physical exertion as a trigger of acute myocardial infarction. N Engl J Med 1993; 329:1684–1690.
22. Curfman GD. Is exercise beneficial—or hazardous—to your heart? (editorial) N Engl J Med 1993; 329:1730–1731.
23. Fernandez Ortiz A, Badimon JJ, Falk E, Fuster V, Meyer B, Mailhac A, Weng D, Shah PK, Badimon L. Characterization of the relative thrombogenicity of atherosclerotic plaque components. J Am Coll Cardiol (in press).
24. Wilcox JN, Smith KM, Schwartz SM, Gordon D. Localization of tissue factor in the normal vessel wall and in the atherosclerotic plaque. Proc Natl Acad Sci 1989; 86:2839–2843.
25. Hackett D, Davies G, Chierchia S, Maseri A. Intermittent coronary occlusion in acute myocardial infarction: value of combined thrombolytic and vasodilator therapy. N Engl J Med 1987; 317:1055–1059.
26. Chesebro JH, Fuster V. Dynamic thrombosis and thrombolysis. Role of antithrombins (editorial). Circulation 1991; 83:1815–1817.
27. Grines CL, Booth DC, Nissen SE, Gurley JC, Bennett KA, O'Connor WN, DeMaria AN. Mechanism of acute myocardial infarction in patients with prior coronary artery bypass grafting and therapeutic implications. Am J Cardiol 1990; 65:1292–1296.
28. Hangartner JRW, Charleston AJ, Davies MJ, Thomas AC. Morphological characteristics of clinically significant coronary artery stenosis in stable angina. Br Heart J 1986; 56:501–508.
29. Rentrop KP, Feit F, Sherman W, Stecy P, Hosat S, Cohen M, Rey M, Ambrose J, Nachamie M, Schwartz W, Cole W, Perdoncin R, Thornton JC. Late thrombolytic therapy preserves left ventricular function in patients with collateralized total coronary occlusion: primary end point findings of the Second Mount Sinai- New York University Reperfusion Trial. J Am Coll Cardiol 1989; 14:58–64.
30. Cohen M, Sherman W, Rentrop KP, Gorlin R. Determinants of collateral filling observed during sudden controlled coronary artery occlusion in human subjects. J Am Coll Cardiol 1989; 13:297–303.
31. Habib GB, Heibig J, Forman SA, Brown BG, Roberts R, Terrin ML, Bolli R, and the TIMI Investigators: Influence of coronary collateral vessels on myocardial infarct size in humans. Circulation 1991; 83:739–746.
32. Theroux P, Waters D, Qiu S, McCans J, Guise P, Juneau M. Aspirin versus heparin to prevent myocardial infarction during the acute phase of unstable angina. Circulation 1993; 88:2045–2048.
33. Kim CB, Braunwald E. Potential benefits of late reperfusion of infarcted myocardium. The open artery hypothesis. Circulation 1993; 88:2426–2436.
34. Glagov S, Weisenberg E, Christopher BA, et al. Compensatory enlargement of human atherosclerotic coronary arteries. N Engl J Med 1987; 316: 1371–1375.
35. Stiel GM, Stiel LSG, Schofer J et al. Impact of compensatory enlargement of atherosclerotic coronary arteries on angiographic assessment of coronary artery disease. Circulation 1989; 80:1603- 1609.

36. Kaski JC, Tousoulis D, Haider AW et al. Reactivity of eccentric and concentric coronary stenoses in patients with chronic stable angina. J Am Coll Cardiol 1991; 17:627–633.
37. Danchin N. Is myocardial revascularisation for tight coronary stenoses always necessary? (viewpoint). Lancet 1993; 342:224–225.
38. Little WC. Angiographic assessment of the culprit coronary artery lesion before acute myocardial infarction. Am J Cardiol 1990; 66:44G-47G.
39. Mizushige K, Reisman M, Buchbinder M, Dittrich H, DeMaria AN. Atheroma deformation during the cardiac cycle: evaluation by intracoronary ultrasound (abstract). Circulation 1993; 88:I-550.
40. Mizuno K, Satomura K, Miyamoto A, et al. Angioscopic evaluation of coronary-artery thrombi in acute coronary syndromes. N Engl J Med 1992; 326:287–291.
41. Brown BG, Zhao X-Q, Sacco DE, Albers JJ. Lipid lowering and plaque regression: new insights into prevention of plaque disruption and clinical events in coronary disease. Circulation 1993; 87:1781–1791.

2

Complex Lesions and Thrombosis:

Experimental Observations

Richard Gallo, MD, Juan J. Badimon, PhD, James H. Chesebro, MD

Introduction

Fissuring or disruption of a complex atherosclerotic plaque in the coronary arteries is pivotal to the development of the acute ischemic syndromes. Several studies of coronary pathology of patients who died shortly after the onset of myocardial infarction or unstable angina have shown disrupted plaques with mural or occlusive thrombi anchored to fissures or ulcerations in the plaque.[1–2] In addition, subclinical plaque disruption with thrombus formation and fibrous organization is an important mechanism of progression of chronic atherosclerosis in patients with or without angina.[3]

The progression of early atherosclerotic lesions to the clinical manifestation of angina, myocardial infarction, or sudden death is more rapid in persons with coronary risk factors and in lesions with certain topographic characteristics.[3] Diabetes, proximal or midvessel location, elevated cholesterol, interval from infarction, and complex lesion morphology were identified as predictors of angiographic progression in the Coronary Artery Surgery Study (CASS).[4] Early progression of plaques

From: Ambrose JA (ed): *Complex Coronary Lesions in Acute Coronary Syndromes*. © Futura Publishing Co., Inc., Armonk, NY, 1996.

develops slowly over decades. However, later in time, growing lesions may progress rapidly. This suggests recurrent minor plaque disruption of the most fatty plaques with subsequent thrombus formation.

Classification of Atherosclerotic Lesions

The morphological studies by Stary have provided many answers about plaque evolution.[5] The first observation made by Stary was that all humans develop focal thickening of the intima due to smooth muscle cell proliferation. The initial atherosclerotic lesion (Stary type I) is only microscopically and chemically perceivable, and consists of isolated groups of macrophages filled with lipid droplets. Type II lesions or fatty streaks are composed of more lipid-laden cells than the initial lesions, and are visible macroscopically as fatty dots or streaks barely raised above the intimal surface. Each lesion is made up of one or more layers of lipid-filled foam cells within the intima. There is evidence that such streaks may be precursors of larger plaques. Transitional forms between fatty streaks and advanced plaques develop in the sites where fatty streaks are more frequent. Progression beyond the fatty streak stage is associated with a sequence of changes starting with the appearance of extracellular lipid, which begins to form a lesion that is more elevated (Stary type III). Multiple scattered pools of extracellular lipid may progress to a large, confluent accumulation of extracellular lipid, forming the lipid core characteristic of Stary type IV lesions. In Stary type V lesions (fibroatheroma) or fibrolipid lesions, smooth muscle cells migrate into and proliferate within the plaque, forming a layer over the luminal side of the lipid core.[1,5] Additional collagen is produced, and plaque size increases. The lipid-rich core is avascular and almost totally acellular, consisting of pultaceous debris, including dead macrophages and mesenchymal cells along with abundant cholesterol crystals (fatty gruel).[6,7] Lesions having visible thrombotic deposits and/or hemorrhage, in addition to lipid and collagen, are Stary type VI lesions (complicated fibroatheroma, or complex lesions). Stary type VII are reserved for advanced, mineralized lesions (calcific lesions). Finally, atherosclerotic lesions consisting almost entirely of fibrotic scar collagen, where the lipid may have regressed, are referred to as Stary type VIII lesions.

By combining pathological and clinical elements, Fuster et al. re-

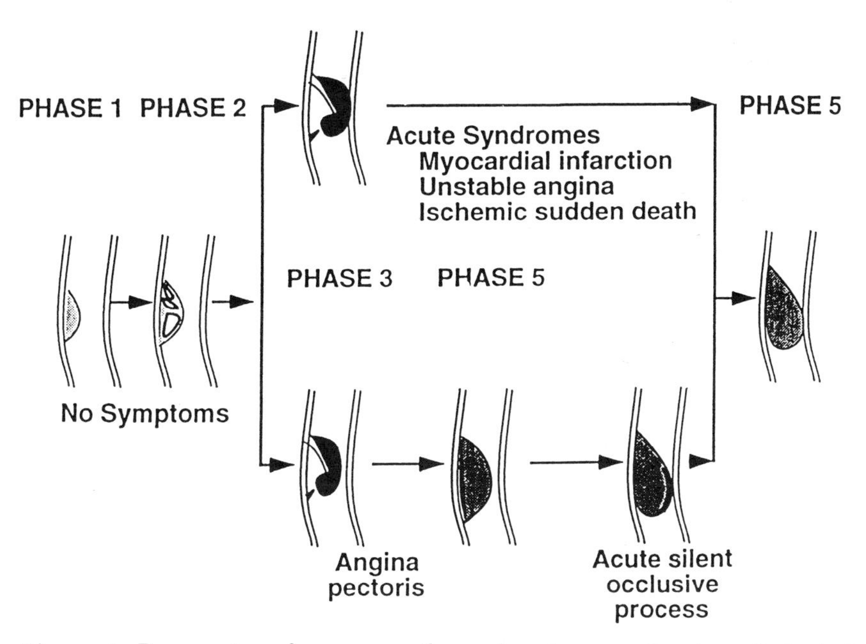

Figure 1: Progression of coronary atherosclerosis, according to pathological and clinical findings. (Reproduced with permission.[3])

cently classified the progression of atherosclerosis into five phases (Figure 1).[3,8–10] The first phase is a small fibrotic plaque, present in the majority of the population, and corresponds histologically to Stary types I, II, and III lesions. Phase 2 is a lipid-rich plaque prone to disruption and corresponds to Stary types IV and V lesions. The disruption of plaque is followed by thrombus formation and a decrease in lumen diameter. Phase 3 morphologically corresponds to the complex lesion, Stary type VI lesions. Clinically this may be quiescent, result in stable angina, or result in an acute ischemic syndrome, phase 4. The mural or occlusive thrombus of phases 3 and 4 with time may become organized by smooth muscle cell infiltration and connective tissue deposition, resulting in phase 5, which corresponds to chronic fibrotic and stenotic plaques or Stary types V and VI lesions (Figure 1).

The process of lipid accumulation, cell proliferation, and extracellular matrix synthesis may be expected to be linear with time. However, angiographic studies show that the progression of coronary artery disease in humans is neither linear nor predictable.[11,12] New high-grade lesions often appear in segments of artery that appeared normal or near normal on previous angiographic examination.[9] Two-thirds or more of the culprit lesions responsible for unstable angina or myocardial infarction were only mildly to moderately stenotic on prior angiograms.[13] Morphological analysis of the new culprit lesions showed complex eccentric stenosis with narrow necks, and overhanging edges or scalloped borders in most cases. This morphology represents plaque disruption with superimposed thrombus.[14]

Pathophysiology of the Acute Coronary Syndromes

Acute coronary syndromes are mainly caused by plaque disruption and coronary thrombi, as confirmed by several clinical and autopsy studies.[1–3,5] Coronary thrombosis may occur acutely in arteries containing atherosclerosis. A fissure or disruption of an atherosclerotic plaque exposes thrombogenic substrates, leads to an acute change in plaque geometry, increased shear stress, generation of thrombin, and increased platelet activation and thrombus formation. The clinical consequences of plaque disruption largely depend on the extent of the thrombotic response.

In *unstable angina,* a smaller fissure or disruption leads to thrombus formation, resulting in a reduction of blood flow and exacerbation of angina. Transient episodes of thrombotic vessel occlusion or near occlusion at the site of plaque injury may occur, leading to angina at rest. The thrombus may be labile and result in temporary obstruction to flow, perhaps lasting minutes. In addition, release of vasoactive substances by platelets and vasoconstriction secondary to endothelial vasodilator dysfunction contributes to further reduction of blood flow.[15] The process may be sufficiently severe to cause total occlusion and myocardial infarction.

In *non-Q-wave myocardial infarction,* the angiographic form of the responsible lesion is similar to that seen in unstable angina.[16] More severe plaque damage would result in more persistent thrombotic occlusion, but the distal myocardial territory is often supplied by collaterals. At early angiography, about one-fourth of patients with non-Q-wave infarction have an infarct-related vessel that is completely occluded, with the distal territory usually supplied by collaterals.[17–19] Resolution of vasospasm may also be pathogenically important in non-Q-wave infarction.[44]

In *Q-wave infarction,* a larger plaque disruption may be associated with deep arterial injury or ulceration, resulting in the formation of a fixed and persistent thrombus. This leads to an abrupt cessation of myocardial perfusion, often for more than 1 hour, and subsequent necrosis of the involved myocardium. As discussed, the coronary lesion responsible for the infarction is frequently only mildly to moderately stenotic,[13,20] which suggests that the severity of the underlying lesion is not the primary determinant of acute occlusion. In patients with longstanding coronary artery disease and severe coronary stenosis, well-developed collaterals prevent or reduce the extent of infarction. In a minority of patients, coronary thrombosis results from superficial injury or blood stasis in areas of high-grade stenosis.[18]

Sudden death related to ischemia probably involves the disruption of a plaque that is rapidly obstructive, resulting in acute occlusion generating a polymeric arrhythmia. Absence of collateral flow, vasoconstriction, or platelet microthrombi to the microcirculation may contribute.[21]

The role of platelets and thrombin in thrombus formation and organization, factors modulating thrombus growth and stabilization, and finally the role of residual thrombus will be discussed in this chapter.

Thrombus Formation and Organization

The pivotal role of endothelial injury in platelet deposition, thrombosis, and the genesis of atherosclerosis dates back over a century.

Plaques at Risk of Disruption and Progression

A fibrolipid lesion (Stary type V) surrounded by a thin fibrous capsule is easily disrupted, leading to thrombus formation. Plaque disruption occurs when the strain within the fibrous cap exceeds the deformability of its component material.[22] Atherosclerotic plaques prone to disruption are commonly composed of a crescentic mass of soft lipids, with abundant cholesterol crystals, separated from the vessel lumen by a thin fibrous cap.[1,6,7] Disrupted plaques contain more extracellular lipids and less collagen and smooth muscle cells than intact plaques. Fissures tend to occur at the margins of plaques where caps are necrotic, very thin, and extensively infiltrated by macrophages.[1,22,23] Plaques in which the extracellular lipid core makes up more than 40% of the overall plaque volume are particularly susceptible to disruption.

Plaque fissuring comes in many shapes and sizes. The tear may be large and the thrombus formed within the lumen may occlude the vessel. It may be partly or largely removed by lysis or may become reorganized. On the other hand, small tears less than 100–200 μm across allow blood to enter and expand the plaque but may not result in intraluminal thrombosis. Plaque expansion produces acute changes in plaque geometry with subsequent alterations in local rheology that may lead to further lesion progression. Pathological studies of patients with coronary artery disease have revealed both fresh thrombi in areas of plaque disruption[1] and old organized coronary thrombi in different stages of organization that later were difficult to differentiate from chronic atherosclerotic changes in the arterial wall. This indicates that thrombus organization contributes to the development of complex coronary plaques. Additionally, thrombi with a layered appearance overlying fissured plaques were commonly seen in fatal cases of unstable angina.[1,22] The layered appearance of the thrombus plus finding small fragments of thrombotic material in the distal intramyocardial circulation suggested that intermittent and recurrent thrombus formation and fragmentation may occur and eventually lead to luminal occlusion. Furthermore utilizing monoclonal antibodies, large amounts of fibrinogen, fibrin, and fibrin degradation products were identified in areas of loose connective tissue, around macrophages, smooth muscle cells, cholesterol deposits, and in thrombi. These findings further support a role for thrombosis and thrombus incorporation as part of plaque progression.[24] Recurrent episodes of plaque disruption and thrombosis may or may not be associated with signs and symptoms of ischemia and may lead to progressive narrowing of the coronary arteries (Figure 2).

Role of Platelets

In normal hemostasis, the initial event is platelet adhesion to the vessel wall. Arterial thrombus formation is initiated mainly by platelet adhesion to disrupted atherosclerotic plaques or injury below the internal elastic lamina (severe injury), and to a lesser degree to areas of denuded endothelium (mild injury). Platelet-vessel wall interaction coats the newly injured vascular wall with platelet-rich thrombus. This involves subendothelial adhesive membrane glycoproteins and numer-

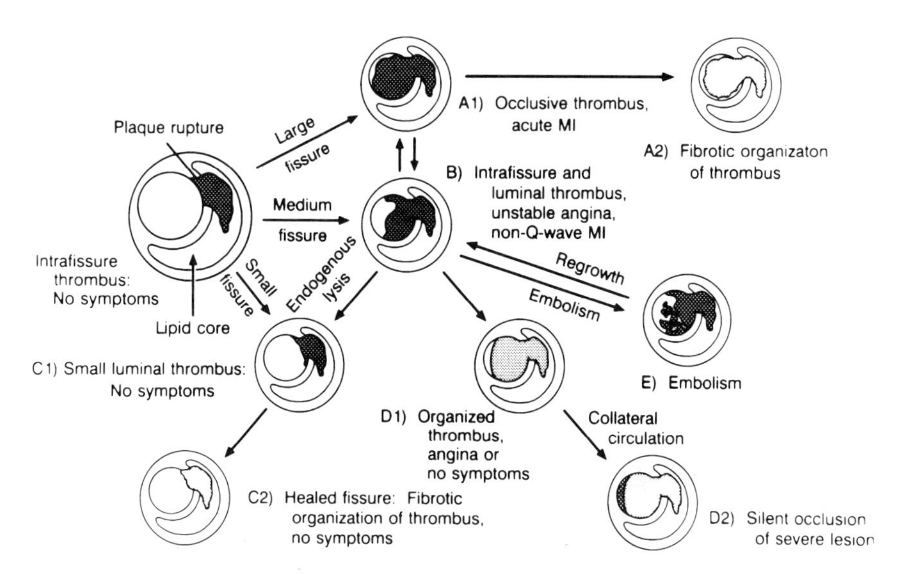

Figure 2: Diagram showing major pathogenic modes of progression of coronary disease. Plaque disruption leads to formation of a fissure with flowing blood contacting intra-arterial structures and forming an intrafissure thrombus. The fissure may be small, medium, or large and may progress immediately to various degrees of luminal obstruction (A1, B, C1). Sudden progression with a large fissure may lead to occlusive thrombus and acute myocardial infarction (A1). Fibrotic organization of the thrombus may occur (A2), or lysis of the thrombus with reopening of the lumen becoming partially obstructive (B). A medium-sized fissure may lead to immediate partial obstruction associated with unstable angina or non-Q-wave myocardial infarction. (B) This may progress to total occlusion (A1), partial embolization (E), fibrotic organization (D1), endogenous lysis to a smaller thrombus (C1), no intraluminal thrombus (E), or fibrotic organization by fibromuscular proliferation (A2, C2, and D1). A severe residual stenosis (D1) may be associated with good collateral circulation and no symptoms. Because of very low antegrade flow and type II injury (endothelial denudation), this may silently occlude with fresh thrombus (D2). A small fissure may lead to a small thrombus without symptoms (C1) and undergo fibrotic organization with progression of disease in the absence of symptoms (C2). (Reproduced with permission.[34])

ous platelet receptors. The initial bond is usually between platelet glycoprotein Ia/IIa complex and collagen. This bond is strengthened by the interaction with other glycoproteins, principally glycoprotein (Gp) Ib/IV complex and von Willebrand's factor (vWF), and between fibronectin and Gp Ic/IIa. vWF binds to a second platelet receptor site on Gp IIb/IIIa, facilitating the stabilization of platelet-vessel wall adhesion and platelet-platelet aggregation.[25]

Severe vessel wall injury exposes components of arterial media or atherosclerotic plaque that in association with local shear stresses trigger platelet aggregation and thrombus formation. Exposed smooth muscle cells, collagen from the vessel wall, circulating $alpha_2$ adrenergic agonists, tissue factor from macrophages, fatty lesions, and adjacent adventia and thrombin generation are powerful platelet activators. Another powerful activator is ADP released from red cells or other blood cells in the area of vascular injury. Occupation by these agonists of specific platelet binding receptors ultimately results in discharge of calcium from the cytoskeleton, promoting release of alpha granule contents: ADP, serotonin, arachidonate derivatives such as thromboxane A_2, along with various growth factors and prostaglandins, which not only promote further platelet activation and aggregation, but also local vasoconstriction.

After activation, previously quiescent platelet receptors undergo measurable conformational changes, signaling activation (e.g., Gp IIb/IIIa). Along with the expression of new receptors (P-selectins), platelets become competent receptors for several adhesive proteins.[26] The simultaneous binding of fibrinogen molecules to clusters of adjacent platelets results in platelet aggregation and subsequent formation of a thrombus (Figure 3).

Platelets and Lysis

Platelets not only contribute to the formation of thrombus but can also inhibit its lysis because of their extremely rich content in plasminogen activator inhibitor type 1 (PAI-1). Platelet-rich thrombus increases the resistance to natural thrombolysis during arterial thrombosis, and may explain the resistance of certain thrombi to exogenous thrombolysis.[27]

Myofibrotic Response

The role of platelets in the myofibrotic response to thrombus organization has been studied in animals. Three phases can be distinguished.[28,29] The first occurs almost immediately after vessel injury and involves the formation of a platelet-containing thrombus. It is during this phase that smooth muscle cells begin to hypertrophy and proliferate, by a mechanism independent of platelet factors.[30] Also during this phase, platelet-derived growth factors (PDGF), which are known

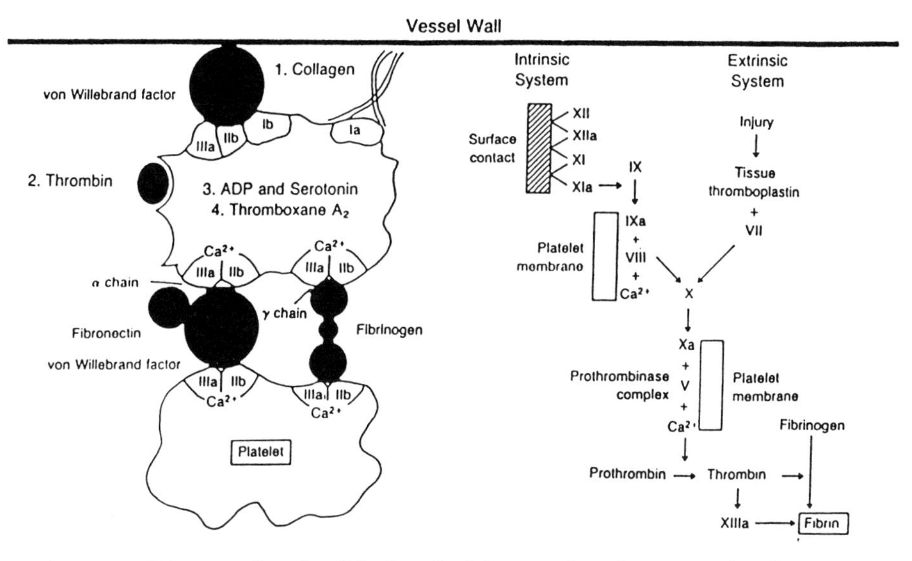

Figure 3: Diagram showing biochemical interactions between platelet membrane receptors, vessel wall, and adhesive macromolecules during platelet adhesion and aggregation. Also depicted are the intrinsic and extrinsic pathways of coagulation with activator complexes which amplify and accelerate thrombin generation and the resultant thrombosis. (Reproduced with permission.[2]

for their chemotactic and mitogenic activity on smooth muscle cells, are released from platelets (paracrine) and synthesized within cells, e.g., smooth muscle cells (autocrine response). The second phase commences a few days after initial injury. During this phase, smooth muscle cells proliferate and migrate into the injured intima. The third phase begins 2 to 3 weeks after the initial injury. It is characterized by the continued proliferation of smooth muscle cells along with the deposition of extracellular matrix (collagen and other proteoglycans) contributing to the fibrotic organization and the growing of atherosclerotic plaques.[31]

Role of Thrombin in Arterial Thrombosis

Thrombin (factor II) is a serine protease generated via the intrinsic and extrinsic coagulation systems.[27] After arterial injury, thromboplastin or tissue factor interacts with factor VII with subsequent activa-

Editor's note: It is now appreciated that tissue thromboplastin (tissue factor) can also activate factor IX and thus activate both systems (see Chapter 7).

tion of factor X in the coagulation cascade. Prothrombin is converted to thrombin by an activator complex (prothrombinase complex), composed of activated factor Xa, activated factor Va, prothrombin, and calcium assembled on a phospholipid membrane such as the platelet, smooth muscle cell, or endothelial cell (Figure 3).

Thrombin is the *most potent activator of platelets*. It converts fibrinogen to fibrin, activates factors V, VIII, and XIII, which crosslinks fibrin for stabilization of the thrombus (Figure 4).[27]

Thrombin also interacts with the vessel wall and is *mitogenic* for smooth muscle cells and fibroblasts and induces oncogenes and tissue factor generation. It is chemotactic for circulating monocytes, and has been implicated in the inflammatory response.[32]

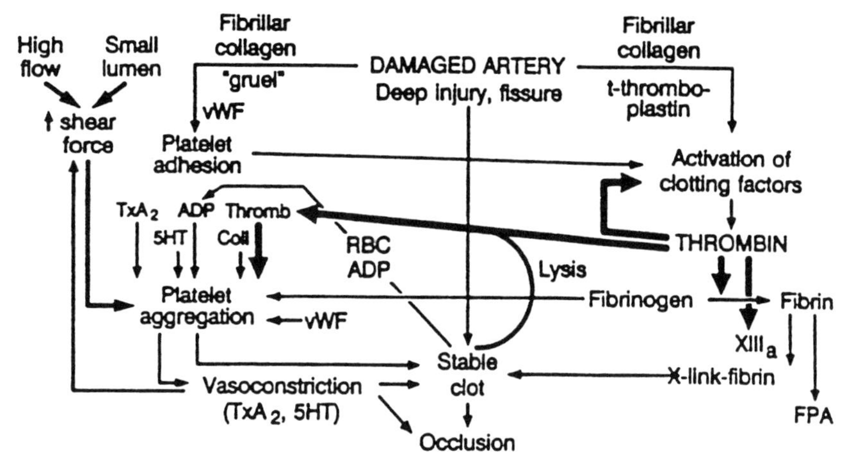

Figure 4: Diagram showing proposed mechanism of arterial thrombosis. Fibrillar collagen from exposed media, "fatty gruel" from atherosclerotic plaque, and tissue factor, which activate factor VII to VIIa; factor VIIa activates factor X to Xa, which helps generate thrombin; thrombin activates platelets, which adhere to the arterial wall via von Willebrand factor; thrombin-activated platelets release thromboxane A_2, serotonin, and ADP, which together cause additional platelet aggregation and vasoconstriction. Activation of the coagulation pathways leads to production of the prothrombinase complex on the platelet and smooth muscle cell phospholipid membranes, which bind Ca^{++} and factors Va and Xa; this accelerates the production of thrombin by 280,000 times. Thrombin is the major activator of platelets and converts fibrinogen to fibrin, releasing fibrinopeptide A (FPA) and fibrin II monomer (which inhibits heparin-antithrombin III inactivation of thrombin). Fibrinogen/fibrin binds to platelet glycoprotein IIb/IIIa receptors and forms bridges between platelets. The activation of factor XIII by thrombin causes a cross-linking of the fibrin strands and a stabilization of the new thrombus. (Reproduced with permission.[34])

Active thrombin *binds to subendothelial extracellular matrix.* After binding, it is protected from inactivation by antithrombin III and heparin but not by direct-acting molecules such as hirudin.[32] Platelet and smooth muscle cell lipid membranes also provide binding sites for the *prothrombinase complex,* which enhances thrombin generation by 300,000 times. Thrombin may bind to deeply injured artery and markedly increased platelet deposition and thrombus formation at this level.[33]

Factors Modulating Thrombus Formation and Stabilization

Angioscopic, intraoperative, and postmortem studies have documented intraluminal thrombi in both unstable angina and acute myocardial infarction.[10] The incidence of thrombi in unstable angina varied greatly depending on the interval between the onset of symptoms and the angiographic study. When angiography was performed immediately after onset of symptoms, thrombi were seen in the majority of cases compared to a very low incidence of thrombi if catheterization was delayed for weeks.

Many variables determine whether a disrupted plaque progresses to a mural or an occlusive thrombus. The major local determinants of the thrombotic response after plaque disruption[34] are the quantity (fissure size), and quality (plaque composition) of thrombogenic substrate exposed, and the rheology of blood flow. Systemic factors such as the fibrinolytic system, catecholamines, and lipoproteins also modulate thrombosis but appear to be less influential than local substrates and rheology. Badimon et al. have developed a physiological extracorporeal perfusion chamber for testing substrate exposure to circulating blood at specific shear rates and during different antithrombotic therapies to discern the effects on thrombus growth and stabilization (Figure 5).[9] The role of some of these variables is discussed below.

Role of Vascular Injury and Substrate

The principal determinant of the severity of the thrombogenic response is the degree of vascular injury, the surface area of exposure, and the types of thrombogenic substrates in the underlying vessel wall (collagen, tissue factor, smooth muscle cells, fatty core) and flow characteristics.[3,8,9]

In order to allow a more uniform description of the mechanisms

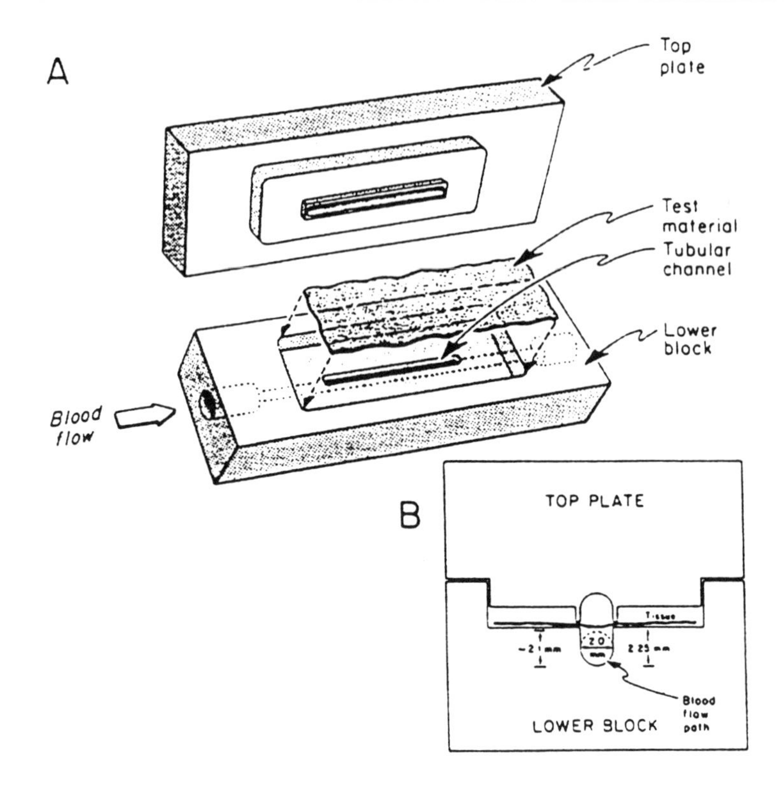

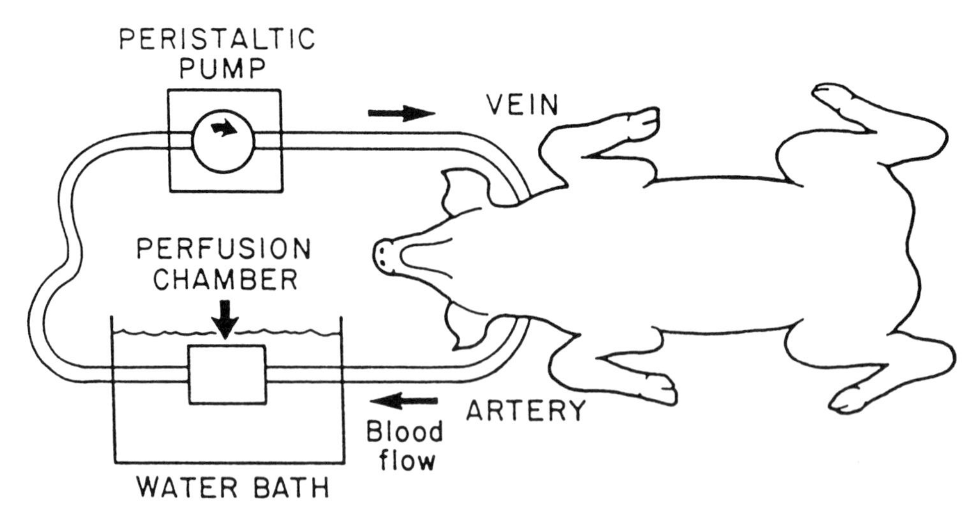

Figure 5: (A) Sketch of the perfusion chamber used to expose material to flowing blood. (B) Cross-section of the perfusion chamber. (C) Sketch of the perfusion system with recirculation. Blood from the carotid artery is passed through the chamber by a peristaltic pump, maintaining a constant shear rate, which then returns blood to the contralateral jugular vein. (Reproduced with permission.[9])

involved in the thrombotic response, Ip et al. proposed a *pathophysiological classification of vascular injury* or damage into three categories representing stages of increasing severity.[29] In type I vascular injury, functional alteration of endothelial cells without substantial morphological changes occurs. In such cases no significant platelet deposition or thrombosis occurs. In type II or mild vascular injury, there is endothelial denudation with superficial intimal damage, but the internal elastic lamina and media remain intact. When type II injury is induced, a monolayer of platelets carpet the injured area with microthrombi However, the thrombus is labile and easily dislodged by the flowing blood.[35] As a clinical counterpart, when the endothelium is denuded, the thrombogenic stimulus is limited resulting in a single layer of platelet deposition (or a possible thrombus if within a stenosis), and mild growth of the plaque via a proliferative response.

In type III vascular injury, deep injury occurs with exposure of highly thrombogenic components of the medial layer, particularly smooth muscle cells and thrombogenic fibrillar collagen (types I and III) and tissue thromboplastin, resulting in marked platelet deposition and visible mural thrombus that is more firmly anchored and not easily dislodged.[3] In the normal artery, tissue thromboplastin is present in the adventia but not in the media. Injury to smooth muscle cells and atherosclerotic plaque both stimulate synthesis of tissue factor in the arterial wall.[36] In a recent study Fernandez-Ortiz et al.[37] studied direct perfusion of the thrombogenicity of fresh blood of various human atherosclerotic plaques including fatty streaks, lipid-rich atheromatous plaques and fibrotic plaques with an abundant collagen matrix. The lipid core exposed in the atheromatous lipid-rich plaques was most thrombogenic with thrombus formation four to six times greater than that of other substrates. This marked thrombogenicity of the lipid-rich plaque may be due to the high levels of procoagulant tissue thromboplastin, lipids which allow assembly of coagulation pathway activator complexes, or platelet activators released in part by exposed macrophages and smooth muscle cells. In another perfusion study using ACD preserved anticoagulated blood, collagen types I and III in atheromatous plaques were shown to be the more thrombogenic component of the plaque.[38] Thus, lipid-rich plaques are both vulnerable to rupture and more thrombogenic.

Role of Fluid Dynamics

When discussing thrombus formation, the effects of blood flow are a necessity. The endothelium is constantly exposed to flowing blood.

In fluid dynamics, rheologic stress is the force per unit area generated during blood flow. When this force is applied at a right angle, it is described as normal stress; when it is applied parallel to a surface, it is referred to as tangential or shear stress.[35] Laminar flow should be parabolic in shape, with the maximal velocities at the center of flow and a fall off to nearly zero at the periphery. Rewriting Poiseuille's law for laminar flow:

$$\text{Shear stress} = 4\mu Q/\pi r^3$$

where μ is viscosity; Q is flow rate; and r is the arterial radius. Thus for regions of laminar flow, shear stress is inversely proportional to the cube of the radius. Small changes in radius will produce a large change in shear stress. In reality, flow into a stenotic area will increase the shear stress beyond that for the anticipated radius change. Acceleration of blood into a stenotic lesion flattens the velocity curve, leading to a much more rapid increase in shear stress.[39]

In normal coronary arteries, the response to increased shear stress is to vasodilate. This compensatory endothelium-dependent vasodilatation does not occur in atherosclerotic segments.[40] Platelet and fibrinogen deposition increase directly with shear stress.[41] With high shear force, red cells force platelets to the periphery and enhance their deposition. ADP also appears to increase at the cell surface in the presence of high shear forces. To investigate the dynamics of platelet deposition and thrombus growth after vascular injury, Badimon et al. have utilized an extracorporeal perfusion system with parallel streamlines, which allows multiple shear rate conditions. Platelet deposition increased significantly with increasing stenosis in the presence of the same vascular injury, indicating a shear rate-induced platelet activation. Furthermore, the maximal platelet deposition was at the maximal stenosis (apex) of the plaque, not in the region of flow separation distal to the plaque.[35,42] These results suggest that the acute thrombotic response to plaque disruption depends in part on the acute geometric changes occurring in the vessel at the time of plaque disruption. Furthermore, the finding that platelet deposition is greatest at the apex of the plaque may result in a platelet-rich thrombus, which may be more resistant to thrombolysis.

Effects of Vasoconstriction

Acute arterial injury is associated with acute vasoconstriction.[43] *Vasoconstriction is endothelium-dependent, platelet-dependent, and cholesterol-endothelin dependent.* Vasospasm was found to be an important contributor to coronary occlusion in patients with acute myocardial infarction.[44]

Endothelial cells are not just an inert barrier but an important regulator of vascular hemostasis and play a central role in the modulation of vascular tone (Figure 6). In a normal artery, acetylcholine vasodilates. However, experimental studies in the pig have shown that endothelial denudation induces acetylcholine-dependent vasoconstriction of that arterial segment.[45,46] After partial regrowth, acetylcholine-induced vasoconstriction persists. Complete endothelial regrowth prevents vasoconstriction to acetylcholine. Therefore, endothelial absence or dysfunction may be associated with vasoconstriction. An intact endothelium is required for acetylcholine to exert its vasorelaxant effect via the release of endothelium-derived relaxing factor (EDRF).[47] Nu-

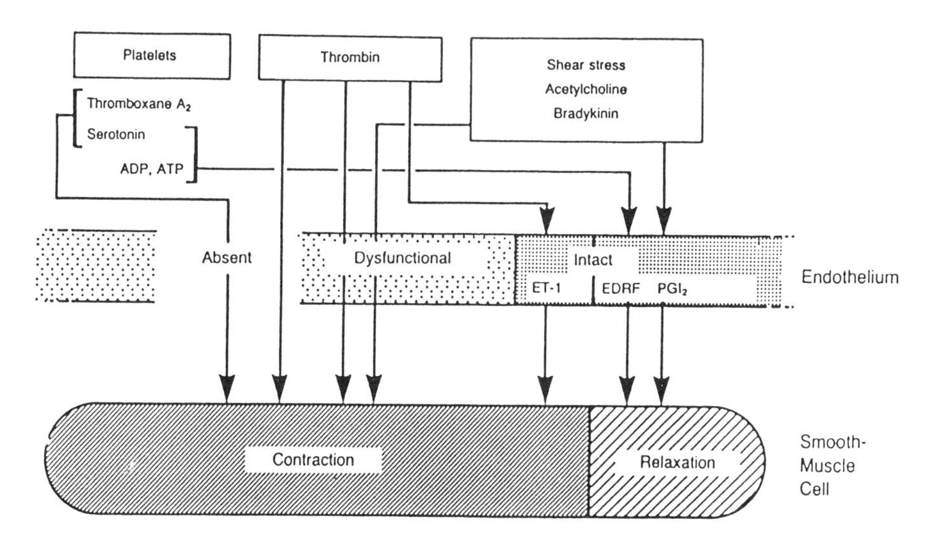

Figure 6: The effects of shear stress, acetylcholine, and bradykinin lead intact endothelium to generate and release endothelium-derived relaxing factor (EDRF) and prostacyclin PGI_2, which in turn causes relaxation of the smooth muscle. The effect of thrombin leads the intact endothelium to generate endothelin-1 (ET-1), which causes vasoconstriction of the smooth muscle. After type I injury or damage, dysfunctional endothelium may not generate relaxing substances; in these circumstances all the above-mentioned stimulants exert a vasoconstrictive effect, either through the enhancement of endothelium-derived contracting factors or directly. As a result of type II or III injury or damage, in areas of de-endothelialization (Absent), thrombin and the platelet products thromboxane A_2 and serotonin induce direct vasoconstriction of the smooth muscle. (Reproduced with permission.[34])

merous other substances including shear stress induce the release of EDRF.[48]

Experimental data suggest that *platelets* contribute to reduction of blood flow. In a porcine model of deep arterial injury by carotid angioplasty, the degree of vasoconstriction proximal and distal to the angioplasty site was directly proportional to the log of the platelet deposition. In this study, vasospasm was reduced but not eliminated with aspirin treatment, suggesting a cyclo-oxygenase-dependent vasospasm.[43] In a canine model with stenosis and probably mild injury, thromboxane A_2 and serotonin inhibitors abolished cyclic flow variations.[49] Platelet-dependent vasoconstriction occurs in the absence of endothelium, suggesting a direct effect of platelet-secreted vasoconstrictors on the underlying smooth muscle cells. This is a possible explanation for the transient vasoconstriction observed in angiograms of patients with acute coronary syndromes and complex plaques.[45] Although inhibition of platelet deposition may reduce vasospasm, it does not totally prevent it, suggesting the presence of a secondary platelet-independent pathway. Vasoconstriction occurs immediately after angioplasty in pigs and 15 minutes after angioplasty in patients, and may be inhibited by intravenous nitroglycerine in both species.[43,45]

Endothelial cells also release contracting factors, such as *endothelin*. Cholesterol feeding, thrombin, and local flow shear stress increase the expression of the proendothelin gene and subsequent release of endothelin. The endothelium modulates vascular tone by releasing relaxing factors such as EDRF and contracting factors such as endothelin.[48,50,51] Under normal conditions, the relaxing factors predominate. An alteration in endothelium as occurs in atherosclerosis may cause a reversal of what is normally seen and set the cells to generate increasingly proconstrictor mediators.[52] Indeed, local secretion of EDRF seems to be diminished and endothelin release increased in atherosclerotic coronary arteries in humans[62] and in animals, respectively.[43]

Local thrombus formation and vasoconstriction are defense mechanisms to prevent bleeding when arteriolar or capillary damage occurs. When injury to larger arteries occurs, as in plaque disruption, the same mechanisms become active but are detrimental and contribute to an acute coronary syndrome. If the downstream vascular bed is intact, the active products of platelet activation such as serotonin, prostacyclins, ADP, and ATP are vasorelaxant, increasing blood flow and limiting the distal myocardium from further ischemia.

The Role of Systemic Factors

Several systemic factors may modulate thrombosis. An *increased adrenergic activation* is associated with acute cardiovascular syndromes.[53–55] The incidence of cardiac events (myocardial infarctions, unstable angina, sudden death), and stroke show circadian variations with significant increase during the early morning hours, which is associated with an increase in sympathoadrenal stimulation.[55,56] There is an increased incidence of myocardial infarction in patients under great stress, such as the increased number of reported myocardial infarctions in Israel during the Gulf war,[57] as well as in patients having undergone heavy physical exertion.[58]

Elevated levels of catecholamines are present in patients with acute myocardial infarcts, but this can be secondary to the myocardial damage, pain, and mental stress. The hypothesis that elevated circulating levels of catecholamines could stimulate the dynamics of arterial thrombus formation in areas at high risk has not been clearly demonstrated. The majority of studies on in vitro platelet aggregation required supraphysiological concentrations of epinephrine to show aggregation, suggesting that epinephrine acted as an indirect platelet activator in concert with other agonists or by its action on the vessel wall. Because of its vasoactive effects, epinephrine may reduce the luminal cross-sectional area, enhancing the local shear stress and indirectly inducing platelet activation. Badimon et al. designed a study to assess a dose-dependent effect of epinephrine on platelet interaction with an immobilized isolated vessel wall component (collagen type I). In this study where vasoreactivity is eliminated and the rheological variables could be directly controlled, it was observed that total catecholamine levels correlated significantly with the extent of platelet deposition at high shear rates.[54]

Elevated lipids appear to increase thrombogenicity mainly via their deposition in the arterial wall. Several lipoprotein fractions are positively associated with atherosclerosis, however, interestingly no specific lipid fraction has been linked directly to increased thrombogenicity. Lipoprotein(a) or Lp(a) is an important inherited risk factor for ischemic heart disease.[59,60] Lp(a) resembles LDL in its content of cholesterol, phospholipid, and apolipoprotein B-100, which is the ligand for the LDL receptor. Apolipoprotein(a) or apo(a) is the distinguishing glycoprotein present in Lp(a). Analysis of cDNA shows a similar structural homology to plasminogen, with both genes closely located on chromosome 6. Although Apo(a) contains terminal sequences similar to the catalytic domain of plasminogen, amino acid substitutions render apo(a) incapable of plasmin-like proteolysis.[61,62] However, the close homology of Lp(a) with plasminogen results in competitive inhibition of the conversion of plasminogen to plasmin and thus of fibrinolytic properties in vitro.[63] Despite substantial in vitro evidence linking Lp(a) to prothrombotic activities, there are no studies in humans that confirm these findings.[62]

Other *metabolic factors* that are linked to an increased thrombogenicity are the renin-angiotensin system, in particular the presence of increased angiotensin converting enzyme activity.[64–66] Increased plasma levels of homocysteine and most importantly diabetes have been linked to increased thrombotic events and platelet reactivity.[67,68] *Hemostatic proteins* such as fibrinogen and factor VII are risk factors for coronary artery disease, however, there are no actual studies linking them directly to increased thrombogenicity.[69]

One social habit that is clearly an independent risk factor for coronary artery disease is *cigarette smoking.*[70] Nicotine increases catecholamines, platelet aggregability, shortens platelet survival, and via adrenergic mechanisms increases coronary vascular tone.[55]

Role of Residual Thrombus

Residual thrombus is the most thrombogenic substrate because of four mechanisms:

1. *Rheologic Factor:* Residual thrombus protrudes into the vessel lumen obstructing flow and decreasing the lumen diameter, which increases shear stress and platelet deposition.[41] The presence of an underlying high-grade stenosis greatly enhances platelet deposition onto the residual thrombus. Without a stenosis, platelet deposition is approximately doubled compared to deeply injured artery. In the presence of an 80% stenosis, platelet deposition is increased three- to fourfold compared to deeply injured artery only.

2. *Substrate Related Factor:* Residual thrombus is a more thrombogenic substrate than deeply injured arterial wall.[35] There is increased thrombin generation via increased activated factor X (FXa) within the thrombus.[34]

3. *Receptors on Thrombin:* Thrombin binding to fibrin masks receptors on thrombin to heparin-antithrombin III complex, but not to direct thrombin inhibitors such as hirudin. Furthermore, fragmentation or embolization of thrombus induces rapid regrowth of a thrombotic mass. Heparin infusion alone or with aspirin does not block this regrowth. However, the specific thrombin inhibitor hirudin completely abolishes thrombus regrowth.[71,72]

4. *Natural Inhibitors of Heparin:* Thrombus with actively generated and bound thrombin increases release of natural inhibitors of heparin activity such as platelet-factor 4 secreted from platelets and fibrin

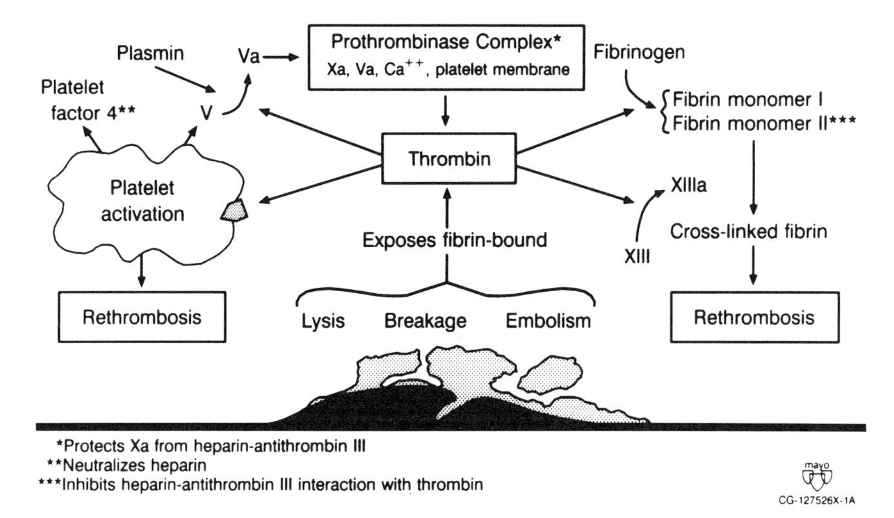

Figure 7: Demonstration of the numerous ways a residual thrombus may reactivate thrombotic mechanisms. See text for more details. (Reproduced with permission.[9])

II monomer generated from fibrinogen. In addition, endogenous or exogenous thrombolysis by plasmin directly activates platelets and increases thrombin generation by activating factor V to Va (Figure 7).[32,73]

Antiplatelet and Antithrombin Agents

Potent antiplatelet agents may offer some promise in preventing the progression of atherosclerotic plaques. The best-studied but modest antiplatelet drug is aspirin. This over-the-counter widely used medication has been shown to be effective in preventing arterial occlusion in unstable angina, acute myocardial infarctions, during and after coronary bypass surgery and angioplasty, as well as in secondary prevention of coronary and cerebrovascular disease, and as primary prevention (reduction of clinical events) in patients with risk factors of coronary artery disease.[74] However, aspirin does not totally block thrombus growth or prevent angiographic progression of coronary disease.

Aspirin interferes with one of the three pathways of platelet activation. It irreversibly inhibits cyclo-oxygenase, and platelet thromboxane production.[74] The other two pathways, one dependent on ADP and collagen and the other thrombin-dependent, remain unaffected. Therefore, aspirin does not completely prevent platelet thrombus formation in vivo. In a prospective angiographic study, patients with coronary artery disease given aspirin and dipyridamole versus placebo showed a reduction in the incidence of myocardial infarction and a trend toward reduced new lesion formation after 5 years of follow-up. There was no angiographic reduction in lesion progression.[34,75]

Other antiplatelet drugs are also limited by their action on one of the three pathways of platelet inhibition. Specific receptor inhibitors to some of these platelet activators delineate their role in thrombosis. Specific receptor inhibitors to thromboxane or thromboxane A_2 synthetase inhibitors reduce the vasoconstriction of acute injury but do not reduce quantitative ^{111}In platelet deposition or the incidence of mural thrombus on deeply injured arteries.[76] Ticlopidine, which acts against ADP, has shown promise in secondary prevention of cerebrovascular disease, in unstable angina, post angioplasty, and in maintaining aortocoronary vein graft patency after bypass surgery, but there are no reports of effects on mural thrombus generation.[77,78] The specific and direct inhibition of thrombin by hirudin documents the pivotal role of thrombin in platelet deposition beyond the first layer of platelet adhesion. Hirudin will be discussed further in the next section. The platelet glycoprotein IIb/IIIa complex (GpIIb/IIIa) has recently been identified as the final common pathway for all agonists.[79] The binding of adhesive proteins, such as fibrinogen to GpIIb/IIIa, causes platelets to aggregate. Monoclonal antibodies to GpIIb/IIIa inhibit platelet aggregation against all known platelet agonists in animals as well as in humans.[80,81]

Hirudin, a specific thrombin inhibitor isolated from the saliva of the European leech, documents the important role of thrombin in the thrombotic response to deep arterial injury. Hirudin has the greatest binding affinity of any antithrombin (kd 2×10^{-13} for recombinant hirudin). It inhibits platelet aggregation to thrombin but not thromboxane, ADP, or collagen. Thrombin inhibition with hirudin reduces fibrin deposition at lower doses (aPTT, 1.7 times control), and at higher doses (aPTT, >2 times control), can totally eliminate mural thrombosis and reduces platelet deposition to a single layer or less. These studies were performed in normal arteries of pigs.[82] Since all mammalian coagulation systems are similar, these results are probably predictive of similar relative outcomes in humans.

Since hirudin forms a 1:1 stoichiometric complex with thrombin, the blood level of hirudin required to totally inhibit intravascular thrombosis for different injuries and thrombogenic stimuli may be considered an index of the thrombin content of each intravascular stimulus for thrombosis. For example, during disseminated intravascular coagulation, the blood level required to inhibit platelet thrombi in pulmonary circulation was five times greater than that necessary to inhibit fibrin thrombi.[34] In comparison, the hirudin level required to inhibit intravascular thrombus in deeply injured arterial tunica media (type III injury) is 10 times greater than that encountered in de-endothelialized or mildly injured artery (type II injury).[83] Utilizing immunohistochemical staining for thrombin within thrombus, Chesebro et al. have shown that thrombus overlying a region of deeply injured artery stains markedly positive for thrombin in comparison to a similar region with mild injury.[34,83] This has functionally coincided with a greater amount of fibrin deposition immediately adjacent to deeply injured artery with lesser deposition more remote from the deep injury or over mild injury.[42]

The powerful and specific antithrombin action of hirudin compared to heparin was shown experimentally by Heras et al. to markedly reduce platelet, fibrin(ogen), and thrombus deposition in deeply injured porcine carotid arteries.[82] Heparin and hirudin prolonged the aPTT to twice the control value. Thrombosis in the heparin-treated animals was present in 57% of segments, whereas no thrombus was found in the hirudin-treated group. Quantitative platelet deposition was markedly decreased and limited to a single layer by hirudin compared to extensive, multilayered platelet deposition in pigs treated with heparin.[82]

Although both heparin and hirudin are antithrombin drugs, their efficacy in arterial thrombosis is very different. Heparin is a co-factor of antithrombin III; heparin-antithrombin III only partially inhibits new thrombin formation and new fibrin polymerization in arteries. Heparin, unlike hirudin, is inhibited by fibrin II monomer and platelet factor 4, released from activated platelets, and is 50 times less effective at partially inhibiting fibrin-bound compared to free thrombin. On the other hand, hirudin totally inhibits fibrin-bound and free thrombin at the same dosage.[84,85]

Hirudin-binding induces conformational changes to thrombin and blocks its coagulant activity. Thrombin activates platelets by binding to Gp Ib on the platelet membrane and producing a proteolytic degradation of Gp V.[86] The site where hirudin binds thrombin is important for the reaction of thrombin with platelets. Hirudin has a high affinity for thrombin and the platelet thrombin receptor and displaces thrombin from platelets.[87] This may explain the efficient endogenous lysis of thrombus with hirudin.[88] The hirudin molecule is about one-tenth the

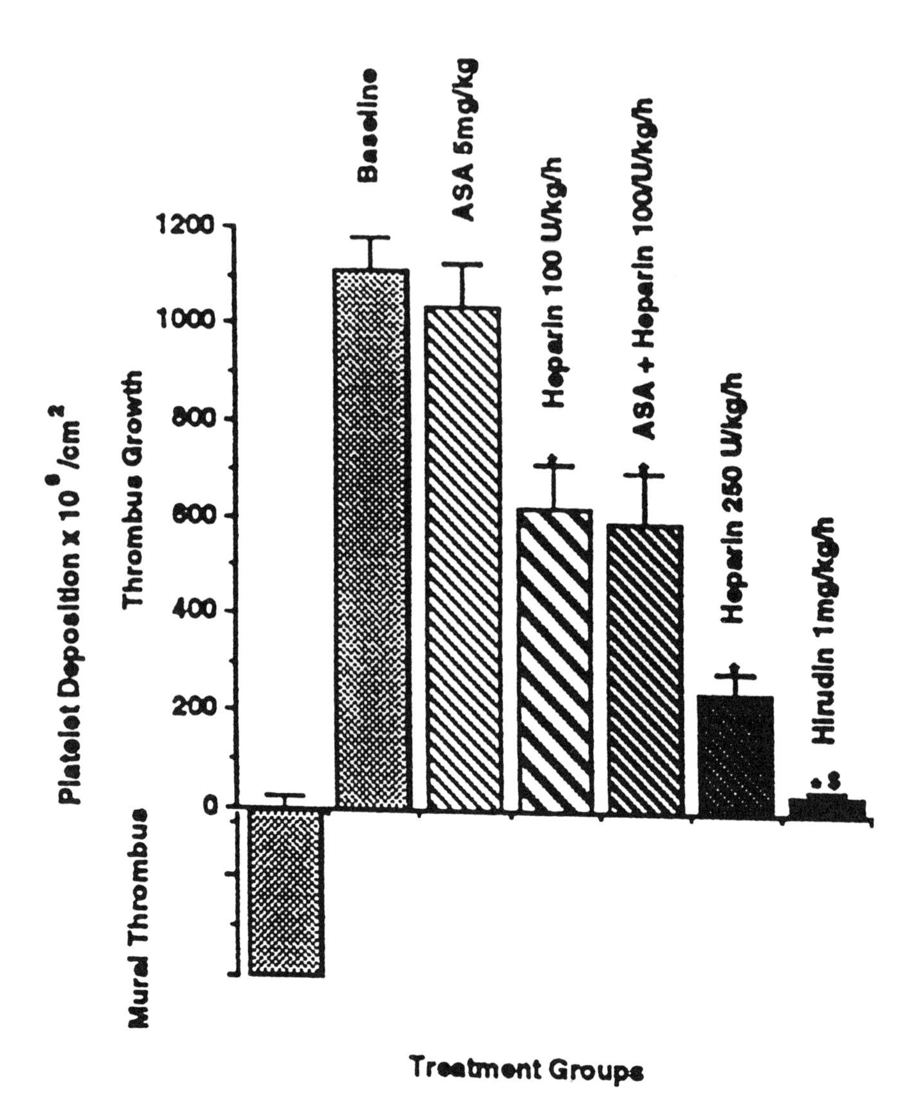

Figure 8: Bar graphs of differential effects of antithrombotic regimens on mean platelet deposition during growth of thrombus triggered by a fresh mural thrombus at high shear rate. Vertical lines indicate SEM. Aspirin (ASA) had no significant effect on growth of thrombus. Heparin showed a dose-dependent effect on growth of thrombus. Platelet deposition in animals treated with hirudin were significantly lower compared with the highest-dose heparin group (*$P<.05$ vs. baseline, $$P<.001$ vs. heparin 250 IU/kg). (Reproduced with permission.[34])

size of the heparin-antithrombin III (AT III) complex, and easily binds thrombin bound to fibrin compared to the masking of receptors to AT III on fibrin-bound thrombin. Since there is no naturally occurring inhibitor of hirudin, its renal elimination is the major limiting factor. The prevention of thrombosis by hirudin documents the pivotal role of thrombin in the activation of platelets. Unlike heparin, hirudin totally blocks growth of mural thrombus (Figure 8) at high and low shear rates.[72] By totally blocking growth of thrombus, hirudin enhances lysis by endogenous tissue-type plasminogen activator (t-PA) or urokinase. This strategy of prolonged antithrombotic therapy to reduce intravascular thrombus and improve lumen diameter may be useful after thrombolysis for myocardial infarction or as primary antithrombotic therapy for patients with unstable angina or non-Q-wave myocardial infarction. Several recent preliminary clinical trials demonstrated a favorable effect of direct thrombin inhibitors in unstable angina, and when used as adjuvant therapy with thrombolysis have shown better rates of arterial patency.[89–92]

References

1. Falk E. Plaque rupture with severe pre-existing stenosis precipitating coronary thrombosis: Characteristics of coronary atherosclerosis plaques underlying fatal occlusive thrombi. Br Heart J 1983; 50:127–134.
2. Fuster V, Stein B, Ambrose JA, Badimon L, Badimon JJ, Chesebro JH. Atherosclerosis plaque rupture and thrombosis: Evolving concepts. Circulation 1990; (Suppl II):II-47-II-59.
3. Fuster V, Badimon L, Badimon JJ, Chesebro JH. The pathogenesis of coronary artery disease and the acute coronary syndromes, Parts 1 & 2. N Engl J Med 1992; 326:242–250,310–318.
4. Alderman EL, Corley SD, Fisher LD, et al. Five-year angiographic follow-up of factors associated with progression of coronary artery disease in the Coronary Artery Surgery Study (CASS). J Am Coll Cardiol 1993; 22: 1141–1154.
5. Stary HC. Composition and classification of human atherosclerotic lesions. Virchows Archiv A Pathol Anat 1992; 421:277–290.
6. Richardson PD, Davies MJ, Born GVR. Influence of plaque configuration and stress distribution on fissuring of coronary atherosclerotic plaques. Lancet 1989; 2:941–944.
7. Davies MJ, Woolf N, Rowles PM, Pepper J. Morphology of the endothelium over atherosclerotic plaques in human coronary arteries. Br Heart J 1988; 60:459–464.
8. Fuster V, Badimon L, Cohen M, Ambrose JA, Badimon JJ, Chesebro J. Insights into the pathogenesis of acute ischemic syndromes. Circulation 1988; 77:1213–1220.
9. Badimon L, Chesebro JH, Badimon JJ. Thrombus formation on ruptured

atherosclerotic plaques and rethrombosis on evolving thrombi. Circulation 1992; 86 (Suppl III):III-74-III-85.

10. Fuster V, Lewis A. Conner Memorial Lecture: Mechanisms leading to myocardial infarction. Insights from studies of vascular biology. Circulation 1994; 90:2126–2146.
11. Moise A, L'esperance J, Theroux P, Taeymans Y, Goulet C, Bourassa MG. Clinical and angiographic predictors of new total coronary occlusion in coronary artery disease: Analysis of 313 nonoperated patients. Am J Cardiol 1984; 54:1176–1181.
12. Ambrose JA, Winters SL, Arora RR, Eng A, Riccio A, Gorlin R, Fuster V. Angiographic evolution of coronary artery morphology in unstable angina. JACC 1988; 12:56–62.
13. Ambrose JA, Tannenbaum MA, Alexopoulos D, et al. Angiographic progression of coronary artery disease and the development of myocardial infarction. J Am Coll Cardiol 1988; 12:56–62.
14. Levin DC, Fallon JT. Significance of the angiographic morphology of localized coronary stenoses: Histopathologic correlations. Circulation 1982; 66: 316–320.
15. Chesebro JH, Fuster V. Thrombosis in unstable angina. N Engl J Med 1992; 327:192–194.
16. Ambrose JA, Hjemdahl-Monsen CE, Borrico S, Gorlin R, Fuster V. Angiographic demonstration of a common link between unstable angina pectoris and non-Q wave myocardial infarction. Am J Cardiol 1988; 61:244–247.
17. De Wood MA, Stifter WF, Simpson CS, et al. Coronary arteriographic findings soon after non-Q wave myocardial infarction. N Engl J Med 1986; 315:417–423.
18. Fuster V, Frye RL, Kennedy MA, Connolly DC, Mankin HT. The role of collateral circulation in the various coronary syndromes. Circulation 1979; 59:1137–1144.
19. Sasayama S, Fujita M. Recent insights into coronary collateral circulation. Circulation 1992; 85(3):1197–1204.
20. Little WC. Angiographic assessment of the culprit lesion before acute myocardial infarction. Am J Cardiol 1990; 66:44G-47G.
21. Falk E. Unstable angina with fatal outcome: dynamic coronary thrombosis leading to infarction and/or sudden death: autopsy evidence of recurrent mural thrombosis with peripheral embolization culminating in total vascular occlusion. Circulation 1985; 71:699–708.
22. Falk E. Why do plaques rupture? Circulation 1992; 86(Suppl III):III-30-III-42.
23. Cheng GC, Loree HM, Kamm RD, Fishbein MC, et al. Distribution of circumferential stress in ruptured and stable atherosclerotic lesions. A structural analysis with histopathological correlation. Circulation 1993; 87:1179–1187.
24. Bini A, Fenoglio JJ, Mesa-Tejada R, Kudryk B, Kaplan KL. Identification and distribution of fibrinogen, fibrin, and fibrin(ogen) degradation products in atherosclerosis: Use of monoclonal antibodies. Arteriosclerosis 1989; 9:109–121.
25. Coleman RW, Cook JJ, Niewiarowski S. Mechanisms of platelet aggregation. In Coleman R, Hirsh J, Marder V, Salzman EW (eds): Hemostasis

and Thrombosis, Basic Principles and Clinical Practice. JB Lippincott, 1994; pp 508–523.

26. Calvete JJ. Clues for understanding the structure and function of a prototypic human integrin: the platelet glycoprotein IIb/IIIa complex. Thromb Hemostasis 1994; 72:1–15.
27. Williams WJ. Sequence of Coagulation Reactions. Hematology 1983, Third edition; part VIII, NY, McGraw Hill, 1983.
28. Steele PM, Chesebro JH, Stanson AW, et al. Balloon angioplasty: natural history of the pathological response to injury in a pig model. Circ Res 1985; 57:105–112.
29. Ip JH, Fuster V, Badimon L, Badimon JJ, Taubman MB, Chesebro JH. Syndromes of accelerated atherosclerosis: role of vascular injury and smooth muscle cell proliferation. J Am Coll Cardiol 1990; 15:1667–1687.
30. Fingerle J, Johnson R, Clowes A, Majesky M, Reidy MA. Role of platelets in smooth muscle cell proliferation and migration after vascular injury in rat carotid artery. Proc Natl Acad Sci USA 1989; 86:8412–8416.
31. Ross R. The pathogenesis of atherosclerosis: a perspective for the 1990s. Nature 1993; 362:801–809.
32. Shuman MA. Thrombin-cellular interactions. Ann NY Acad Sci 1986; 485: 228–239.
33. Bar-Shavit R, Eldor A, Voldavsky I. Binding of thrombin to subendothelial extracellular matrix: protection and expression of functional properties. J Clin Invest 1989; 84:1096–1104.
34. Chesebro JH, Webster MWI, Zoldhelyi P, Roche PC, Badimon L, Badimon JJ. Antithrombotic therapy and progression of coronary artery disease: antiplatelets versus antithrombins. Circulation 1992; 86:III-100-III-111.
35. Badimon JJ, Badimon L. Mechanism of arterial thrombosis in nonparallel streamlines: platelet thrombi grow at the apex of stenotic severely injured vessel wall. Experimental study in the pig model. J Clin Invest 1989; 84: 1134–1144.
36. Taubman MB. Tissue factor regulation in vascular smooth muscle: a summary of studies performed using in vivo and in vitro models. Am J Cardiol 1993; 72:55C-60C.
37. Fernandez-Ortiz A, Badimon JJ, Falk E, Fuster V, Meyer B, Mailhac A, Weng D, Shah PK, Badimon L. Characterization of the relative thrombogenicity of atherosclerotic plaque components: Implications for consequences of plaque rupture. J Am Coll Cardiol 1994; 23:1562–1569.
38. van Zanten GH, de Graaf S, Slootweg PJ, Heijnen HFG, Connolly TM, de Groot PG, Sixma JJ. Increased platelet deposition on atherosclerotic coronary arteries. J Clin Invest 1994; 93:615–632.
39. MacIsaac A, Thomas JD, Topol EJ. Toward the quiescent coronary plaque. J Am Coll Cardiol 1993; 22:1228–1241.
40. Rubanyi GM, Romero JC, Vanhoutte PM. Flow-induced release of endothelium-derived relaxing factors. Am J Physiol 1986; 250:H1145–1149.
41. Lassila R, Badimon JJ, Vallabhajosula S, Badimon L. Dynamic monitoring of platelet deposition on severely damaged vessel wall in flowing blood: effects of different stenosis on thrombus growth. Atherosclerosis 1990; 10: 306–315.
42. Mailhac A, Badimon JJ, Fallon JT, Ortiz AF, Meyer B, Chesebro JH, Fus-

ter V, Badimon L. Effect of an eccentric severe stenosis on fibrin(ogen) deposition on severely damaged vessel wall in arterial thrombosis. Circulation 1994; 90:988–996.

43. Lam JYT, Chesebro JH, Steele PM, Badimon L, Fuster V. Is vasospasm related to platelet deposition? Relationship in a porcine preparation of arterial injury in vivo. Circulation 1987; 75:243–248.
44. Maseri A, L'Abbate A, Parodi G. Coronary vasospasm as a possible cause of myocardial infarction: a conclusion derived from the study of "preinfarction" angina. N Engl J Med 1978; 317:1055–1059.
45. Penny WJ, Chesebro JH, Heras M, Badimon L, Fuster V. In vivo identification of normal and damaged endothelium by quantitative coronary angiography and infusion of acetylcholine and bradykinin in pigs. J Am Coll Cardiol 1988; 11:29A.
46. Webster MWI, Chesebro JH, Reeder GS, Mock MB, Grill DE, Bailey KR, Steichen S, Fuster V. Antiplatelet therapy reduces acute complications but not restenosis. Circulation 1989; 80(Suppl):II-64.
47. Furchgott RF, Zawadzki JV. The obligatory role of endothelial cells in the relaxation of arterial smooth muscle by acetylcholine. Nature 1980; 299: 373–376.
48. Luscher TF. Endothelium-derived relaxing and contracting factors: potential role in coronary artery disease. Eur Heart J 1989; 10:847–857.
49. Ashton JH, Benedict CR, Fitzgerald C. Serotonin as a mediator of cyclic flow variations in stenosed canine coronary arteries. Circulation 1986; 73: 572–578.
50. Vanhoutte PM, Shimokawa H. Endothelium-derived relaxing factor and coronary vasospasm. Circulation 1988; 78:1323–1324.
51. McClellan G, Weisberg A, Rose D, Winegrad S. Endothelial cell storage and release of endothelin as a cardioregulatory mechanism. Circ Res 1994; 75:85–96.
52. Chester AH, O'Neill GS, Moncada S, Tadjkarimi S, Yacoub MN. Low basal and stimulated release of nitric oxide in atherosclerotic epicardial coronary arteries. Lancet 1990; 336:897–900.
53. Hjemdahl P, Larson PT, Waller NH. Effects of stress and beta-blockade on platelet function. Circulation 1991; 84(III):44–61.
54. Badimon L, Lassila R, Badimon J, Fuster V. An acute surge of epinephrine stimulates platelet deposition to severely damaged vascular wall. J Am Coll Cardiol 1990; 15(Suppl):181A.
55. Muller JE, Toefler GH, Stone PH. Circadian variations and triggers of onset of acute cardiovascular disease. Circulation 1989; 79:733–743.
56. Goldberg RJ, Brady P, Muller JE, et al. Time of onset of symptoms of acute myocardial infarction. Am J Cardiol 1990; 66:140–144.
57. Meisel SR, Kutz I, Dayan KI, et al. Effect of Iraqi missiles on incidence of acute myocardial infarction and sudden death in Israeli civilians. Lancet 1991; 338:660–661.
58. Mittleman MA, Maclure M, Tofler GH, Sherwood JB, et al. Triggering of acute myocardial infarction by heavy physical exertion. N Engl J Med 1993; 329:1677–1683.
59. Loscalzo J. Lipoprotein(a): a unique risk factor for atherothrombotic disease. Arteriosclerosis 1990; 10:672–679.

60. Nachman RL. Stratton Lecture: thrombosis and atherogenesis: molecular connections. Blood 1992; 79.1897–1906.
61. Liu AC, Lawn RM. Lipoprotein(a) and atherogenesis. Tr Cardvas Med 1994 4; 1:40–44.
62. Berg K. Lp(a) lipoprotein: an overview. Chem Phys Lipids 67/68, 1994; 9–16.
63. Anglés-Cano E, Hervio L, Rouy D, Fournier C, Chapman JM, Laplaud M, Koschinsky ML. Effects of lipoprotein (a) on the binding to fibrin and its activation by fibrin-bound tissue-type plasminogen activator. Chem Phys Lipids 67/68, 1994; 369–380.
64. Meade TW, Cooper JA, Peart WS. Plasma renin activity and ischemic heart disease. N Engl J Med 1993; 329:616–619.
65. Ridker PM, Gaboury CL, Conlin PR, et al. Stimulation of plasminogen activator inhibitor in vivo by infusion of angiotensin II: evidence of a potential interaction between the renin-angiotensin system and fibrinolytic function. Circulation 1993; 87:1969–1973.
66. Vaughan DE, Shen C, Lazos SA. Angiotensin II induces plasminogen activator inhibitor (PAI-1) in vitro. Circulation 1992; 86(Suppl I): I-557.
67. Genest JJ, McNamara JR, Upson B, et al. Prevalence of familial hyperhomocyst(e)inemia in men and premature coronary artery disease. Arterioscler Thromb 1991; 11:1129–1136.
68. Schneider DJ, Sobel BE. Effect of diabetes on the coagulation and fibrinolytic systems and its implications for atherogenesis. Coronary Artery Dis 1992; 3:26–32.
69. Wilhilmsen L, Svadsudd K, Korsan-Bengtsen K, Larsson B, Welin L, Tibblin G. Fibrinogen as a risk factor for stroke and myocardial infarction. N Engl J Med 1984; 311:501–505.
70. Kimura S, Nishinaga M, Ozawa T, Shimada K. Thrombin generation as an acute effect of cigarette smoking. Am Heart J 1994; 128: 7–11.
71. Badimon L, Badimon JJ, Lassila R, Merino A, Chesebro JH, Fuster V. Rethrombosis on an evolving thrombus is mediated by thrombus-bound thrombin that is not inhibited by systemic heparin. Thromb Haemost 1991; 65(Suppl): 321.
72. Meyer B, Badimon JJ, Mailhac A, Fernandez-Ortiz A, Chesebro JH, Fuster V, Badimon L. Inhibition of growth of thrombus on fresh mural thrombus: Targeting optimal therapy. Circulation 1994; 90:2432–2438.
73. Owen J, Freidman KD, Grossman BA, Wilkens C, Berke AD, Powers ER. Thrombolytic therapy with tissue plasminogen activator or streptokinase induces transient thrombin activity. Blood 1988; 72:616–620.
74. Patrono C. Aspirin as an antiplatelet drug. N Engl J Med 1994; 330: 18.1287–1294.
75. Chesebro JH, Webster MWI, Smith HC, et al. Antiplatelet therapy in coronary disease progression: reduced infarction and new lesion formation. Circulation 1989; 80(Suppl II):II-266.
76. Lam JYT, Chesebro JH, Badimon L, Fuster V. Serotonin and thromboxane A_2 receptor blockage decrease vasoconstriction but not platelet deposition after deep arterial injury. Circulation 1986; 74(Suppl II):II-97.
77. Flores-Runk P, Raasch RH. Ticlopidine and platelet therapy. Ann Pharmacother 1993; 27(9):1090–1098.

78. Salomon DH, Hart RG. Antithrombotic therapies for stroke prevention. Current Opinions Neurol 1994; 7(1)48–53.
79. Mousa SA, Bozarth JM, Forsythe MS, Jackson SM, Leamy A, Diemer MM, Kapil RP, Knabb RM, Mayo MC, Pierce SK, De Grado WF, Thoolen MJ, Reilly TM. Antiplatelet and antithrombotic efficacy of DMP 728, a novel platelet GPIIb/IIIa receptor antagonist. Circulation 1994; 89:3–12.
80. Coller BS, Folts JD, Scrudder LE, Smith SR. Antithrombotic effect of a monoclonal antibody to the platelet glycoprotein IIb/IIIa receptor in an experimental animal model. Blood 1986; 68;783–786.
81. Gold HK, Gimple LW, Yasuda T, Leinbach RC, Werner W, Holt R, Jordon R, Berger H, Collen D, Coller BS. Pharmacologic study of $F(ab')_2$ fragments of murine monoclonal antibody 7E3 directed against human platelet glycoprotein IIb/IIIa in patient with unstable angina pectoris. J Clin Invest 1990; 86:651–659.
82. Heras M, Chesebro JH, Webster MWI, Mruk JS, Grill DE, Penny WJ, Walter Bowie EJ, Badimon L, Fuster V. Hirudin, heparin, and placebo during deep arterial injury in the pig. The in vivo role of thrombin in platelet-mediated thrombosis. Circulation 1990; 82:1476–1484.
83. Badimon L, Badimon JJ, Lassila R, Heras M, Chesebro JH, Fuster V. Effects of thrombin inhibition in porcine platelet interaction with severely damaged vessel wall, mildly damaged vessel wall and isolated fibrillar collagen type I. Hirudin and r-hirudin versus heparin in arterial thrombosis. Blood 1991; 78:423–434.
84. Markwardt F, Kaiser B, Novak G. Studies on antithrombotic effects of recombinant hirudin. Thromb Res 1989; 54:377–388.
85. Massel DR, Hudoba M, Weitz JI. Clot-bound thrombin is protected from heparin inhibition: a potential mechanism for rethrombosis after lytic therapy. Circulation 1989; 80(Suppl II):II-420.
86. Seiss W. Molecular mechanisms of platelet activation. Physiol Rev 1989; 69:58–178.
87. Tam SW, Fenton JW, Detweiler TC. Dissociation of thrombin from platelets by hirudin. J Biol Chem 1979; 254:8723–8725.
88. Chesebro JH, Rao AK, Schwartz D, Bear PA, Kleiman NS, Harrington RA, Henis M, Fuster V. Endogenous thrombolysis and recanalization of occluded aortocoronary vein grafts with recombinant hirudin in patients with unstable angina. Circulation 1994; 90:I-568.
89. Lidon-Corbi RM, Theroux P, Juneau M, Adelman B, Maraganore J. Initial experience with a direct antithrombin, hirulog, in unstable angina. Anticoagulant, antithrombotic and clinical effects. Circulation 1993; 88(4): 1495–1501.
90. Lidon-Corbi RM, Theroux P, Lesperance J, Adelman B, Bonan R, Duval D, Levesque J. A pilot, early angiographic patency study using a direct thrombin inhibitor as adjunctive therapy to streptokinase in acute myocardial infarction. Circulation 1994; 89(4):1557–1566.
91. Topol EJ, Fuster V, Harrington RA, Califf RM, Kleinman NS, Kerelakes DJ, Cohen M, Chapekis KA, Gold HK, Tannenbaum MA, Rao AK, Debowey D, Schwartz D, Henis M, Chesebro J. Recombinant hirudin for un-

stable angina pectoris: A multicenter, randomized trial. Circulation 1994; 89:1557–1566.

92. Cannon CP, McCabe CH, Henry TD, Schweiger MJ, et al. A pilot study of recombinant desulfatohirudin compared with heparin in conjunction with tissue-type plasminogen activator and aspirin for acute myocardial infarction: Results of the Thrombolysis in Myocardial Infarction (TIMI) 5 trial. J Am Coll Cardiol 1994; 23:993–1003.

3

Angiographic Correlations of Complex Lesions in Acute Coronary Syndromes

Douglas Israel, MD, John A. Ambrose, MD

Pathophysiology

Development of the Atherosclerotic Plaque

The angiographic features of coronary stenosis associated with the acute coronary syndromes of unstable angina, non-Q-wave and Q-wave infarction are best understood by exploring the pathophysiology of stable and unstable coronary disease. Therefore, we begin this chapter on angiographic correlations with a brief review of the evolution of atherosclerotic heart disease and its transition to the unstable state.

Early pathological studies demonstrated the ubiquitous presence of fatty streaks in the aorta of infants and children.[1,2] These lesions progressively appear within the coronary tree by the age of 20 years. Microscopically, these fatty streaks are composed of lipid-laden macrophages.[3] As fatty streaks progress, lipid uptake can be demonstrated to occur in intimal smooth muscles cells as well. Droplets of extracellular lipid presumably derived from dead lipid-engorged cells begin to accumulate along with smooth muscle cells that have migrated and proliferated in the intima. The formation of fatty streaks has a predilec-

From: Ambrose JA (ed): *Complex Coronary Lesions in Acute Coronary Syndromes*.

tion for specific anatomic sites such as angulated segments and bifurcations, particularly on the wall opposite a flow divider. This has been observed in the coronary tree as well as in the brachiocephalic and carotid bifurcations.[4–6] This early localization of atherosclerotic lesions is presumably related to hemorheologic factors. Locations prone to lesion development are sites with low shear stress and/or oscillations in shear stress.

The further evolution of the lesions described above is variable in its timing and occurrence. Progression does not occur in all individuals and is related to the presence of risk factors for vascular disease as well as geographic and ethnic factors which likely reflect variable genetic susceptibility.[7] When further progression occurs, a lipid core is formed by coalescence and fusion of separate extracellular lipid pools. Progression to the fibrofatty plaque occurs over time. A variable amount of extracellular lipid in the form of cholesterol or cholesteryl ester is present and the lipid core is covered by a fibrous cap composed of variable amounts of smooth muscle cells and connective tissue.[8,9] The gradual development of luminal narrowing is related to the continued elaboration of the cellular components, extracellular matrix, and the lipid pool as well as thickening of the overlying cap. While some lesions are lipid-rich, others even in the same individual are devoid of lipid and rich in connective tissue and ground substance. Progression may occur both gradually and rapidly.[10] The rapid form of progression may lead to an acute syndrome as described below or intermittent fissuring/disruption with mural thrombus formation may lead to episodic increases in luminal narrowing following incorporation of thrombus into the wall of the artery.[11] For a more detailed discussion of atherosclerosis in general and the mechanisms involved in its progression, we refer you to Chapter 2 and to recently published reviews.[12,13]

Transition to the Unstable State: Role of Plaque Disruption and Thrombosis in the Acute Coronary Syndromes

The pathophysiology of the acute coronary syndromes has been a source of controversy throughout this century. More recently, a large body of evidence partially reviewed in Chapters 1 and 2 has suggested that a common pathogenetic mechanism related to the occurrence of minor or major plaque fissuring complicated by intraintimal and/or intraluminal thrombosis may explain these syndromes.[12–16] These acute syndromes appear as a continuum—the clinical presentation being the end result of multiple factors including the severity and acuteness of obstruction, the presence and/or duration of total coronary occlusion, the ability to acutely recruit collaterals, and perhaps, to a lesser extent, myocardial oxygen demands.[17–19]

In unstable angina, plaque fissuring or disruption leads to an abrupt increase in luminal obstruction. A mural thrombus largely composed of platelets forms initially within the intima which in itself may increase luminal obstruction. Thrombus may extend into the lumen and transiently decrease myocardial blood flow. Episodic embolization may also occur. Total coronary occlusion is infrequent but has been described in 10% to 20% of patients.[20] However, total occlusion followed by spontaneous opening of the artery is a possible mechanism of ischemia/necrosis in unstable angina as well as in non-Q-wave infarction.[21] Ischemia at rest in unstable angina may be related to either transient decreases in myocardial oxygen supply related to vasoconstriction or enhanced vasomotion at or distal to the site of coronary narrowing as well as to changes in the thrombus.[22] As a new lesion has formed in the coronary artery causing a new imbalance between myocardial supply and demand, ischemic rest pain may also be precipitated by transient increases in myocardial oxygen demand.[23]

The syndrome of non-Q-wave myocardial infarction occupies an intermediate position in the continuum of the acute coronary syndromes between unstable angina and Q-wave infarction. A severely stenotic but patent infarct-related artery is found in 60% to 80% of cases. In the remaining 20% to 40%, total coronary occlusion is demonstrated angiographically.[20,24] In many cases of non-Q-wave infarction where total occlusion is not found, it has been postulated that spontaneous reperfusion occurs. This has been suggested by the frequent finding of ST segment elevation on the ECG during infarction and an early peak of creatine kinase following infarction.

In patients who present with Q-wave myocardial infarction, there is total coronary occlusion in 80% to 90% of cases as determined by angiography performed within 6 hours of the onset of acute myocardial infarction.[25,26] A thrombus rich in fibrin and red cells extends from the intima obstructing the lumen of the artery. In a majority of cases of Q-wave infarction, a deep tear into the intima of a lipid-rich plaque can be demonstrated.[27] The amount of thrombus that forms following plaque disruption is a complex phenomenon and depends at least in part on the degree of plaque disruption as well as the hypercoagulability of the blood and hemodynamic factors that may potentiate vasospasm following plaque disruption. The latter may lead to the formation of a fibrin-rich, stasis thrombus[28,29] (Figure 1).

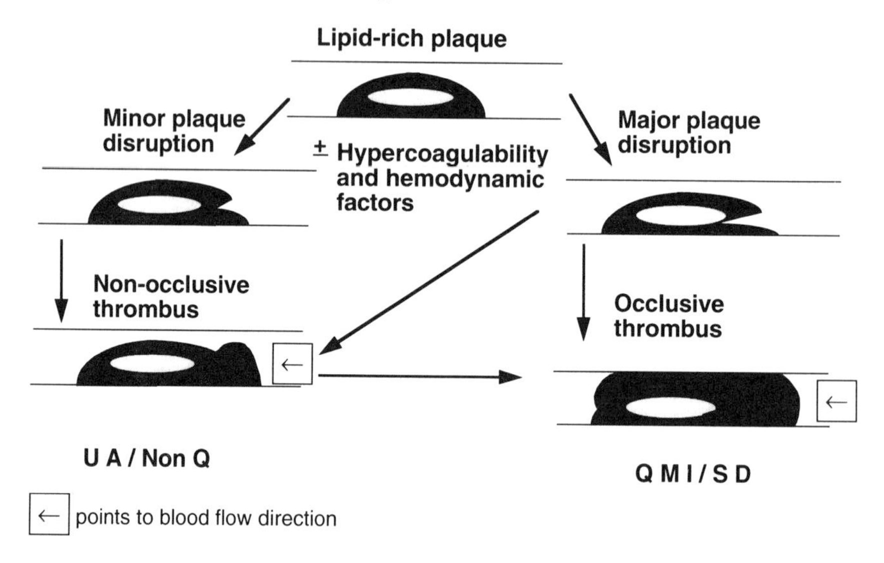

Figure 1: Schematic representation of the determinants of thrombus formation following clot disruption. UA = unstable angina; non-Q = non-Q-wave myocardial infarction; QMI = Q-wave myocardial infarction; SD = sudden death.

Recent data also suggest a potential role for inflammation in the pathogenesis of unstable angina.[30,31] Increased expression of granulocyte and monocyte adhesion receptors can be demonstrated in the coronary sinus of patients with unstable angina. Activated monocytes capable of expressing a tissue factor-like procoagulant activity have also been demonstrated in unstable but not in stable syndromes. Inflammatory cell infiltrates in the fibrous cap are a trigger for plaque disruption in acute syndromes.[32] Epicardial "streaks" on the surface of the heart containing inflammatory cells have also been seen at autopsy in patients dying following an episode of unstable angina.[33] Whether the presence of these inflammatory mediators indicates an additional pathophysiological mechanism for inflammation in unstable angina and acute myocardial infarction is unknown at present. However, thrombosis and inflammation are not incompatible, and neutrophil-platelet interactions as well as the release of inflammatory mediators occur commonly at sites of thrombosis.[34,35] Inflammatory infiltrates may also develop in the microcirculation or myocardium secondary to prolonged ischemia.

Pathological-Angiographic Correlations in Acute Coronary Syndromes

The angiographic features of such disrupted or complex plaques were first described by Levin and Fallon who examined the heart and coronary arteries and performed postmortem angiography on patients who died following acute myocardial infarction or after coronary bypass surgery.[36] They found a strong relationship between complicated stenoses as determined angiographically and histologic features of plaque rupture, plaque hemorrhage, superimposed partially occluding thrombi, or recannalized thrombi. These pathological features corresponded to a distinctive angiographic appearance characterized by eccentric, irregular, and shaggy borders with intraluminal haziness. Among 35 lesions with none of these angiographic features and only stenoses with smooth borders, 11.4% were complicated histologically. Among stenoses manifesting one or more of these complex angiographic morphologies, 79% were complicated histologically. Postmortem angiography had a sensitivity of 88% and a specificity of 79% for detecting a complicated stenosis on the basis of these angiographic findings. In a more recent study, Onodera et al. re-examined the relationship between postmortem coronary angiographic morphology and coronary histology in patients who died after intracoronary thrombolysis.[37] This study reaffirmed the correlation between atheromatous plaque rupture and hemorrhage with the angiographic features of irregular stenosis borders and filling defects. Eighty percent of such irregular lesions manifested these histologic characteristics. More recently, angiographic-histologic correlations have been made at the time of directional atherectomy.[38–40] These data have been considered separately in another chapter.

Angiographic Correlations in Unstable Angina

Early studies on the angiographic findings in unstable angina found no significant difference in the number of diseased vessels, the stenosis severity, or left ventricular function when compared to patients with stable angina.[41,42] It was only until certain morphological characteristics of lesions were compared between syndromes that significant differences were noted between coronary syndromes.[15,43–47]

Angiographic morphology refers to the assessment of lesion shape rather than the severity of stenosis. In general, two lesion characteristics are identified that are usually easy to ascertain. These characteristics are lesion symmetry and the regularity or irregularity of lesion borders. The assessment of morphology requires high-resolution image intensifiers or digital subtraction. This analysis could not have been performed in the early days of angiography when resolution on cine film was suboptimal.

Concerning the qualitative assessment of coronary morphology, one must realize that it is subjective. There are multiple shapes and forms of atherosclerotic lesions as demonstrated by angiography. Yet with careful attention to detail, this analysis of symmetry and irregularity can be very reproducible. We can consistently obtain an inter- and intraobserver reproducibility above 90% for the detection of complex lesions. To qualitatively assess coronary morphology, one must view the lesion in multiple projections without foreshortening or overlap of vessels. This analysis is performed best both in stop frame and in motion since the eye appears to integrate images better while in motion. It is also helpful to magnify the images by projecting the cine film on a white wall with magnification of about four times normal. It is not sufficient to view lesions in a single projection. Orthogonal views are often necessary since in one view a lesion may look rather smooth while complex features are seen only in the other projection (Figure 2).

In general, lesions that are less than 100% occluded can be divided qualitatively into simple and complex (Figure 3). There are four aspects to defining a lesion as being complex. These include overhanging edges or irregular borders, ulcerations, abrupt faces (≥90%), or filling defects proximal or distal to a stenosis. (Figures 4–6). A lesion with one or more of these features is designated as complex.

Angiographic Studies in Unstable Angina and Acute Infarction

In our initial study of coronary morphology in unstable angina, we evaluated the morphological features of 110 patients with either stable or unstable angina.[15] Unstable angina was defined as rest pain or crescendo angina. In all cases there was an abrupt change or onset of symptoms. This definition would include most but not all patients with a diagnosis of unstable angina. In these patients, the presence of an asymmetric or eccentric stenosis with a narrow neck and/or irregular borders was seen in 54% of vessels compared to 7% with stable angina. When the lesion responsible for symptoms could be identified by clinical, electrocardiographic, and ventriculographic criteria, this

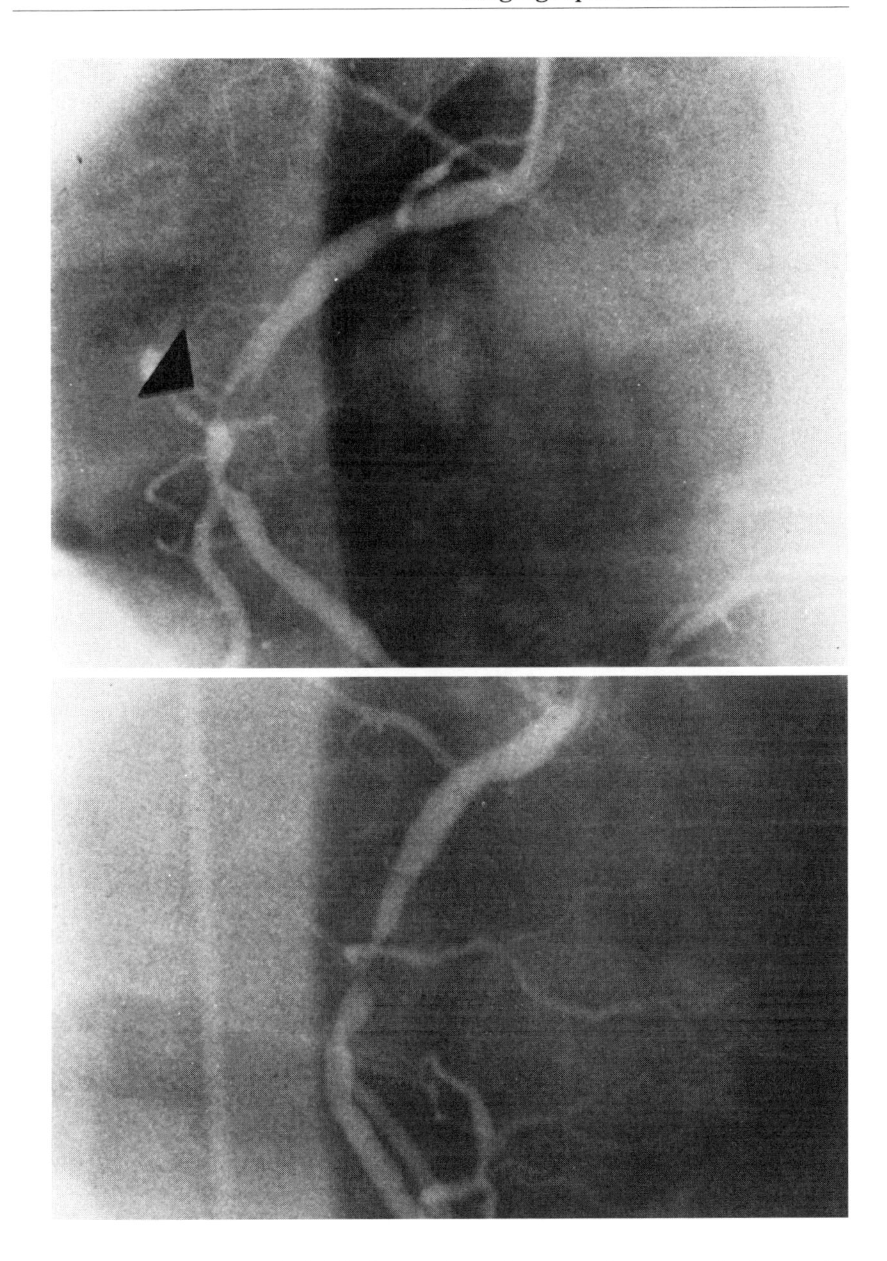

Figure 2: LAO (top) and RAO (bottom) angiogram of a severe lesion in the mid-right RCA of a patient presenting with unstable angina. Only the LAO view shows an overhanging edge in the proximal portion of the stenosis. In the RAO, the lesion is eccentric but has a smooth border.

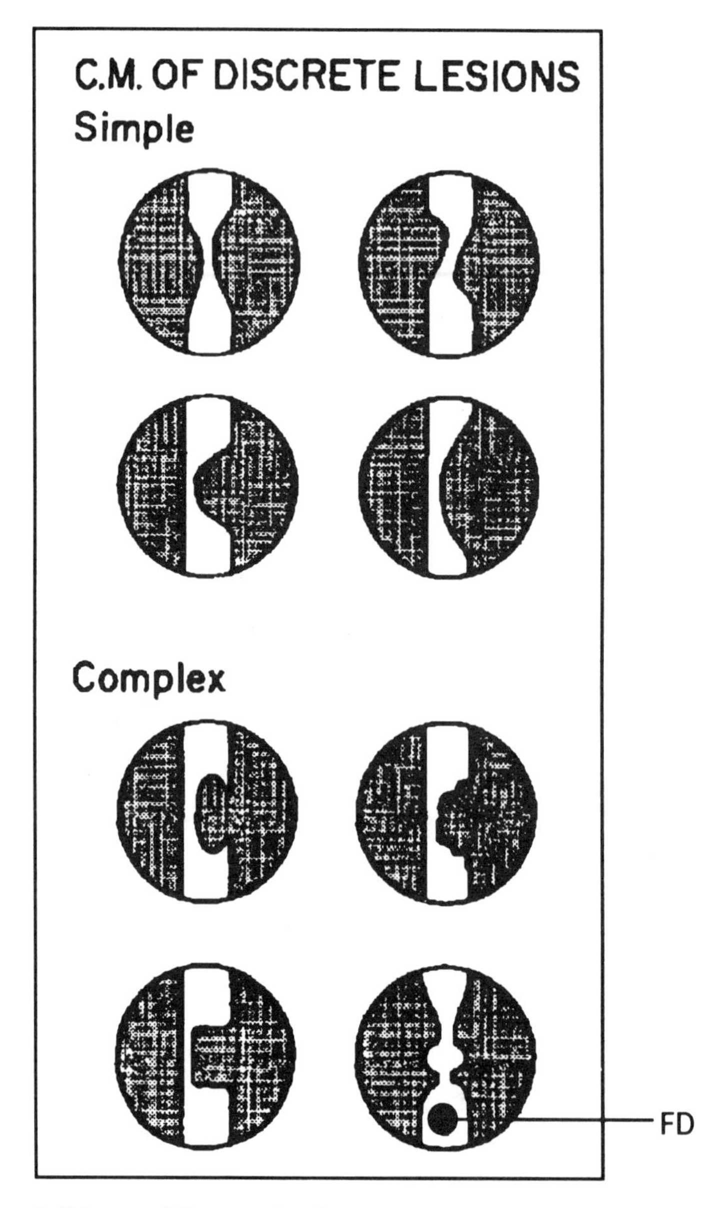

Figure 3: Schema of discrete simple versus complex lesions showing the most frequent lesion geometries noted. A filling defect (FD) may be seen proximal or distal to any lesion and if present in a lesion with simple morphology automatically changes the classification to complex. (Modified from Ambrose JA, Israel D: Am J Cardiol 1991; 68:78B–84B by permission of the American Journal of Cardiology.)

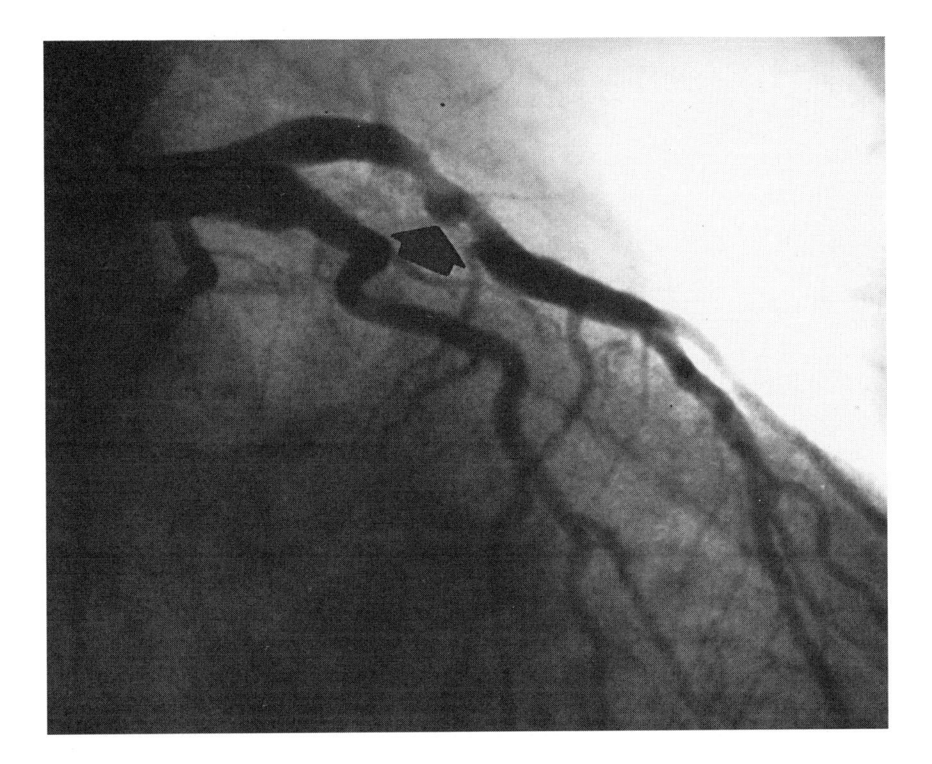

Figure 4: Left coronary artery in the RAO projection showing a significant proximal left anterior descending lesion (arrow). There is an ulcer in the middle of the lesion.

specific type II morphology was identifiable in 71% of "culprit" lesions with unstable angina but in only 16% of lesions with stable angina. Our initial nomenclature classified these lesions as type II eccentric to distinguish them from eccentric or concentric stenoses with smooth borders. As mentioned above, we now tend to classify these type II lesions as complex or complicated lesions. As lesion complexity may also be associated with concentric as opposed to eccentric stenosis, this newer designation seemed appropriate.

These qualitative observations have been corroborated by other investigators who have characterized similar-appearing lesions as "T" lesions, intracoronary thrombi, or complex plaques.[15,43–47] In several studies, these angiographic features were found in a majority of patients with unstable angina while in only a minority of patients with stable angina (Table 1). It should be noted that the term *complex lesion*

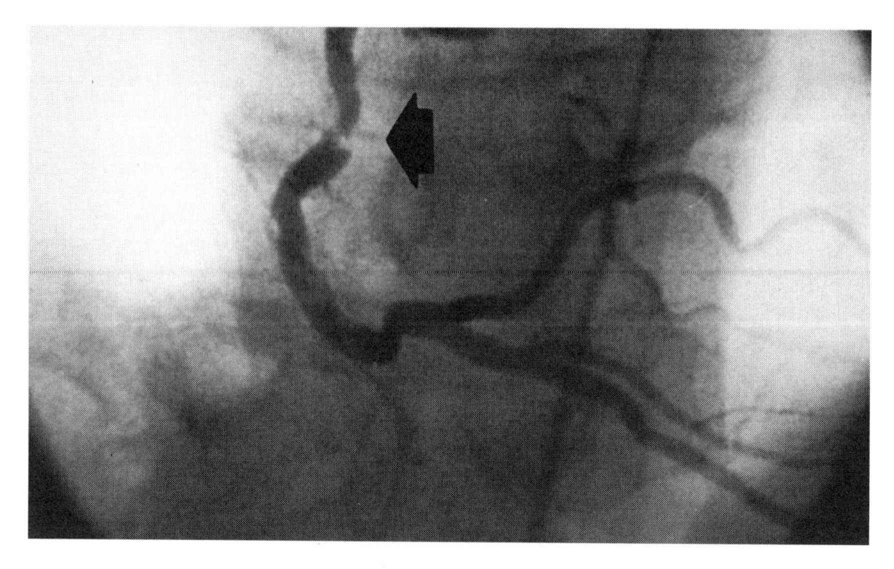

Figure 5: There is a severe midlesion in the right coronary artery as visualized in the LAO projection. The arrow points to a complex lesion with overhanging edges on its proximal and distal aspect.

has also been used to characterize lesions at risk for adverse ischemic events during coronary intervention. Here, the complexity refers to certain anatomic characteristics such as lesion tortuosity, calcification, etc. that decrease success and/or increase complications.[48] The reader should realize the distinction between these two designations of complex. The quantification of coronary morphology has been reported[49,50] and will be covered in a separate chapter.

In patients with recent non-Q-wave infarction or with a Q-wave myocardial infarction and a patent infarct-related artery, these angiographic features are also commonly seen with an incidence similar to that found in unstable angina. However, while 80% to 90% of culprit lesions are less than 100% occluded in patients with unstable angina, this percentage is significantly less in patients who present with myocardial infarction. Within the first 6 hours of myocardial infarction, total coronary occlusion is found in about 90% of patients with Q-wave myocardial infarction. The incidence of total coronary occlusion in non-Q-wave infarction varies between 20% and 40%.[24] Angiographic signs of acute thrombotic coronary occlusion include either dye staining of the occlusion, convex borders to the occlusion, or multiple filling defects without distal filling or when distal filling of the artery is markedly delayed and incomplete (TIMI 0 or 1 flow).[51]

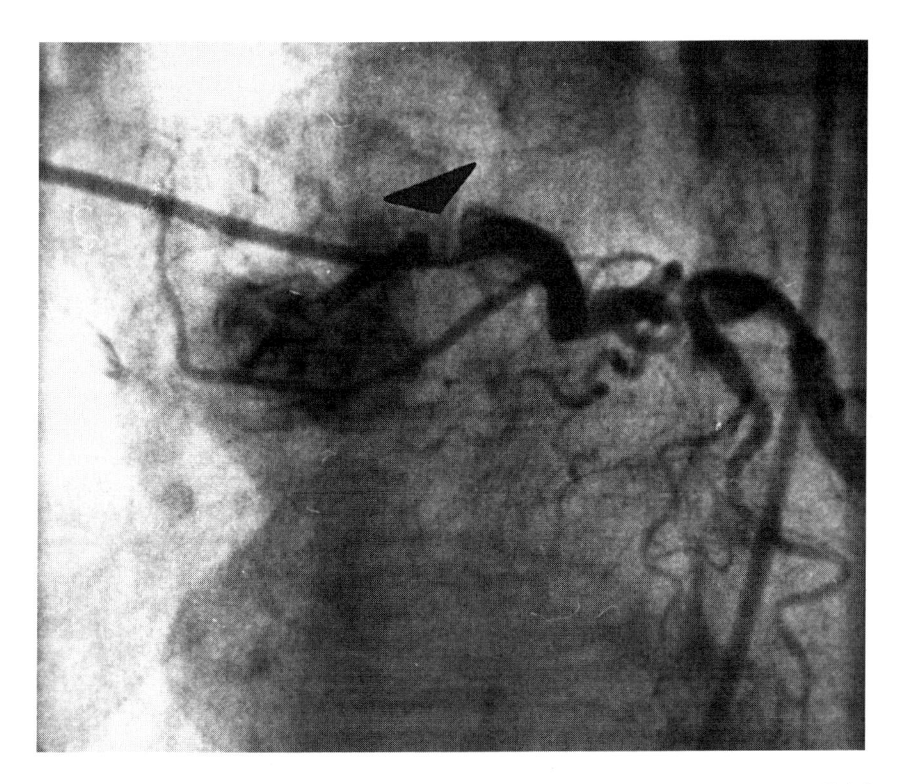

Figure 6: The left main and proximal circumflex are visualized in an LAO projection. The arrow points to a complex lesion with abrupt proximal and distal faces.

The incidence of complex lesions on angiography is similar in patients with unstable angina and myocardial infarction with a patent vessel but there are differences between the appearance of lesions in these syndromes. It has been our experience that multiple filling defects or distal filling defects are seen more frequently following myocardial infarction than unstable angina. Other investigators have reported similar findings. Patients presenting with non-Q-wave infarction are more likely to exhibit thrombotic features on angiography than patients with unstable angina.[52] Furthermore, serial angiographic studies following myocardial infarction often reveal a gradual decrease in the degree of complexity on subsequent angiography suggesting ongoing thrombolysis.[53,54] In one of these studies, nearly half of the lesions that were classified as complex early after successful thrombolysis changed to smooth lesions in the following 3 months.[54] These progressive and significant changes in morphology on serial angiography ap-

Table 1
Complex Lesions or Intracoronary Thrombi in Unstable Angina

		Unstable Angina	*Stable Angina*
	Number	*Complex Lesions/ICT*	*Complex Lesions/ICT*
Ambrose et al.	41 U 29 S	71%	16%
Capone et al.	119 U	52% last pain <1 day	0%
	35 S	28% last pain 1–14 days	
Bresnahan et al.	67 U 201 S	35%	2.5%
Haft et al.	73 U 36 S	73%	47%
Williams et al.	93 U	62%	—
Rehr et al.	50 U 42 S	70%	21%

U = unstable angina; S = stable angina; complex lesions/ICT = complex lesion morphology or the presence of intracoronary thrombus.

pear less frequently in unstable angina, possibly due to a lesser amount of fibrin thrombus in lesions in unstable angina than in myocardial infarction. In fact, in one study, 57% of complex lesions detected angiographically remained complex on follow-up.[55] This progressive decrease in the degree of lesion complexity after myocardial infarction has not been observed by all investigators. Nakagawa et al. showed that once there was dissolution of overlying mural thrombus, one may see features of plaque disruption (ulceration, overhanging edges, etc.) on subsequent angiography after myocardial infarction.[56]

While lesion complexity and severity may decrease after myocardial infarction, the opposite may be seen after unstable angina. In a preliminary investigation assessing progression of ischemia-related stenosis in unstable angina, Chen et al. noted differences between the progression of culprit and nonculprit lesions in unstable angina.[57] At restudy following medical stabilization, 25% of culprit lesions progressed by >20% or to total occlusion in comparison to only 7% of nonculprit lesions (P = 0.001). In addition, 18 of 53 culprit lesions with complex morphology progressed compared to only 3 of 31 smooth lesions (34% vs. 10%, P = 0.02).*

* Editor's note: These observations have been published in a full article recently (Chen et al. Circulation 1995; 91:2319).

Thus, a majority of lesions in unstable angina show these angiographic characteristics suggesting a complex plaque, but why do approximately 20% to 30% of lesions in culprit vessels not exhibit an angiographic morphology suggesting a complex lesion? There are several possibilities. First of all, angiography may be performed long enough after the episode of unstable angina for the lesion to have undergone some remodeling and healing. This is more likely to occur following myocardial infarction than unstable angina as mentioned before. This remodeling is likely related to organization of mural thrombus. In the experimental model, the surfaces of mural thrombi become endothelialized as fibrin and platelets are replaced by smooth muscle cells, fibroblasts, and connective tissue.[58] The original thrombus is no longer recognized as such histologically and the complex features are correspondingly obscured angiographically. The incidence of complex features on angiography are seen more frequently when angiography is performed soon after an episode of unstable angina than when performed days or weeks later.[59] Perhaps, the most important reason for this relative insensitivity of angiography to pick up complex plaques is related to the limitations of angiography itself. Angiography only visualizes the lumen of the artery. The details of the intima cannot be seen by even the most high resolution of systems. It has been clearly shown that angioscopy is a more sensitive technique than angiography for assessing the presence of thrombus.[60,61] Thus, many patients with unstable angina may have a smooth-appearing angiographic culprit lesion yet angioscopy will detect intracoronary thrombus or other features of a complex plaque. Angioscopy is discussed in Chapter 6 of this book. Of course, it is also possible that clinical instability may occur without plaque disruption and thrombus formation and may be related to other processes including vasospasm, increased myocardial oxygen demand, or secondary factors related to conditions such as anemia or congestive heart failure.[18,23]

Conversely, why are complex lesions and thrombi as detected angiographically seen in 7% to 21% of patients with stable angina? This finding supports the hypothesis of intermittency of acute plaque disruption and thrombus formation as an important mechanism of plaque progression. Particularly in patients with new onset of stable angina, these angiographic features of complex lesions may be commonly seen. However, its exact incidence in this group of patients has not been adequately assessed.

Intracoronary Thrombus

The angiographic detection of intracoronary thrombus is extremely variable in studies on unstable angina being reported between 1% and 85% of cases.[43–47,62–65] This dramatic variation depends on numerous factors including the definition of angiographic thrombus, the timing of angiography in relationship to the last episode of pain, and the medical therapy prior to angiography. The most important factor in our opinion, relates to the definition of intracoronary thrombus. There is no standardized angiographic definition of intracoronary thrombus in a nonoccluded vessel. Thrombus is often defined in angiographic studies as a filling defect surrounded by contrast on at least three sides. Other definitions employed to define thrombus have been identical to criteria used to define complex or type II eccentric lesions. Lesion translucency has also been used to define thrombus. Therefore, there is considerable overlap in angiographic definitions of thrombus versus complex lesions which clouds the distinction between complex lesions and intracoronary thrombi. This distinction is, in part, semantics since most complex lesions undoubtedly contain some thrombus as shown in pathological studies and by angioscopy. The thrombotic component in the lesion may consist of platelet-rich intimal thrombi only, but often includes laminar mural thrombus anchored to the intimal component or a free intraluminal fibrin-rich tail that may be anchored to the site of intimal disruption. It is likely that this latter feature is what is detected when filling defects are clearly visualized angiographically proximal or distal to a significant stenosis (Figure 7). The study by Nakagawa et al. provides strong evidence for the coexistence of mural thrombus within complex lesions and demonstrates the difficulties in making an angiographic diagnosis of mural thrombus overlying a complex lesion.[56] In spite of these difficulties and lack of a clear distinction between a complex lesion and an intraluminal thrombus, we have tried to standardize the definition of intracoronary thrombus. We define an intracoronary thrombus as a clear-cut filling defect located proximal or distal to a significant narrowing in a coronary artery. Translucency or a filling defect at the site of a lesion are considered in the definition of a complex plaque (Figure 8).

A second important factor in the detection of intracoronary thrombus is the timing of angiography in relationship to the onset of unstable angina or the last ischemic episode.[59] When patients are studied late after the onset of unstable angina, the thrombus may undergo endogenous lysis or may organize and become incorporated into the plaque. In either case, this might lead to failure to detect a prior thrombus by

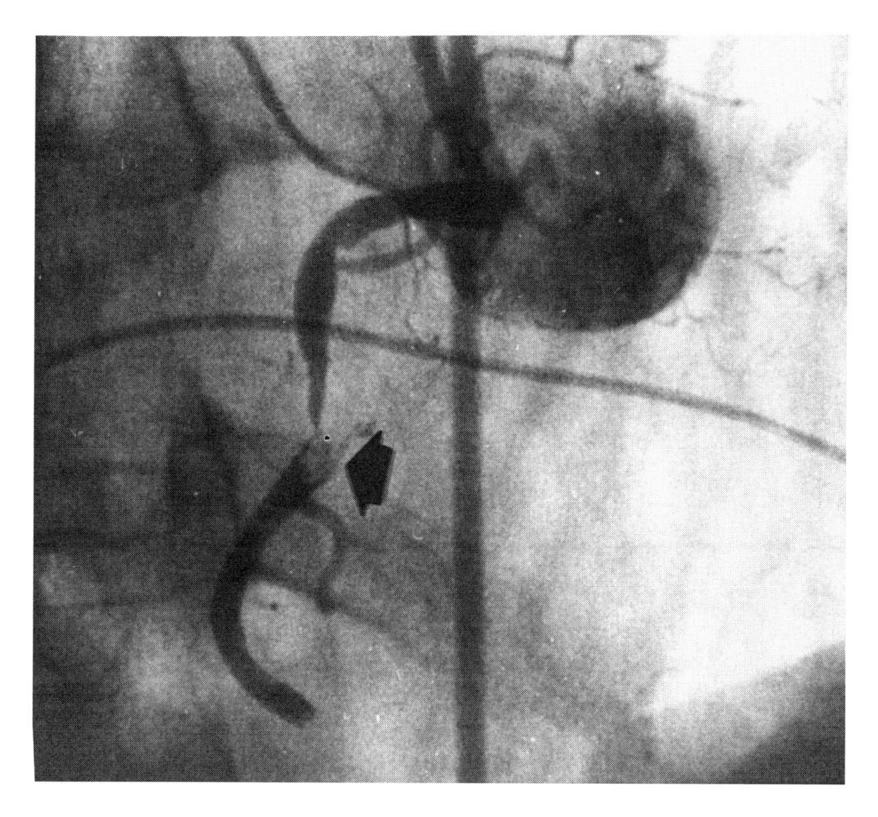

Figure 7: The arrow points to a large filling defect, distal to a severe narrowing of the right coronary artery in the RAO projection. The distal artery is not completely visualized due to TIMI-2 flow.

angiographic techniques. In studies where patients were studied within hours or days of the onset of unstable angina, the angiographic appreciation of thrombus was made in 40% to 50% of the cases.[43,44]

Angiographic Evolution of Coronary Lesion in Acute Coronary Syndromes

Several angiographic studies in which more than one angiogram was performed on a patient who subsequently developed an acute syn-

---

Editor's note: In a multivariate model, Ahmed et al. (*Am J Cardiol* 1993; 72: 544) recently showed that increasing unstable angina score as defined by the Braunwald classification of unstable angina was the most important predictor of angiographic intracoronary thrombus (P = 0.01) and lesion complexity (P

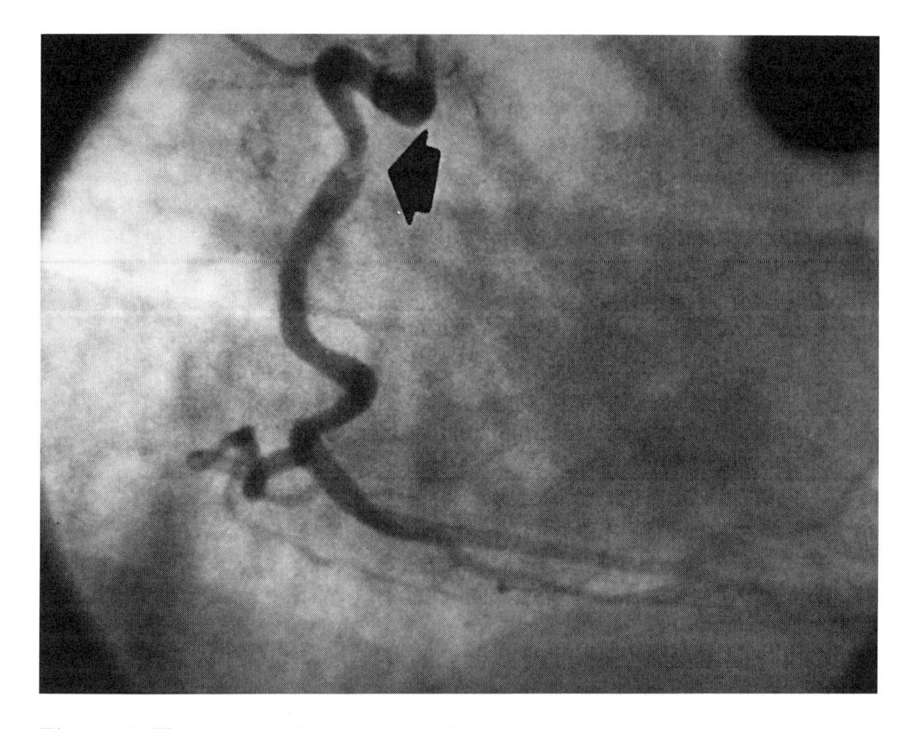

Figure 8: The arrow points to a translucent lesion in the mid-right coronary artery, RAO projection. This projection is the orthogonal view of the complex right coronary lesion seen in Figure 5.

drome have shown that a majority of these syndromes develop from atherosclerotic plaques that did not cause severe obstruction on the initial angiogram (Table 2).[66–71] In a majority of patients who developed unstable angina or acute myocardial infarction, the culprit lesion was <70% narrowed on the initial angiogram. In retrospective studies of acute myocardial infarction 78% to 97% of lesions were <70% or 75% obstructed on the initial angiogram while only 3% to 23% were >70% or 75% narrowed initially. Less than 50% narrowing was found in 48% of myocardial infarctions by Ambrose et al.[67] and in 66% by Little et al.[68] In a more recent prospective study of the effects of lipid-lowering therapy on progression of coronary atherosclerosis, Brown et al. found that in 69% of patients the lesion subsequently responsible

= 0.004) of the culprit artery. This supports the fact that increasing acuity predicts the thrombus or lesion complexity.

Table 2
Angiographic Evolution to Acute Coronary Syndromes

	Initial Angiographic Stenosis		
Syndrome	*≤50%*	*51%–70%*	*>70%*
• Unstable angina, %			
Ambrose et al.	72	16	12
• Acute Myocardial Infarction, %			
Ambrose et al.	48	30	22
Little et al.	66	31	3
Nobuyoshi et al.	59	15	26
Giroud et al.	78	9	13
Hackett et al.	90	10	0

for either unstable angina, myocardial infarction or death was <70% narrowed on the first angiogram.[72] Although all of these studies have selected out a population of patients in whom serial angiography was performed, these results differ significantly from patients who had been restudied and found to have had a new total coronary occlusion but without an intervening infarction. In this latter group, a severe lesion with >70% narrowing was found on the first angiogram in the majority.[67,73]

In addition to the above, angiographic studies after successful thrombolysis often show only moderate coronary stenoses in the infarct-related artery. Of 32 patients studied by Brown et al. after successful thrombolysis, in 32% the underlying stenoses were <50% obstructive and in 66% the lumen was narrowed by <60%.[74] Other angiographic studies post-thrombolysis indicate that moderate stenoses causing a 50% to 70% diameter reduction are the rule rather than the exception in the infarct-related artery.[75,76] Furthermore, particularly in patients with acute myocardial infarction in whom thrombolysis was given, there is remodeling of the infarct-related lesion in the first week to 10 days following myocardial infarction.[53] This remodeling is associated with an increase in minimal lumen diameter and a decrease in the degree of irregularity of the lesion. Undoubtedly, this is related to endogenous thrombolysis which continues to dissolve residual thrombus even after thrombolytic therapy has opened an occluded artery. This observation of continued thrombolysis of the culprit lesion has been reconfirmed in the APRICOT trial and reported recently in a preliminary publication.[54] A progressive decrease in lesion irregularity and severity of stenoses was found at 3 months following myocardial infarction and this effect was potentiated by the use of antithrombotic and anticoagulant therapy following infarction.

While these angiographic observations are extremely interesting and potentially important, we must realize that angiography often underestimates the degree of atherosclerosis. From studies of intravascular ultrasound and pathological studies in pressure-fixed arteries, angiography will consistently underestimate the amount of atherosclerotic narrowing since it does not visualize the arterial wall.[77,78] Therefore, in all of these angiographic studies that assessed the degree of luminal narrowing prior to an acute syndrome even with the most sophisticated of quantitative coronary angiographic techniques, the amount of narrowing of the artery may be unpredictably underestimated in some cases.

Furthermore, not all angiographic data support the notion that acute syndromes develop from less than severe lesions.[79,80] These studies suggest that in about one-third of cases, infarction developed from a lesion that was severe (>70% obstructed) on the first angiogram. However, even in these studies, the data are not completely consistent with the concept that a severe lesion is a sensitive and specific indicator of subsequent infarction. Moise et al. found new coronary occlusion in 31% of 313 patients restudied after medical therapy for coronary disease.[79] A new occlusion was strongly associated with an interim infarction. The best predictor of infarction on initial study was the presence of at least an 80% narrowing of an artery supplying a nonakinetic left ventricular segment. However, in 54% of arteries, the site of occlusion appeared to be distal to or at a different segment of the same artery remote from the 80% narrowing. Similar observations have been reported by Neill et al. who found a new total occlusion in 30% of severely stenotic lesions on follow-up angiography.[80] This finding was associated in a large percentage with an interim infarction. However, six additional patients with progression of coronary disease to a new total occlusion did not develop a Q-wave infarction after occlusion. In these patients as in the other angiographic studies where a severe narrowing was present on the initial angiogram, new total occlusion did not result in infarction probably because the acute recruitment of collaterals prevented or limited the amount of the damage.

Conclusion

We have traced the development of the early atherosclerotic plaque and described how the plaque grows slowly with progressive incorporation of lipid and matrix material or episodically with intermittent episodes of plaque fissuring or disruption and thrombosis. The latter leads to subsequent thrombus organization and incorporation into the lumen wall. When such an episode of plaque disruption leads acutely to critical luminal narrowing or occlusion, unstable angina or myocardial infarction may occur. The acutely disrupted plaques responsible for these syndromes have a distinctive angiographic morphology characterized by either irregularity, overhanging edges, ulcerations, and/or filling defects. The prognostic and therapeutic significance of these lesions will be discussed in other chapters.

References

1. Holman RL, McGill HC Jr. The natural history of atherosclerosis: the early aortic lesions as seen in New Orleans in the middle of the 20th century. Am J Pathol 1958; 34:209–230.
2. Strong JP, McGill HC Jr. The natural history of coronary atherosclerosis. Am J Pathol 1962; 40:37–49.
3. Stary HC. Evolution and progression of atherosclerotic lesions in coronary arteries of children and young adults. Arteriosclerosis 1989; 9(Suppl I): 19–32.
4. Fox B, James K, Morgan B, Seed A. Distribution of fatty and fibrous plaques in young human coronary arteries. Arteriosclerosis 1983; 48: 139–145.
5. Kjaernes M, Svindland A, Walloe L, Wille SO. Location of early atherosclerotic lesions in an arterial bifurcation in humans. Acta Pathol Microbiol Immunol Second Sect A1981; 89:35–40.
6. Zairns CK, Giddens DP, Bharadvaj BK, Sottiurai VS, Mabon RF, Glagov S. Carotid bifurcation atherosclerosis. Quantitative correlation of plaque location with flow velocity profiles and wall shear stress. Circ Res 1983; 53:502–514.
7. McGill HC Jr. The Geographic Pathology of Atherosclerosis. Baltimore, Williams & Wilkins, 1968.
8. Davies MJ. Thrombosis and coronary atherosclerosis. In Julian DG, Kubler W, Norris RM, et al. (eds): Thrombolysis in Cardiovascular Disease. NY, Marcel Dekker, 1989, pp 25–33.
9. Mitchison MI, Ball RY. Macrophages and atherogenesis. Lancet 1987; 2: 147–149.
10. Ambrose JA, Hjemdahl-Monsen C. Acute ischemic syndromes: coronary pathophysiology and angiographic correlations. In Gersh BJ, Rahimtoola SH (eds): Acute Myocardial Infarction. NY, Elsevier, 1991.
11. Duguid JB. Thrombosis as a factor in the pathogenesis of coronary atherosclerosis. J Pathol Bacteriol 1946; 58:207–213.
12. Ross R. The pathogenesis of atherosclerosis. In Braunwald E (ed): Heart Disease. Philadelphia, W.B. Saunders Co., 1992, pp 1106–1124.

13. Fuster V, Badimon L, Badimon JJ, Chesebro JH. Coronary artery disease. Progression and acute coronary syndromes. Parts 1 & 2. N Engl J Med 1992; 326:242–250, 310–318.
14. Falk E. Unstable angina with fatal outcome. Dynamic coronary thrombosis leading to infarction and/or sudden death. Circulation 1985; 71:699–708.
15. Ambrose JA, Winters SL, Stern A, Eng A, Teicholz LE, Gorlin R, Fuster V. Angiographic morphology and the pathogenesis of unstable angina pectoris. J Am Coll Cardiol 1985; 5:609–616.
16. Davies MJ, Thomas AC. Plaque fissuring: the cause of acute myocardial infarction, sudden ischaemic death, and crescendo angina. Br Heart J 1985; 53:363–373.
17. Ambrose JA. Coronary angiographic findings in the acute coronary syndromes in unstable angina. In Bleifeld W, Braunwald WE, Hamm C (eds): Unstable Angina. Berlin/Heidelberg, Springer-Verlag, 1990.
18. Ambrose JA, Monsen C. Arteriographic anatomy and mechanisms of myocardial ischemia in unstable angina (editorial). J Am Coll Cardiol 1987; 9:1397–1402.
19. Gorlin R, Fuster V, Ambrose JA. Anatomic-physiological links between the acute coronary syndromes. Circulation 1986; 74:6–9.
20. Ambrose JA, Monsen C, Borrico S, Gorlin R, Fuster V. Angiographic demonstration of a common link between unstable angina pectoris and non-Q wave acute myocardial infarction. Am J Cardiol 1988; 61:244–247.
21. Huey BL, Gheorghiade M, Crampton RS, Beller GA, Kaiser DL, Watson DD, Nygaard TW, Craddock GB, Sayre SL, Gibson RS. Acute non-Q wave myocardial infarction associated with early ST segment elevation: evidence for spontaneous coronary reperfusion and implications for thrombolytic trials. J Am Coll Cardiol 1987; 9:18–25.
22. Willerson JT, Hills LD, Winniford M, Buja LM. Speculation regarding mechanisms responsible for acute ischemic heart disease syndromes. J Am Coll Cardiol 1986; 8:245–50.
23. Langer A, Freeman MR, Armstrong PW. ST segment shift in unstable angina. Pathophysiology and association with coronary anatomy and hospital outcome. J Am Coll Cardiol 1989; 13:1495–1502.
24. DeWood MA, Stifler WF, Simpson CS, et al. Coronary arteriographic findings soon after non-Q wave myocardial infarction. N Engl J Med 1986; 315:417–423.
25. DeWood MA, Spores J, Notske RN, et al. Prevalence of total coronary occlusion during the early hours of transmural myocardial infarction. N Engl J Med 1980; 303:897–902.
26. Rentrop KP, Feit F, Blanke H, Stecy P, Schneider R, Rey M, Horowitz S, Goldman M. Effects of intracoronary streptokinase and intracoronary nitroglycerin infusion on coronary angiographic patterns and mortality in patients with acute myocardial infarction. N Engl J Med 1984; 311: 1456–1463.
27. Richardson PD, Davies MJ, Born GVR. Influence of plaque configuration and stress distribution on fissuring of coronary atherosclerotic plaques. Lancet 1989; 2:941–944.
28. Ambrose JA. Plaque disruption and the acute coronary syndromes of un-

stable angina and myocardial infarction: If the substrate is similar, why is the clinical presentation different? J Am Coll Cardiol 1992; 19:1653–1658.
29. Mizuno K, Satomuro K, Miyamato A, et al. Angioscopic evaluation of the character of coronary thrombi in acute coronary syndromes. N Engl J Med 1992; 326:287–291.
30. Mazzone A, DeServi S, Ricevuti G, et al. Increased expression of neutrophil and monocyte adhesion molecules in unstable coronary artery disease. Circulation 1993; 88:358–363.
31. Neri Serneri GG, Albate R, Gori AM, et al. Transient intermittent lymphocyte activation is responsible for the instability of angina. Circulation 1992; 86:790–797.
32. Van der Wal A, Becker AE, Van der Loos CM, Das PK. Site of intimal rupture or erosion of thrombosed coronary atherosclerotic plaques is characterized by an inflammatory process irrespective of the dominant plaque morphology . Circulation 1994; 89:36–44.
33. Kohchi K, Takebayashi S, Hiroki T, Nobuyoshi M. Significance of adventitial inflammation of the coronary artery in patients with unstable angina: results at autopsy. Circulation 1985; 71:709–716.
34. Entman ML, Ballantyne CM. Inflammation in acute coronary syndromes. Circulation 1993; 88:800–803.
35. Bazzoni G, Dejana E, Del Maschio A. Platelet-neutrophil interactions: possible relevance in the pathogenesis of thrombosis and inflammation. Haematologica 1991; 76:491–499.
36. Levin DC, Fallon JT. Significance of the angiographic morphology of localized coronary stenoses: histopathologic correlations. Circulation 1982; 66: 316–320.
37. Onodera T, Fujiwara H, Tanaka M, Wu DJ, Matsuda M, Takemura G, Ishida M, Kawamura A, Kawai C. Cineangiographic and pathological features of the infarct related vessel in successful and unsuccessful thrombolysis. Br Heart J 1989; 61:385–389.
38. Sharma SK, Israel DH, Fyfe B, Lotvin A, Torre SR, Kushner AL, McMurtry K, Marmur J, Cocke T, Almeida OD, Ambrose JA. Coronary thrombus: Clinical and angiographic correlates in 185 lesions undergoing directional coronary atherectomy (abstract). Circulation 1993; 88:I-208.
39. Christou CP, Haft JI, Goldstein JE, Carnes RE. Correlation of ischemic coronary syndromes with angiographic morphology and lesion histology. J Am Coll Cardiol 1992; 19:375A.
40. Isner JM, Brinker JA, Gottlieb RS, Leya F, Masden RR, Shani J, Kearney M, Topol EJ, for CAVEAT. Coronary thrombus: Clinical features and angiographic diagnosis in 370 patients studied by directional atherectomy (abstract). Circulation 1992; 86:I-649.
41. Alison HW, Russell RO Jr. Mantle JA, Kouchoukos NT, Moraski RE, Rackley CE. Coronary anatomy and arteriography in patients with unstable angina pectoris. Am J Cardiol 1978; 41:204–209.
42. Fuster V, Frye RL, Connolly DC, Danielson MA, Elveback LR, Kurkland LT. Arteriographic patterns early in the onset of the coronary syndromes. Br Heart J 1975; 37:1250–1255.
43. Capone G, Wolf NM, Meyer B, Meister SG. Frequency of intracoronary

filling defects by angiography in angina pectoris at rest. Am J Cardiol 1985; 56:403–406.
44. Bresnahan DR, Davis DR, Holmes DR Jr, Smith HC. Angiographic occurence and clinical correlates of intraluminal coronary artery thrombus: Role of unstable angina. J Am Coll Cardiol 1985; 6:285–289.
45. Haft JI, Goldstein JE, Niemiera ML. Coronary arteriographic lesion of unstable angina. Chest 1987; 92:609–612.
46. Williams AE, Freeman MR, Chisholm RJ, et al. Angiographic morphology in unstable angina pectoris. Am J Cardiol 1988; 62:1024–1027.
47. Rehr R, Disciascio G, Vevtrovec G, Cowley M. Angiographic morphology of coronary artery stenosis in prolonged rest angina: Evidence of intracoronary thrombosis. J Am Coll Cardiol 1989; 14:1429–1437.
48. Ellis SG, Vandormael MG, Cowley MJ, et al. Coronary morphology & clinical determinants of procedural outcome with angioplasty for multivessel coronary disease: Implications for patient selection. Circulation 1990; 82: 1193–1202.
49. Wilson FR, Holida MD, White CW. Quantitative angiographic morphology of coronary stenoses leading to myocardial infarction or unstable angina. Circulation 1986; 73:286–293.
50. Kalbfleisch SJ, McGillen MJ, Simon SB, et al. Automated quantitation of indexes of coronary lesion complexity: Comparison between patients with stable and unstable angina. Circulation 1990; 82:439–447.
51. The TIMI Study Group. Comparison of invasive and conservative strategies following intravenous tissue plasminogen activator in acute myocardial infarction: Results of the thrombolysis in myocardial infarction (TIMI)II trial. N Engl J Med 1989; 320:618–628.
52. Rivera W, Sharaf BL, Miele NJ, Thompson B, McKendall GR, Riley RS, Drew TM, Thomas ES, Williams DO, for the TIMI III investigators: Coronary anatomy in patients who present with non-Q wave myocardial infarction differs from unstable angina pectoris: A report from TIMI 3B (abstract). Circulation 1994; 90 (no. 4, part 2):I-438.
53. Davies SW, Marchant B, Lyons JP, Timmis AD, Rothman MT, Layton CA, Balcon R. Coronary lesion morphology in acute myocardial infarction: demonstration of early remodelling after streptokinase treatment. J Am Coll Cardiol 1990; 16:1079–1086.
54. Veen G, Meijer A, Werter CJPJ, et al. Dynamic changes of culprit lesion morphology and severity after successful thrombolysis for acute myocardial infarction: an angiographic follow-up study. J Am Coll Cardiol 1994; 23:147A.
55. Haft JI, al-Zarka AM. The origin and fate of complex coronary lesions. Am Heart J 1991; 121:1050–1061.
56. Nakagawa S, Hanada Y, Koiwaya Y, Tanaka K. Angiographic features in the infarct-related artery after intracoronary urokinase followed by prolonged anticoagulation: Role of ruptured atheromatous plaque and adherent thrombus in acute myocardial infarction, in vivo. Circulation 1988; 78:1335–1344.
57. Chen L, Chester MR, Huang J, Leatham E, Tousolis D, Kaski JC. Progression of ischaemia-related stenoses in unstable angina (abstract). Circulation 1994; 90 (no. 4, part 2):I-438.

58. Van Axen PJ, Emeis JJ. Organization of experimentally induced arterial thrombosis in rats from two weeks until ten months. The development of an arteriosclerotic lesion and the occurence of rethrombosis. Artery 1983; 11:384–399.
59. Freeman MR, Williams AE, Chisholm RJ, Armstrong PW. Intracoronary thrombus and complex morphology in unstable angina: Relation to timing of angiography and in hospital cardiac events. Circulation 1989; 80:17–23.
60. Sherman CT, Litvack F, Grundfest W, et al. Coronary angioscopy in patients with unstable angina pectoris. N Engl J Med 1986; 315:913–919.
61. White CJ, Ramee SR, Mesa J, Collins TJ. Percutaneous coronary angioscopy in patients with restenosis after coronary angioplasty. J Am Coll Cardiol 1991; 17(Suppl B):46–49B.
62. Ambrose JA: Coronary arteriographic analysis and angiographic morphology (editorial). J Am Coll Cardiol 1989; 13:1492–1494.
63. Vetrovec GW, Cowley MJ, Overton H, Richardson DW. Intracoronary thrombus in syndromes of unstable myocardial ischemia. Am Heart J 1981; 102:1202–1208.
64. Mandlekorn JB, Wolf NM, Singh S, et al. Intracoronary thrombus in nontransmural myocardial infarction in unstable angina pectoris. Am J Cardiol 1983; 52:1–6.
65. Cowley MJ, DiSciascio G, Rehr RB, Vetrovec GW. Angiographic observations and clinical relevance of coronary thrombus in unstable angina pectoris. Am J Cardiol 1989; 63:108 E-113E.
66. Ambrose JA, Winters SL, Arora RR, Riccio A, Gorlin R, Fuster V. Angiographic evolution of coronary morphology in unstable angina. J Am Coll Cardiol 1986; 7:472–478.
67. Ambrose JA, Tannenbaum MA, Alexopoulos D, Hjemdahl-Monsen CE, Leavy J, Weiss M, Borrico S, Fuster V. Angiographic progression of coronary artery disease and the development of myocardial infarction. J Am Coll Cardiol 1988; 12:56–62.
68. Little WC, Constantinescu M, Applegate RJ, Kutcher MA, Burrows MT, Kahl FR, Santamore WP. Can coronary angiography predict the site of a subsequent myocardial infarction in patients with mild to moderate coronary artery disease? Circulation 1988; 78:1157–1166.
69. Nobuyoshi M, Tanaka M, Mosaka H, et al. Progression of coronary atherosclerosis: Is coronary spasm related to progression? J Am Coll Cardiol 1991; 18:904–910.
70. Giroud D, Jian ML, Urban P, Meier B, Rutishauser W. Relation of the site of acute myocardial infarction to the most severe coronary arterial stenosis at prior angiography. Am J Cardiol 1992; 69:729–732.
71. Hackett D, Verwilghen J, Davies G, Maseri A. Coronary stenoses before and after acute myocardial infarction. Am J Cardiol 1989; 63:1517–1518.
72. Brown BG, Zhao XQ, Sacco DE, Albers JJ. Lipid lowering and plaque regression: New insights into prevention of plaque disruption and clinical events in coronary disease. Circulation 1993; 87:1781–1791.
73. Webster MWI, Chesebro JH, Smith HC, Frye FL, Holmes DR, Reeder GS, Breshnan DR, Nishimura RA, Clements IP, Bradley WT, Grill DE, Bailey KR, Fuster V. Myocardial infarction and coronary artery occlusion: A prospective 5-year angiographic study. J Am Coll Cardiol 1990; 15:218A.

74. Brown BG, Gallery CA, Badger RS, et al. Incomplete lysis of thrombus in the moderate underlying atherosclerotic lesion during intracoronary infusion of streptokinase for acute myocardial infarction: Quantitative angiographic observations. Circulation 1986; 73:653–661.
75. Hackett D, Davies G, Maseri A. Pre-existing coronary stenoses in patients with first myocardial infarction are not necessarily severe. Eur Heart J 1988; 9:1317–1323.
76. Serruys PW, Arnold AER, Brower RW, DeBono DP, Bokslag M, Lusben J, Reiber JHC, Rutsch WR, Uebis R, Vahanian A, Verstraete M, for the European co-operative study group for recombinant tissue-type plasminogen activator: Effect of continued rt-PA adminstration on the residual stenosis after initially successfull recanalization in acute myocardial infarction: a quantitative coronary angiography study of a randomized trial. Eur Heart J 1987; 8:1172–1181.
77. Porter TR, D'Sa A, Turner C, Jones LA, Minisi AJ, Mohanty PK, Vevtrovec GW, Nixon JV. Myocardial contrast echocardiography for the assessment of coronary blood flow reserve: validation in humans. J Am Coll Cardiol 1993; 21:349–355.
78. Stiel GM, Stiel LSG, Schofer J, Donath K, Mathey DG. Impact of compensatory enlargement of atherosclerotic coronary arteries on angiographic assessment of coronary artery disease. Circulation 1989; 80:1603–1609.
79. Moise A, Lesperance J, Theroux P, et al. Clinical and angiographic predictors of a new total coronary occlusion in coronary artery disease: Analysis of 313 non-operated patients. Am J Cardiol 1984; 54:1176–1181.
80. Neil WA, Wharton TP, Fluri-Lundeen J, Cohen IS. Acute coronary insufficiency: Coronary occlusion after intermittent ischemic attacks. N Engl J Med 1980; 302:1157–1162.

4

Atherectomy and Complex Coronary Lesions

Jacob I. Haft, MD, Christos P. Christou, MD, Jonathan E. Goldstein, MD, Raymond E. Carnes, MD

The acute coronary syndromes, unstable angina, and myocardial infarction are currently believed to be due in most cases to rupture of an atherosclerotic plaque.[1–3] If the area of denuded endothelium or the material extruded from the plaque stimulates the formation of an overlying totally occlusive thrombus and there is not sufficient collateral circulation, an acute myocardial infarction will result. If there is no thrombus formed or if the thrombus is not totally occlusive or if there are sufficient collaterals feeding the area of myocardium usually perfused by the artery with the ruptured plaque, or if an occlusive overlying thrombus is rapidly lysed by endogenous fibrinolytic proteins, a myocardial infarction will not occur but the patient may develop unstable angina. This concept was determined from pathological studies performed in the 1950s[4] but was not accepted until the early 1980s after the report of DeWood et al.[5] documenting that thrombus was almost always present as part of the acute occlusion that resulted in myocardial infarction. It was further supported by the frequently repeated demonstration that thrombolysis with intracoronary streptokinase could abort a myocardial infarction in progress by opening the vessel.[6]

From: Ambrose JA (ed): *Complex Coronary Lesions in Acute Coronary Syndromes.* © Futura Publishing Co., Inc., Armonk, NY, 1996.

Levin and Fallon,[7] using arteriograms of barium-filled coronary arteries post mortem, demonstrated that lesions histologically having characteristics of ruptured plaque had specific morphological characteristics that could be recognized on x-ray examination.

Ambrose et al.[8] examined clinical coronary cinearteriograms of living patients and found similar lesions in the majority of patients who had a history of unstable angina and found the lesions rarely in patients who had a history of stable angina. We confirmed their findings soon after,[9] though the incidence of these complex, eccentric narrowings with irregular borders occasionally associated with outpocketing ("ulcers") or filling defects was somewhat higher in our patients with stable angina than reported by Ambrose et al. Subsequently, in a cooperative endeavor with us, Ambrose et al.[10] demonstrated that the lesion underlying the clot in patients with myocardial infarction who had responded to fibrinolysis with intracoronary streptokinase was also usually a typical complex lesion. These findings strongly supported the concept that there is a continuum between unstable angina and myocardial infarction: that both are usually the result of a ruptured plaque.

Further evidence that these morphologically complex lesions recognized on coronary angiography are due to ruptured plaques has come from studies of the natural history of these lesions.[11,12] In a series of studies, the coronary arteriograms of patients who had repeat coronary arteriograms over years were studied and the early films were compared with later arteriograms. Complex lesions were identified on the initial films and their fate or evolution was followed on the later films. Similarly, the sites of complex lesions found on the later films were checked on the earlier films to determine the precursors of these complex lesions. We found that complex lesions on the earlier films were usually stable over years. Many of the complex lesions that were 90% or more occlusive frequently went on to total occlusion; however, although the less severe complex lesions went on to further occlusion more often than did smooth lesions of similar severity, most of the complex lesions did not change. Evolution of complex lesions into smooth lesions almost never occurred (two "ulcers" filled). This suggested that the presence of a complex lesion was a sign that a plaque had ruptured, but that it had not necessarily ruptured recently.

The more interesting findings were in the precursor data; most of the new complex lesions on the later films occurred in areas of the coronary tree that had appeared normal or that had had minimal nonocclusive disease (lesions less than 30% occlusive). Some areas had had less severe smooth lesions (50%–75% occlusive) on the earlier arteriogram, and a few complex lesions became apparent when totally occluded arteries recanalized. Totally occluded areas of vessels also frequently occurred in minimally diseased segments of coronaries or were preceded by complex lesions. These findings supported the concept that a relatively flat plaque, appearing as a normally patent or minimally diseased artery on arteriography can rupture and result in either a more occlusive coronary lesion or a totally occluded vessel. Some lesions may go on to total occlusion in two steps: first by rupturing and causing a severe but not totally occlusive complex lesion and then subsequently by going from 90% to total occlusion. These findings gave further anatomic support to the observation that the artery that subsequently causes a myocardial infarction can rarely be identified on a prior coronary arteriogram[13] and that at least 50% of progression of coronary atherosclerosis is catastrophic, occurring in normal or minimally diseased coronary segments.[14,15]

However, although the coronary arteriographic morphological findings of complex lesions have initiated and supported concepts concerning the importance of ruptured plaques in the evolution of coronary atherosclerosis and in the etiology of the acute syndromes complicating coronary atherosclerosis, the anatomic basis on which a complex lesion on coronary arteriography is considered indicative of a ruptured plaque is very slim. Levin and Fallon[7] had only a few patients who had both postmortem arteriography and histological correlation. There have been a few cases reported where complex lesions on coronary arteriography were correlated with angioscopic findings suggestive of ruptured plaque and thrombus.[16] With the advent of the Simpson atherectomy device,[17,18] anatomic material from atherosclerotic lesions has become available. We have used this opportunity to correlate coronary morphology with histology of lesions,[19] and more recently we have also correlated histology and angiographic morphology with clinical history.

Methods

One hundred forty patients had atherectomy performed. All had selective arteriograms prior to atherectomy and these were reviewed by two of the authors. Lesions were classified based on whether they were complex (eccentric, jagged, irregular, roughened edges with overhanging borders or filling defects) or smooth (concentric or eccentric lesions with smooth walls).

Atherectomy was performed using the Simpson atherocath.[17,18]

Briefly, this device is a catheter that has a small chamber at its tip that has an opening approximately 1 cm long on one side. On the side opposite the opening, there is a balloon. The catheter is advanced into the coronary artery and the opening of the chamber is positioned over the lesion. The balloon is filled, pushing the chamber opening against the plaque. At the proximal part of the chamber, there is a fine rotating blade that is attached by a long wire to a motor held by the operator. The motor is turned on and the blade is advanced from the proximal part of the chamber to the distal part, shaving off the part of the lesion that is in the opening of the chamber. The tissue cut from the lesion is pushed by the back of the rotating blade into a reservoir at the tip of the chamber. After a number of passes of the rotating blade, the device is removed from the patient, and the material shaved from the lesion is harvested from the filled tip reservoir. The device can then be replaced through the guiding catheter into the vessel and further material can be removed. The procedure is fairly safe and perforation or rupture of vessels has been rarely reported. Acute closure with a massive clot occasionally occurs and restenosis develops at the same incidence as with conventional angioplasty. The device is stiff and fairly long and is used mainly on lesions in proximal straight segments of coronary arteries or vein grafts.

The material removed from the coronary artery is immediately harvested from the atherectomy device and placed in 10% formalin. It is processed by the pathology department and all the material is fixed, sectioned, mounted, and stained with H&E. All of the slides were reviewed by at least two of the authors, and the presence of fibrous tissue, cholesterol clefts, calcification, thrombus, and inflammatory cells were recorded. A ruptured plaque was considered present when there was thrombus intermingled with debris, fibrous material, and the other components of the plaque (Figure 1).

Adequate clinical data were available on 81 patients who had atherectomy. Patients were classified as having stable angina pectoris if they had typical exertional angina relieved by rest or nitroglycerin or had slowly progressive effort angina without pain at rest.

Unstable angina pectoris was defined in patients if they experienced new-onset chest pain with minimal work or at rest, or if an abrupt increase or change in character and frequency of angina occurred in a previously stable patient.

The correlations of clinical history with complex and smooth lesions and with histology were compared using chi square analysis.

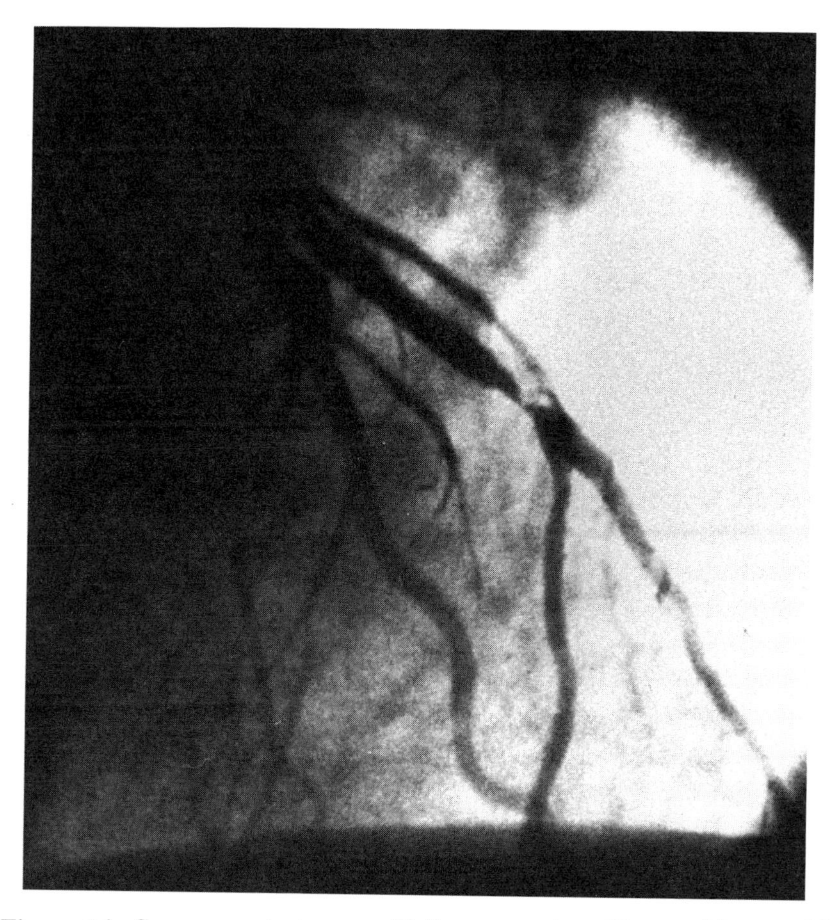

Figure 1A: Coronary arteriogram of left coronary in a 62-year-old man with a history of hypertension who was admitted to hospital after 1 hour of chest pain at rest. Myocardial infarction was ruled out and on catheterization he was found to have a 95% complex lesion in the left anterior descending coronary artery.

Results

Of a total of 81 patients, 66 males, mean age 57 ± 11 years (range 30–80) underwent successful directional coronary atherectomy; adequate clinical information was readily available. Fifty-seven patients presented with episodes of unstable angina pectoris or postmyocardial

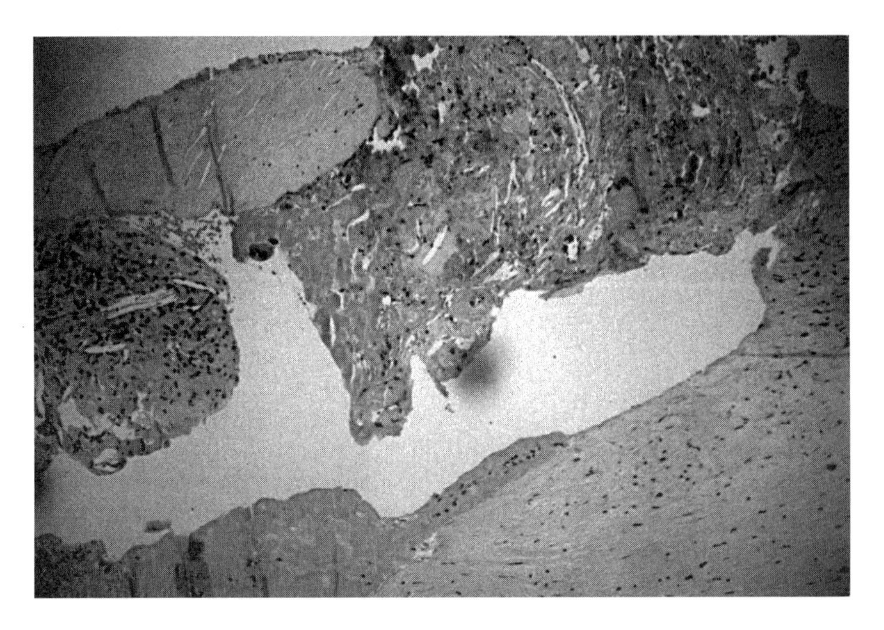

Figure 1B: Histological specimen obtained at atherectomy of the complex LAD lesion. Note the presence of thrombus, calcification, cholesterol clefts inflammatory cells, fibrous tissue, and evidence of plaque rupture.

infarction with or without thrombolysis (20 patients). Twenty-four patients presented with symptoms of stable angina pectoris and/or had a positive exercise stress test.

Among the 57 patients with unstable angina pectoris, 49 (86.0%) had arteriographic complex lesions and 8 (14.1%) had smooth lesions. In the 24 patients who presented with symptoms of stable angina pectoris, arteriography revealed complex morphology in 17 (70.8%) lesions and smooth in 7 (29.8%) (P = NS).*

In patients with irregular complex morphology on arteriography, histology revealed thrombus in 54 patients, ruptured plaques in 42, calcification in 42, inflammatory cells in 43, fibrous tissue in 63, and cholesterol clefts in 59 (Table 1).

In 15 patients with smooth morphology on arteriography, histology

* Editor's note: The incidence of complex morphology in stable angina is higher in this report than in all other studies (see Chapter 3).

Table 1
Histological Findings in Irregular and Smooth Lesions

	Total Series	
	Irregular	*Smooth*
Number	66	15
Cholesterol Clefts	59 (89.4%)	10 (66.6%)[x]
Calcification	42 (63.6%)	4 (26.7%)[xx]
Fibrous Tissue	63 (95.5%)	15 (100%)*
Inflammatory Cells	43 (65.2)	8 (53.3%)*
Thrombus	54 (81.8%)	3 (20.0%)[xxx]
Ruptured Plaque	42 (63.6%)	2 (13.3%)[xxx]

* = NS.
xxx = $P < .001$.
xx = $P < .01$.
x = $P < .05$.

revealed thrombus in 3 patients, ruptured plaque in 2, calcification in 4, inflammatory cells in 8, cholesterol clefts in 10, and fibrous tissue in all 15 (Table 1).

The incidence of thrombus, ruptured plaque, and calcification was significantly higher in patients with complex lesions than among those patients with smooth morphology ($P < .01$).

In patients with unstable angina, thrombus was present in 50 patients (47 irregular, 3 smooth), ruptured plaque in 38 patients (36 irregular, 2 smooth), calcification in 35 patients (33 irregular, 2 smooth) (Table 2).

In patients with stable angina, histology revealed thrombus in 7 patients (all irregular), ruptured plaque in 6 (all irregular) and calcification in 11, (9 irregular, 2 smooth) (Table 2).

In patients with symptoms of unstable angina pectoris, the incidence of thrombus and ruptured plaque was statistically significantly higher than in patients with stable angina pectoris ($P < .001$) (Table 2), especially among those with irregular lesion morphology.

Discussion

Our findings confirm that coronary lesion morphology correlates with lesion histology. As shown in our previous work,[19] irregular lesions on coronary angiography usually are due to plaque rupture and/

Table 2
Histological and Morphological Findings in Patients with Unstable vs. Stable Angina

	Stable AP			*Unstable AP*		
	Irregular	*Smooth*	*Total*	*Irregular*	*Smooth*	*Total*
Number	17 (70.8%)*	7	24	49 (86%)*	8	57
Cholesterol Clefts	14 (82.3%)*	4 (57.1%)*	18 (75%)*	45 (91.8%)*	6 (75%)*	47 (89.5%)*
Calcification	9 (53%)*	2 (28.5%)*	11 (45.8%)*	33 (67.3%)*	2 (25%)*	35 (61.4%)*
Fibrous Tissue	15 (88.2%)*	7 (100%)*	22 (91.7%)*	48 (98.0%)*	8 (100%)*	56 (98.2%)*
Inflammatory Cells	9 (52%)	5 (71.4%)	14 (58.3%)*	34 (69.4%)*	3 (37.5%)	37 (64.9%)*
Thrombus	7 (41.2%)^{XXX}	0*	7 (29.2%)^{XXX}	47 (95.9%)^{XXX}	3 (37.5%)*	49 (86.0%)^{XXX}
Ruptured Plaque	6 (35.3%)^{XX}	0*	6 (25%)^{XXX}	36 (73.5%)^{XX}	2 (25%)*	38 (66.7%)^{XXX}

* = NS.
XXX = $P < .001$.
XX = $P < .01$.
X = $P < .05$.

or thrombus, and smooth lesions rarely are associated with thrombus. Interestingly, we found that although there was a trend toward a higher incidence of irregular lesions in our patients with unstable syndromes, there were many patients who presented with "stable" angina who had complex lesions. This may be partly due to the fact that lesions selected for atherectomy are usually eccentric[18] and eccentric lesions are frequently complex. Patients with smooth concentric lesions (the frequent finding in patients with stable angina) usually did not have atherectomy. However, in a previous study,[9] we also observed complex lesions to occur frequently in patients with stable angina. These findings fit with observations of the natural history of complex lesions.[11,12] Many complex lesions, although frequently developing over a short period of time, will thereafter remain stable for years. The presence of a complex lesion suggests that there has been instability (rupture of a plaque with or without thrombus) in the past, but not necessarily in the very recent past. On histology, the presence of evidence of thrombus and plaque rupture was much higher in complex lesions compared to smooth, but in addition, there was a higher incidence of evidence of thrombus and plaque rupture in the complex lesions from patients with symptoms of unstable angina than in those with stable angina. Moreover, thrombus and plaque rupture was found only in smooth lesions when there was a history of instability.

These histological findings in "biopsies" of complex lesions support the use of coronary arteriographic lesion morphology in diagnosing that a plaque has ruptured. From the histology we tried to determine if plaque constituents were different in those that had ruptured compared to the smooth plaques. We were hoping to find an overabundance of inflammatory cells in irregular lesions,[20] confirming a hypothesis that proteolytic enzymes emanating from leukolytes played a critical role in weakening the plaque wall so that it ruptured. Although we found inflammatory cells to be common in irregular lesions that showed plaque rupture histologically they were also common in smooth lesions that had no plaque rupture. This suggests that leukolytes are almost always present in plaques and their accumulation is not necessarily etiologic in plaque rupture.

In comparing irregular lesions with smooth lesions, aside from the presence of thrombus and evidence of ruptured plaque, there were more lesions with calcification and cholesterol clefts among the irregular lesions, suggesting that the underlying plaque that had ruptured and caused thrombosis was probably a more mature plaque, (even if possibly flat and not obstructive before rupture), and that it had been present a long time, able to have accumulated much cholesterol and able to have calcified. Moreover, the irregular lesions in patients with unstable angina had the highest incidence of calcification and cholesterol.

The presence of a high incidence of cholesterol clefts in complex lesions may offer a clue to a possible approach to prevention of plaque rupture that also may find support from some of the recently reported prospective serial coronary arteriographic studies that have randomized patients to cholesterol-lowering agents or placebo. It is possible that a large amount of cholesterol crystals in lesions makes the plaque more prone to rupture or is an identifying marker that a lesion is prone to rupture (see also Chapter 14). Patients with hypercholesterolemia may have endothelial dysfunction with an impairment of normal nitrous oxide (EDRF) production.[21] Patients with coronary lesions often have a paradoxical response to acetylcholine with vasoconstriction rather than with vasodilation.[22] It is not clear whether local presence of cholesterol plays a role in this vascular abnormality, but apparently cholesterol in plaques is metabolically active, moving in and out of plaques, and it has been suggested that lowering systemic hypercholesterolemia levels will restore normal vascular reactivity in patients with CAD.[23]

There have been interesting data emanating from a number of serial coronary arteriographic studies that suggest that cholesterol lowering might stabilize plaques. In these randomized controlled studies, various methods for lowering serum cholesterol were utilized and progression or regression was assessed by comparison of arteriograms after years of cholesterol-lowering therapy. Cholesterol lowering was effected by lifestyle change,[24] colestipol and nicotinic acid,[25] surgery with ileal bypass (POSCH),[26] lovastatin/colestipol/niacin (FATS),[27] SCOR,[28] diet plus cholestyramine (STARS),[29] or lovastatin (MARS)[30] (C CAIT).[31] All of these studies reported that although there was only a minimal degree of regression of atherosclerotic lesions as measured by lumen diameter in the area of a lesion, there was much less progression. There is a suggestion in these studies that much of the progression that was prevented (that occurred less frequently in patients on cholesterol-lowering regimens than on placebo) was in the development of new significant lesions. It is very likely that most of these new lesions, especially over the relatively short periods that encompassed these studies, are due to new complex lesions in areas of minimal or no apparent coronary occlusion, i.e., are due to the development of plaque rupture. Unfortunately, the investigators in these studies did not note lesion morphology in their evaluation of the study arteriograms. An interesting opportunity has been missed, but even so we can extrapolate from their data that less plaque rupture had probably occurred and that lowering of serum cholesterol with any effective regimen may indeed result in plaque stabilization.

Interestingly, another serial arteriogram study may have shown that a pharmacological intervention might stabilize plaques. Lichtlen et al.[32] showed that patients treated with nifedipine over 3 years had less frequent development of new coronary lesions (INTACT) (103 new lesions in patients on nifedipine vs. 144 new lesions in patients on placebo). There was minimal regression in plaque occlusive severity, and minimal lack of progression in pre-existing lesions in the nifedipine-treated group compared to the placebo group. As in the cholesterol-lowering trials, this decrease in new lesions suggests fewer plaque ruptures. However, once more, an opportunity to say this more definitively was missed because lesion morphology was not assessed, only severity of lumen occlusion. The mechanism of benefit of nifedipine is unknown; it may be related directly to its calcium channel blocking effect, such that less calcium enters the atherosclerotic cell (thereby possibly making it less prone to rupture; most of our irregular lesions had calcification), via a direct other pharmacological effect, or indirectly via its vasodilating and spasm prevention effects. In any event, it appears that nifedipine might have its beneficial effect of preventing new lesions via a plaque stabilizing effect.

In summary, we have studied the histology of material removed from coronary atherosclerotic lesions and have correlated it with the morphology of lesions on coronary arteriography and with the clinical presentation. Irregular lesions were associated with thrombus, plaque rupture, cholesterol clefts, and calcification significantly more frequently than were smooth lesions. Clinically, thrombus and ruptured plaques were found significantly more often in patients with unstable than with stable angina, although the incidence of irregular lesions was only minimally increased. Although not completely sensitive, we have demonstrated that irregular lesions suggest that a plaque has ruptured, acutely in patients with symptoms of unstable angina, and remotely in patients with stable angina. Evaluation of lesion morphology can be a surrogate for diagnosing plaque rupture. Use of lesion morphology evaluation in arteriographic studies of pharmacological interventions may aid in understanding the mode of action of these agents and may support that they work via plaque stabilization.

Editor's Note:

Two other studies have been preliminarily reported correlating lesion morphology at angiography with histologic findings at the time of atherectomy [Isner et al: Circulation 1992; 86 (abstract) 2583 and Sharma et al: Circulation 1993; 88 (abstract) 1112]. Particularly in the latter study, complex lesions on angiography were highly correlated with the presence of intracoronary thrombus at atherectomy.

References

1. Davies MJ, Thomas AC. Plaque fissuring: the cause of acute myocardial infarction, sudden ischemic death, and crescendo angina. Br Heart J 1985; 53:363–373.
2. Falk E. Plaque rupture with severe pre-existing stenosis precipitating coronary thrombosis. Characteristics of coronary atherosclerotic plaques underlying fatal occlusive thrombi. Br Heart J 1983; 50:127–134.
3. Ridolfi RL, Hutchins GM. The relationship between coronary artery lesions and myocardial infarcts: ulceration of atherosclerotic plaques precipitating coronary thrombus. Am Heart J 1977; 93:468–486.
4. Friedman M. The pathogenesis of coronary plaques, thromboses, and hemorrhages: an evaluative review. Circulation 1975; 52:III-34–40.
5. DeWood MA, Spores J, Notske R, et al. Prevalence of total coronary occlusion during the early hours of transmural myocardial infarction. N Engl J Med 1980; 303:897–902.
6. Rentrop P, Blanke H, Karsch KR, Kaiser H, Kostering H, Leitz K. Selec-

tive intracoronary thrombolysis in acute myocardial infarction and unstable angina pectoris. Circulation 1981; 63:307–317.
7. Levin DC, Fallon JT. Significance of the angiographic morphology of localized coronary stenoses: Histopathologic correlations. Circulation 1982; 66: 316–320.
8. Ambrose JA, Winters SL, Stern A, Eng A, Teichholz LE, Gorlin R, Fuster V. Angiographic morphology and the pathogenesis of unstable angina pectoris. J Am Coll Cardiol 1985; 5:609–616.
9. Haft JI, Goldstein JE, Niemiera ML. Coronary arteriographic lesion of unstable angina. Chest 1987; 92:609–612.
10. Ambrose JA, Winters SL, Arora RR, Haft JI, Goldstein JE, Rentrop P, Gorlin R, Fuster V. Coronary angiographic morphology in myocardial infarction: a link between pathogenesis of unstable angina and myocardial infarction. J Am Coll Cardiol 1985; 6:1233–1238.
11. Haft JI, Al-Zarka AM. The origin and fate of complex coronary lesions. Am Heart J 1991; 121:1050–1061.
12. Haft JI, Al-Zarka AM. Comparison of the natural history of irregular and smooth coronary lesions: Insights into the pathogenesis, progression, and prognosis of coronary atherosclerosis. Am Heart J 1993; 126:551–561.
13. Little WC, Costninescu M, Applegate RJ, Kutcher MA, Burrows MT, Kahl FR, Santamore WP. Can coronary angiography predict the site of a subsequent myocardial infarction in patients with mild-to-moderate coronary artery disease? Circulation 1988; 78:1157–1166.
14. Ambrose JA, Tannenbaum MA, Alexopoulos D, et al. Angiographic progression of coronary artery disease and the development of myocardial infarction. J Am Coll Cardiol 1988; 12:56–62.
15. Haft JI, Haik BJ, Goldstein JE. Development of significant coronary artery lesions in areas of minimal disease: a common mechanism for coronary disease progression. Chest 1988; 94:731–736.
16. Sherman CT, Litvack F, Grundfest W, Lee M, Hickey A, Chaux A, Kass R, Blanche C, Matloff J, Morgenstern L, Ganz W, Swan HJC, Forrester J. Coronary angioscopy in patients with unstable angina pectoris. N Engl J Med 1986; 315:913–919.
17. Simpson JB, Robertson GC, Selmon MR. Percutaneous coronary atherectomy (abstract). Circulation 1988; 78(Suppl 2):II82.
18. Safian RD, Gelbish JS, Erny RE, Schnitt SJ, Schmidt DA, Baim DS. Coronary atherectomy. Circ 1988; 78:1157–1166.
19. Haft JI, Christou CP, Goldstein JE, Carnes RE. Correlation of atherectomy specimen histology with coronary arteriographic lesion morphology. Am Heart J (in press).
20. Jonasson L, Holm J, Skalli O, Bonjers G, Hansson GK. Regional accumulation of T cells, macrophages, and smooth muscle cells in the human atherosclerotic plaque. Arteriosclerosis 1986; 6:131–138.
21. Flavahan NA. Atherosclerosis or lipid-induced endothelial dysfunction. Potential mechanisms underlying reduction in EDRF/nitric oxide activity. Circulation 1992; 85:1927–1938.
22. Ludmer Pl, Selwyn AP, Shook TL, Wayne RR, Mudge GH, Alexander RW, Ganz P. Paradoxical vasoconstriction induced by acetylcholine in atherosclerotic coronary arteries. N Engl J Med 1986; 315:1046.

23. Anderson TJ, Meredith IT, Yeung AC, Lieberman EH, Selwyn AP, Ganz P. Cholesterol lowering therapy improves endothelial function in patients with coronary atherosclerosis. Circulation 1993; 88:(Suppl to #4):I-368.
24. Ornish D, Brown SE, Scherwitz LW, Billings JH, Armstrong WT, Porrs TA, McLanahan SM, Kirkeeide RL, Brand RJ, Gould KL. Can lifestyle changes reverse coronary heart disease? The Lifestyle Heart Trial. Lancet 1990; 336:129–133.
25. Blankenhorn DH, Nesim SA, Johnson RL, Sanmarco ME, Azen SP, Cashin-Hemphill I. Beneficial effects of combined colestipol-niacin therapy on coronary atherosclerosis and coronary venous bypass grafts. JAMA 1987; 257:3233–3240.
26. Buchwald II, Varco RL, Matts JP, Long JM, Fitch LL, Campbell GS, Pearce MB, Yellin AE, Edmiston WA, Smink RD Jr. Effect of partial ileal bypass surgery on mortality and morbidity from coronary heart disease in patients with hypercholesterolemia: report of the Program on the Surgical Control of the Hyperlipidemias (POSCH). N Engl J Med 1990; 323:946–955.
27. Brown G, Albers JJ, Fisher LD, Schaefer SM, Lin JT, Kaplan C, Zhao XQ, Bisson BD, Fitzpatrick VF, Dodge HT. Regression of coronary artery disease as a result of intensive lipid-lowering therapy in men with high levels of apolipoprotein B. N Engl J Med 1990; 323:1289–1298.
28. Kane JP, Malloy MJ, Ports TA, Phillips NR, Diehl JC, Havel RJ. Regression of coronary atherosclerosis during treatment of familial hypercholesterolemia with combined drug regimens. JAMA. 1990; 264:3007–3012.
29. Watts GF, Lewis B, Brunt JN, Lewis ES, Coltart DJ, Smith LD, Mann JI, Swan AV. Effects on coronary artery disease of lipid-lowering diet, or diet plus cholestyramine, in the St Thomas' Atherosclerosis Regression Study (STARS). Lancet 1992; 339:563–569.
30. Blankenhorn DH, Azen SP, Kramsch DM, Mack WJ, Cashin-Hemphill L, Hodis HN, DeBoer LWV, Mahrer PR, Masteller MJ, Vailas LI, Alaupovic P, Hirsch LJ, and the MARS Research Group. Coronary angiographic changes with lovastatin therapy: the Monitored Atherosclerosis Regression Study (MARS). Ann Intern Med 1993; 119:969–976.
31. Waters D, Lesperance J, Craven TE, Hudon G, Gillam LD. Advantages and limitations of serial coronary arteriography for the assessment of progression and regression of coronary atherosclerosis: implications for clinical trials. Circulation 1993; 87(Suppl II):II38–II47.
32. Lichtlen PR, Hugenholtz PG, Rafflenbeul W, Hecker H, Jost S, Deckers JW. Retardation of angiographic progression of coronary artery disease by nifedipine. Lancet (INTACT). 1990; 335:1109–1113.

5

Quantifying Lesion Morphology

Craig E. Hjemdahl-Monsen, MD

Introduction

Lesion morphology encompasses a variety of features that characterize a coronary artery stenosis. Many of these features are subjective and relate to what seem to be primarily qualitative features of a lesion. As is the case with stenosis severity, which can be measured by percent diameter reduction, many of these qualitative features are subject to quantification. Quantification of these descriptive parameters allows for more objective characterization of the lesion. This is important in order to reduce inter- and intraobserver variability. It is also important to allow broader application of morphological measurements to improve our understanding of the pathophysiology of coronary artery disease by using the quantitative measures in clinical studies.

Rational for Quantification of Coronary Morphology

Quantitative analysis of a coronary lesion refers to the assignment of a numeric parameter to substitute for an otherwise descriptive characterization of a stenosis. In the early days of coronary arteriography,

From: Ambrose JA (ed): *Complex Coronary Lesions in Acute Coronary Syndromes.* © Futura Publishing Co., Inc., Armonk, NY, 1996.

descriptive terminology was used to characterize coronary stenoses.[1] A stenosis might be graded as mild, moderate, severe, or result in an occlusion of the artery. Initially, qualitative indices of stenosis severity were correlated with the presence or absence of clinical cardiac disease, and a history of angina and/or myocardial infarction. Quantification of stenosis severity followed when studies were performed that related the severity seen by coronary arteriography with that seen by postmortem examination.[2] The quantitative parameter that gained popularity was the percent diameter reduction or percent stenosis. This was conveniently estimated from the angiogram by comparison of the lumen remaining within the stenosis to the lumen seen in the "normal" adjacent segment. In addition to the clinical and pathological correlations with this quantitative parameter, physiological flow measurements by Gould et al.[3] showed the effect of stenosis on flow through a stenotic segment. Coronary flow reserve was maintained until a stenosis reached a value of approximately 50% diameter reduction. Flow at rest was affected when the stenosis attained a severity of about 85%.

Despite the broad acceptance of percent stenosis as a valuable parameter in the characterization of a coronary stenosis, there are significant limitations in its estimation. Subjective determination of the percent stenosis made by visual estimation was found to be quite variable due to inter- and intraobserver variation.[4,5] The magnitude of this variation could result in a stenosis estimation varying by more than 20%. That is, one observer might estimate a lesion as 50% diameter stenosis while another might estimate it at 70%. This observation was further confounded by the observation that the maximum variation occurs in lesions that are of "borderline" significance (Figure 1).[6] Numerous efforts to automate the process of stenosis severity determination have been attempted in order to reduce the inter- and intraobserver variability. Gensini et al.[7] developed one of the first caliper-based methods for measuring the percent stenosis of a coronary lesion from cineangiograms. This resulted in an improvement in reproducibility of stenosis severity measurements.

In addition to the difficulty in accurately determining the percent diameter stenosis by visual estimation, there are other important limitations in the quantitative characterization of a coronary stenosis. Mathematical models depicting fluid flow through arterial stenoses have shown that it is the area within the stenosis that determines the flow resistance, not the percent diameter reduction.[8,9] Clinical correlation between coronary blood flow and percent diameter reduction has also been shown to be poor. White et al.[10] examined the flow velocity ratios induced by a brief period of ischemia in stenosed coronary arter-

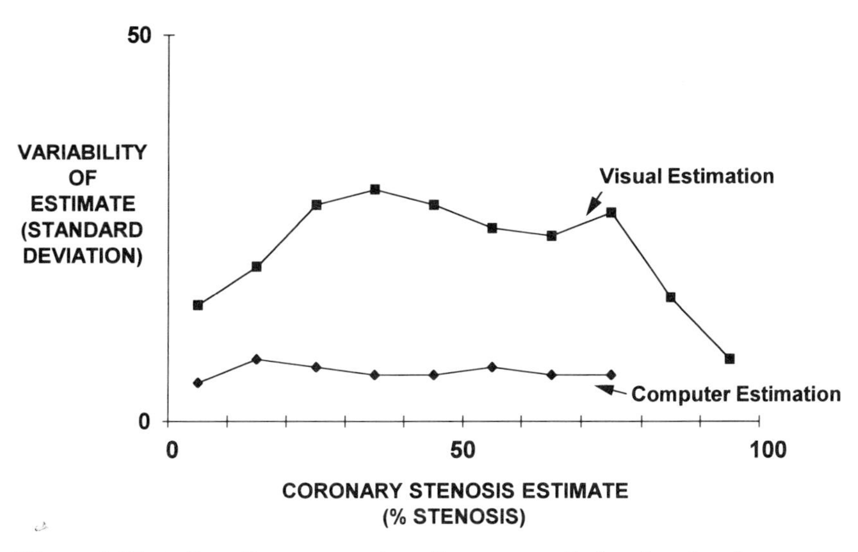

Figure 1: Variation of coronary artery disease severity by visual and computer-derived estimates. (Adapted from Brown et al.[6])

ies by means of a Doppler flow probe. These measurements of physiological flow reserve bore a poor correlation to the percent diameter stenosis that were measured for each of the stenoses. This study indicated that the physiological consequences of a coronary stenosis were poorly predicted from quantification of the coronary stenosis severity as represented by percent diameter stenosis. The coronary stenosis morphology has been shown to affect distal flow reserve in a study comparing simple to complex coronary artery stenoses.[11] Model stenoses implanted in swine with a complex morphology consisting of multiple lumina compared to a simple morphology consisting of a single lumen showed a twofold difference in flow reserve measurements.

More recent developments in quantitation of coronary stenosis have included minimal lesion diameter determination, which is more directly related to the stenosis area. Numerous computer-based systems have been developed that make determination of these quantitative parameters of coronary stenosis severity more objective and reproducible.[12–16] Since they are somewhat time-consuming and require specialized equipment that is not widely available, quantitative coronary arteriography has still not become commonplace in all cardiac catheterization laboratories.

Even with accurate assessments of coronary stenosis severity by percent stenosis or minimum lumen diameter measurements, the clinical utility of these measurements may have limitations. In addition to the poor correlation with coronary flow reserve measurements, the percent stenosis of a coronary stenosis does not correlate well with the clinical status of the patient. Several studies have shown that neither the number of diseased vessels nor the severity of the coronary artery disease measured by the percent stenosis correlates with the clinical presentation of the patient.[17,18] Thus, the percent diameter stenosis cannot by itself help to distinguish the patient with stable or unstable angina. Despite these limitations, quantification of coronary stenoses by percent diameter determination remains the single most broadly applied quantitative technique to assess coronary morphology.

To better define the angiographic characteristics that distinguish among the various clinical subsets, other morphological features must be analyzed. This approach has led to the identification of specific morphological features that are associated with various clinical disease states.[19]

Qualitative Parameters Comprising Lesion Morphology

In addition to the basic morphological characterization of a coronary stenosis by percent diameter reduction, there are numerous other morphological features that may be used to characterize a coronary lesion angiographically (Table 1).

The length or extent of a lesion is a morphological parameter that is commonly described. Although lesion length lends itself readily to quantitative measurements, deciding where a lesion begins and ends is sometimes difficult. The length of a lesion may be defined as where

Table 1
Some Lesion Characteristics Subject to Quantification

Severity	Translucencies
Length	Contrast inhomogeneity
Symmetry	Location of lesion
Roughness	Calcification
Shape	

the shoulders of the lesion appear to be, or in terms of the length of the stenosis exceeding 30%, 50%, or 70% diameter stenosis.[20] In addition, luminograms obtained by contrast angiography do not demonstrate the often diffuse nature of coronary disease involvement. Therefore, the length or extent of coronary disease may appear more focal than is seen by pathological or intravascular ultrasound examination.

Angiographic analysis can also be used to determine the symmetry or eccentricity of coronary stenoses. Angiograms obtained using multiple views can define whether a coronary stenosis is concentric or eccentric. Pathological studies indicate that the majority of coronary lesions result in obstructions that leave the artery narrowed in an eccentric fashion.[21] It is important in determining eccentricity that adequate angiographic images be obtained in order to be certain of the symmetry of a lesion. That is, a lesion may appear concentric in one view but be eccentric by viewing it from another angiographic angle. Quantitative determination of axis symmetry requires knowledge of the location of the vessel lumen with respect to the location of the vessel walls. This is at times difficult due to the natural curvature of coronary arteries throughout their course that makes estimation of the normal vessel wall difficult.

Examination of the appearance of the vessel edges outlined by contrast can also yield important morphological information. This qualitative parameter may be called lesion roughness or shape. Roughness can be thought of as the small perturbations in the vessel lumen edges that may be seen not only within a coronary stenosis but also along the "nondiseased' segments. When the variations of the vessel edge invaginate into the lumen beyond a certain point, a coronary lesion is identified. The shape or conformation of the lesion may also be subject to characterization. Quantification of vessel roughness or shape requires rather sophisticated analysis of the vessel edges. Roughness determinations can be made by comparing the local variation of a vessel edge from a smooth line to the average variation over a longer segment of the vessel. Shape may be measured quantitatively by breaking the vessel edge into small segments. The radius of the curves generated by these small segments can be determined by a process known as curvature analysis. Another process to characterize vessel shape depends on determining the fractal nature of the vessel wall edge. The coronary lesion may also be quantified in part by measuring the angle that the lesion creates to the flow of blood both into and out of the lesion. Inflow angles and outflow or exit angles can be used to characterize the lesion shape. These and other approaches to analysis of vessel roughness and shape may be used quantitatively.

Examination of the area within the contrast-filled lumen is another site for potential morphological characterization. Filling defects may occur proximal, within, or distal to a coronary stenosis. These filling defects may create a lucency within the contrast-filled lumen. They can be identified as a filling defect when contrast is seen surrounding the lucency on at least three sides.[22] Filling defects may represent the angiographic equivalents to intracoronary thrombus, and therefore are of importance in the characterization of a particular coronary lesion. Other invaginations into the vessel lumen by coronary lesions may make the lumen appear nonhomogeneous. Such variations in appearance may make the lesion seem translucent. This may commonly be observed with a lesion that has a cross-sectional area that departs significantly from a circle. Haziness of the vessel lumen may also be noted qualitatively under certain circumstances, such as following coronary angioplasty when an intimal dissection is created. Quantitation of these morphological features requires analysis of the cross-sectional features of the contrast bolus. This can be carried out by computer measurements of the videodensity of the x-ray image. If the brightness values from a grid of picture elements (pixels) across a coronary lumen are examined, a videodensity curve is generated that can be used to quantitatively characterize the contrast bolus within the coronary lumen. Inhomogeneities within the lumen alter the curve and can be quantified by analysis of these curves.

Other qualitative features of coronary morphology may also be defined. These include the location of the stenosis within the artery, such as ostial, proximal, mid, or distal. The location of the stenosis relative to branch points in the artery may be noted. Also the presence and extent of vessel wall calcium may be measured. These and other features may be defined and quantified to add to the specific characterization of the coronary stenosis. Applying these quantitative parameters of coronary morphology may be useful in clinical studies of coronary artery disease.

Clinical Studies

The application of quantitative analysis to coronary morphological features other than the severity of a coronary stenosis has been limited. Because of the need to improve the reproducibility of qualitative analysis and the importance of angiographic features other than percent stenosis, quantitative analysis of coronary morphology has been developed to some extent.

One of the early efforts to quantitate morphology of human atherosclerosis was a technique developed by Crawford et al.[23] This technique was initially applied to studies involving vessel roughness measurements from postmortem angiograms of femoral arteries. The technique involved determining the vessel edges of the femoral arteries by computer analysis of digitized images of the femoral arteries. The derived vessel edges were then smoothed by the use of digital filters. Using filters of different lengths resulted in vessel edges having different degrees of smoothing. The root-mean-square difference of images obtained using two different filters was determined. The difference was used to define a roughness parameter. It was found that this roughness value correlated well with the cholesterol content in the arterial wall. In another study applying the same type of quantitative analysis, the edge irregularity parameter was also correlated with the presence of raised atheromatous plaques.[24]

Another approach to quantitative analysis of vessel lumen irregularity was developed by Wilson et al.[25] They studied coronary angiograms from three groups of patients with recent myocardial infarction, unstable angina, and stable angina without prior myocardial infarction. Coronary stenoses were measured by serial coronary artery diameter determination throughout the length of the coronary stenosis. An ulceration index was derived (Figure 2), which was defined as the ratio

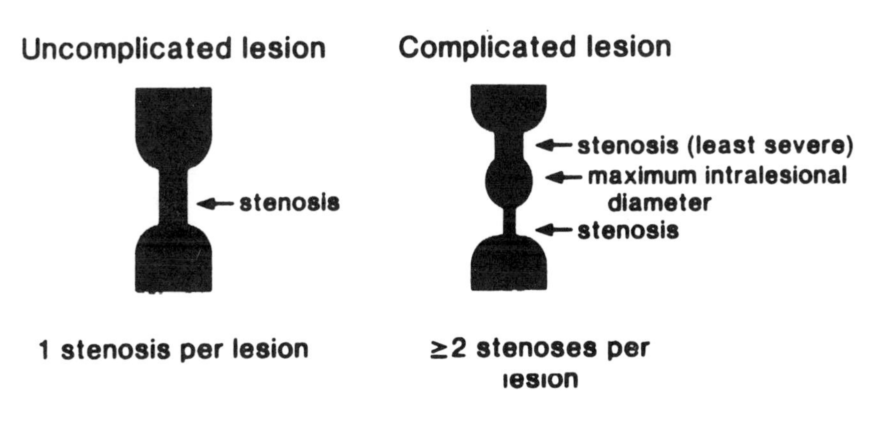

Figure 2: Method for classification of stenoses and calculation of the ulceration index. (Reproduced with permission from Wilson et al.[25])

of the least severe stenosis within the measured stenotic segment to the maximal intralesional diameter. They found that there was poor correlation of the percent stenosis to the clinical status of the patient. However, the ulceration index was significantly different in lesions responsible for unstable angina or myocardial infarction as compared to stable angina or noninfarct-related lesion. This may be related to disruption of a plaque or lysis of a superimposed thrombus that results in an ulcerated appearance to the plaque (Figure 3). The lower ulceration index in the clinically unstable patients was postulated to be related to either disruption of the atherosclerotic plaque and/or intraluminal thrombus.

Lesion length is an important morphological feature that has been used in various clinical studies. Lesion length has been shown to be a predictor of anterior myocardial infarction in left anterior descending

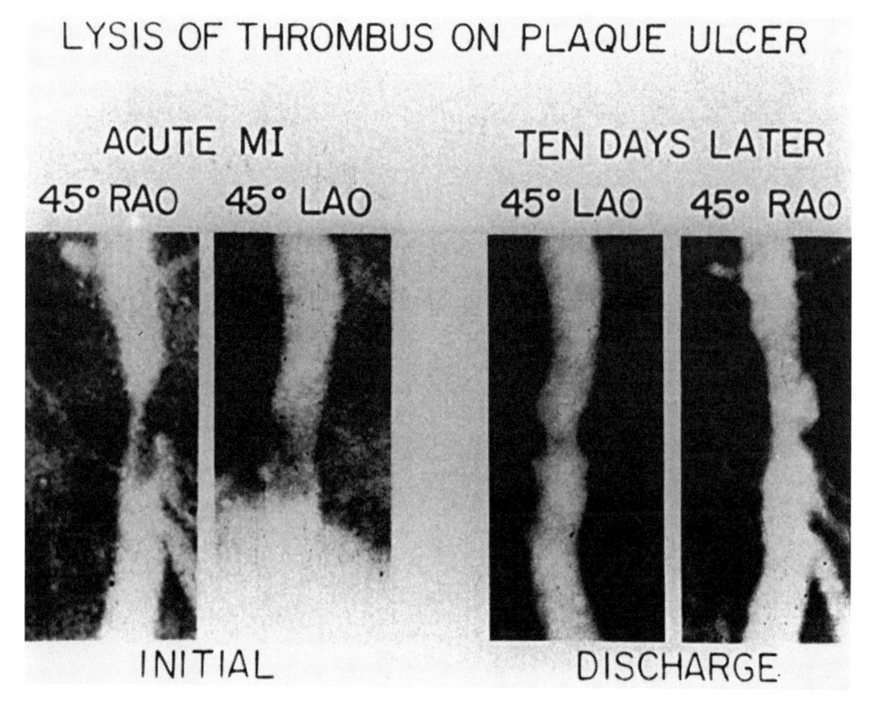

Figure 3: Coronary angiograms obtained from a patient with acute myocardial infarction and 10 days later. Initially a thrombus is adherent to the vessel wall that subsequently lyses revealing an apparent plaque ulceration. (Reproduced with permission from Wilson et al.[25])

artery lesions.[20,26] Ellis et al. showed that acute closure following coronary angioplasty was dependent on numerous factors including the length of the coronary stenosis. Other studies have shown that among several angiographic variables, lesion length is an important predictor of complications following angioplasty.[27,28] Therefore, lesion length is a principal factor in risk stratifying patients for coronary angioplasty. The length of a lesion can be determined quantitatively by computer analysis of the vessel edges. The coronary angiography analysis system (CAAS) makes use of curvature analysis to define the length of a lesion.[29] Other morphological parameters such as plaque area may also be determined by this computerized system.

Perhaps the most rigorous approach to quantification of lesion morphology was undertaken by Kalbfleisch et al.[30] Cineangiograms of patients with unstable and stable angina were digitized to allow for computer edge detection. Five computer-derived parameters were calculated from the vessel edges that provided a measure of the amount of vessel irregularity at the site of a lesion. Four of these parameters were derived from curvature analysis of the vessel edges. This was done by thinking of each point along a vessel edge line as lying on the edge of a circle and determining the radius of the circle at that point. By determining the inverse of the radius of the curve for all points along a vessel edge line, a curvature signature could be derived (Figure 4). A straight line would have a curvature signature line of zero. The more irregular the vessel edge, the more it deviated from zero. Four quantitative parameters were based on the curvature signature of the vessel edge line. The parameters included the number of peaks of the curve per centimeter, the sum of the maximum error or deviation in the curvature line per centimeter, the integrated error per centimeter, and the number of features per centimeter, as defined by a characteristic triplet shape of the curvature signature. In patients with unstable angina, there was more irregularity as determined by the curvature parameters than in patients with stable angina. Another parameter derived form the vessel edges was measured by a variation of fractal analysis. Roughness of a line or vessel edge can be determined by comparing the lengths of a curved line measured by applying a ruler of different lengths (Figure 5). The ratio of the lengths determined by two rulers of different lengths reflects the roughness of the line. In this study, however, this measure of lesion morphology was not shown to distinguish lesions in patients with or without unstable angina.

The strength of this type of quantitative morphological analysis is the high reproducibility that is derived. In addition, the defined parameters allow assessment of lesion morphology in a continuous scale

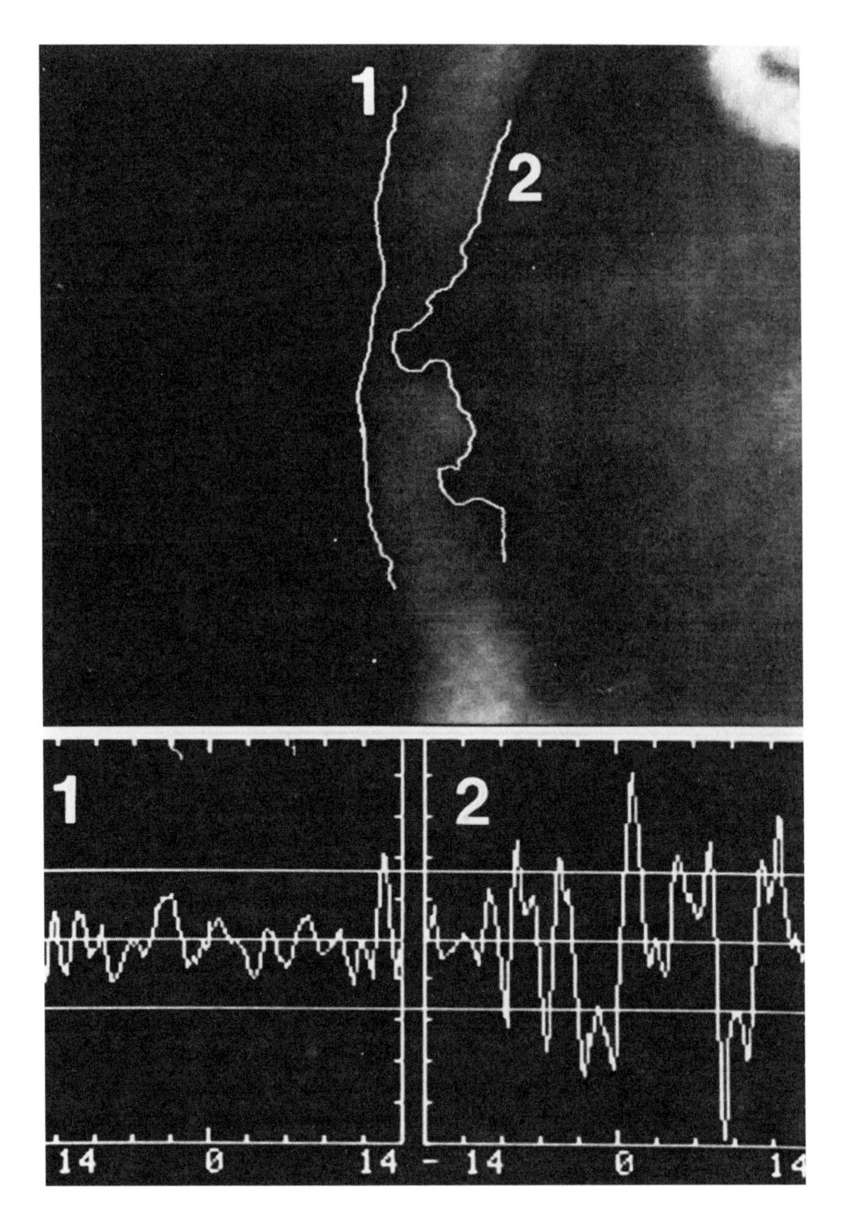

Figure 4: Digitally defined vessel edges are used to determine curvature signatures 1 and 2 in a patient with unstable angina. Edge 2 shows numerous complex features. (Reproduced with permission from Kalbfleisch et al.[30])

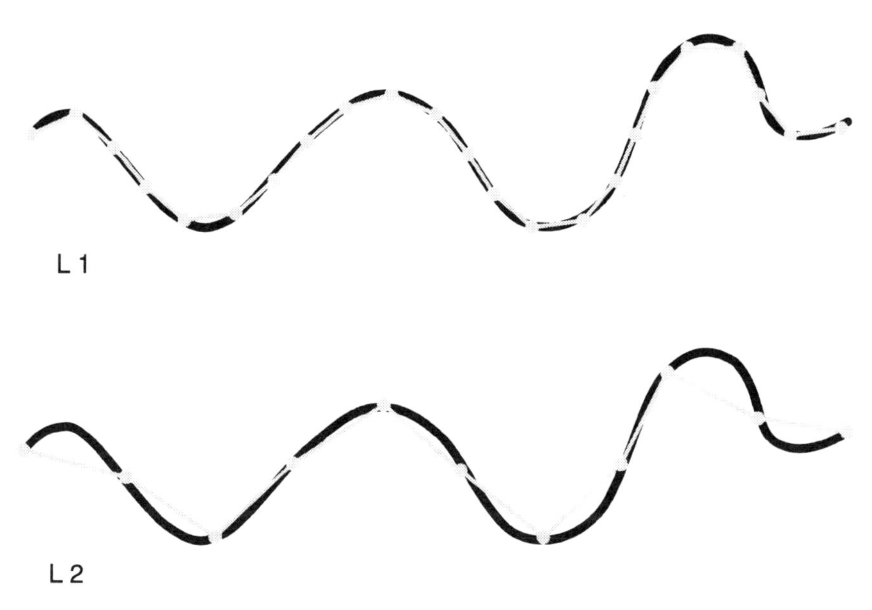

Figure 5: Scaled edge length ratio is the ratio of the length of arterial border measured by two different rulers (L1/L2). This can be used to quantify vessel roughness. (Adapted with permission from Kalbfleisch et al.[30])

fashion rather than by a categorical representation. The limitation of this particular study is that it only accounts for a portion of the factors that constitute coronary lesion morphology. Such factors as lesion shape and symmetry about the lumen axis are not accounted for by roughness determination alone. Also, lumen haziness and filling defects are not quantified by this technique. Therefore, many of the factors that may be related to the pathophysiological state of the coronary lesion may be missing from this analysis method.

Quantitative measures of the inflow and outflow angles of a coronary lesion have also been made. In a study of 38 coronary artery lesions that occluded within a 3-year time period to cause a myocardial infarction, Taeymans et al.[31] found that the inflow and outflow angles of the stenosis were significantly greater in those lesions that subsequently led to myocardial infarction compared to 64 control segments. Gould et al.[32] used quantitative coronary angiography to determine the effect of a low-cholesterol, low-fat, vegetarian diet, stress management, and exercise on lesion characteristics. One of the parameters used to characterize the lesions in this study was the exit angle of the lesion. This parameter was used to calculate the stenosis flow reserve

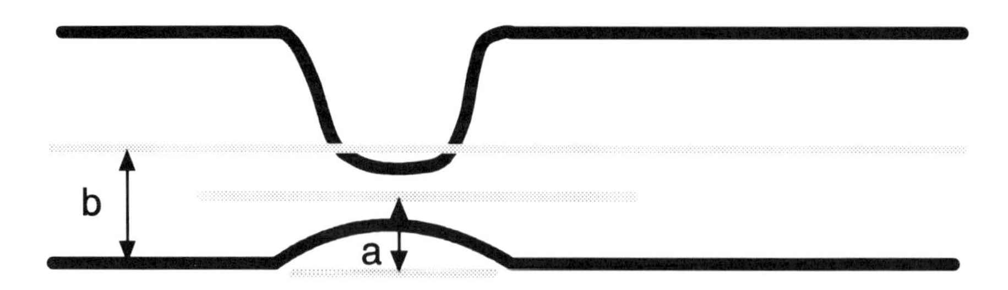

$$a/b \leq 0.5 = \text{Eccentric}$$
$$a/b > 0.5 = \text{Concentric}$$

Figure 6: Eccentricity index as defined by the ratio of difference of centerline of lesion and estimated normal edge and centerline of adjacent segment and normal wall. (Adapted with permission from Fischell et al.[33])

of a lesion. The study showed an improvement in the stenosis flow reserve for treated patients with severe lesions.

Several studies have incorporated quantitative measures of lesion symmetry. Symmetry measures depend on estimating, usually by interpolation, a normal vessel wall. Umans et al.[29] defined symmetry as the coefficient of the distance between the vessel contour and the estimated reference edge of one side of a stenosis and the distance between the vessel contour and the reference edge of the other side. The symmetry index ranged from 0 (totally eccentric stenosis) to 1 (totally symmetrical). These data were used to study the effects of directional atherectomy and balloon angioplasty.

Lumen eccentricity can also be quantified by comparing the ratio of the difference of the lengths between the centerline of the lesion and the estimated vessel wall (a) and the length of the centerline and normal wall at the adjacent segment (b)[33] (Figure 6). This definition was used to determine whether eccentricity of a lesion had any effect on vasoconstriction after coronary angioplasty. Lesions with low a/b ratios were called eccentric.

Future Directions

Analysis of coronary morphology has uncovered important pathophysiological mechanisms that have been critical to our understanding of clinical coronary artery disease. The use of quantitative measures of morphology provides a means of standardizing the morphological features to enable better reproducibility of studies of coronary artery disease. The limited application of these techniques is compounded by the inherent limitations of cineangiography.

Atherosclerosis affects the coronary vessel wall in a three-dimensional fashion. Yet cineangiography is limited to representing the artery in several two-dimensional views. Vessel overlap and foreshortening can modify the appearance of a coronary stenosis making it difficult to measure by any quantitative approach. The luminograms obtained by contrast angiography provide no clear definition of the normal vessel wall. Therefore, when knowledge of the location of the normal vessel wall is necessary for measurement purposes, it must be estimated. The spatial and temporal limitations of the imaging system used for angiography also compromise the ability of contrast angiography to determine lesion morphology.

In the future, other measures of coronary morphology will have to be defined and quantified in order to provide further insights as to the pathophysiology of coronary artery disease and the response to therapy. This is beginning to be seen by the use of other modalities such as intravascular ultrasound and coronary angioscopy.

At present these modalities are being used in an observation mode without extensive efforts to quantify the qualitative aspects of lesions observed by these devices. These features that may better reflect the true three-dimensional nature of coronary disease may provide further important morphological parameters that can be quantified and used to better characterize coronary artery disease.

References

1. Robbins SL, Rodriguez FL, Wragy AL, Fish SJ. Problems in the quantitation of coronary arteriosclerosis. Am J Cardiol 1966; 18:153–159.
2. Kemp HG, Evans H, Elliott WC, Gorlin R. Diagnostic accuracy of selective coronary cinearteriography. Circulation 1967; 36:526–533.
3. Gould KL, Lipscomb K, Hamilton GW. Physiologic basis for assessing critical coronary stenosis. Instantaneous flow response and regional distribution during coronary hyperemia as measures of coronary flow reserve. Am J Cardiol 1974; 33:87–94.
4. Zir LM, Miller SW, Dinsmore RE, Gilbert JP, Harthorne JW. Interobserver variability in coronary angiography. Circulation 1976; 53:627–632.
5. DeRouen TA, Murray JA, Owen W. Variability in the analysis of coronary arteriograms. Circulation 1977; 55:324–328.
6. Brown BG, Bolson EL, Dodge HT. Coronary arteriography and the objec-

tive assessment of coronary artery pathology. In Kalsner S (ed): The Coronary Artery. New York, Oxford University Press, 1982, p 523.

7. Gensini GG, Kelly AE, DaCosta BC, Huntington PP. Quantitative angiography: The measurement of coronary vasomobility in the intact animal and man. Chest 1971; 60:522–530.
8. Young DF, Tsai FY. Flow characteristics in models of arterial stenosis: I. Steady flow. J Biomech 1973; 6:395–410.
9. Young DF, Tsai FY. Flow characteristics in models of arterial stenosis: II. Unsteady flow. J Biomech 1973; 6:547–559.
10. White CW, Wright CB, Doty DB, et al. Does visual interpretation of the coronary arteriogram predict the physiologic importance of a coronary stenosis? N Engl J Med 1984; 310:819–824.
11. Fedele FA, Sharaf B, Most AS, Gewirtz H. Details of coronary stenosis morphology influence its hemodynamic severity and distal flow reserve. Circulation 1989; 80:636–642.
12. Brown BG, Bolson EL, Frimer M, Dodge HT. Quantitative coronary arteriography. Estimation of dimensions, hemodynamic resistance, and atheroma mass of coronary artery lesions using the arteriogram and digital computation. Circulation 1977; 55:329–337.
13. Brown BG, Bolson EL, Dodge HT. Quantitative computer techniques for analyzing coronary arteriograms. Prog Cardio Dis 1986; 6:403–418.
14. Spears JR, Sandor T, Als AV, et al. Computerized image analysis for quantitative measurement of vessel diameter from cineangiograms. Circulation 1983; 68:453–461.
15. Reiber JHC, Serruys PW, Kooijman CJ, et al. Assessment of short-, medium, and long-term variations in arterial dimensions from computer-assisted quantitation of coronary cineangiograms. Circulation 1985; 71: 280–288.
16. Nichols AB, Gabrielli CFO, Fenolio JJ, Esser PD. Quantification of relative coronary arterial stenosis by cinevideodensitometric analysis of coronary arteriograms. Circulation 1984; 69:512–522.
17. Alison HW, Russell RO Jr, Mantle JA, Kouchoukos NT, Moraski RE, Rackleu CE. Coronary anatomy and arteriography in patients with unstable angina pectoris. Am J Cardiol 1978; 41:204–209.
18. Fuster V, Frye RL, Connolly DC, Danielson MA, Elveback LR, Kurkland LT. Arteriographic patterns early in the onset of the coronary syndromes. Br Heart J 1975; 37:1250–1255.
19. Ambrose JA, Hjemdahl-Monsen CE. Angiographic morphology of unstable plaque. In Rutherford JD (ed): Unstable Angina. New York, Marcel Dekker, 1992, pp 49–67.
20. Ellis SG, Roubin GS, King SB, et al. Angiographic and clinical predictors of acute closure after native vessel coronary angioplasty. Circulation 1988; 77:372–379.
21. Freudenberg H, Lichtlen PR. The normal wall segment in coronary stenosis: a postmortem study. Z Kardiol 1981; 70:863–869.
22. Ambrose JA, Hjemdahl-Monsen CE. Acute ischemic syndromes: coronary pathophysiology and angiographic correlations. In Gersh BJ, Rahimtoola SH (eds): Acute Myocardial Infarction. New York, Elsevier, 1991, pp 64–77.

23. Crawford DW, Brooks SH, Selzer RH, Barndt R Jr, Beckenbach ES, Blankenhorn DH. Computer densitometry for angiographic assessment of arterial cholesterol content and gross pathology in human atherosclerosis. J Lab Clin Med 1977; 89:378–392.
24. Blankenhorn DH, Brooks SH, Selzer RH, Crawford DW, Chin HP. Assessment of atherosclerosis from angiographic images. Proceed Soc Exper Biol Med 1974; 145:1298–1300.
25. Wilson RF, Holida MD, White CW. Quantitative angiographic morphology of coronary stenoses leading to myocardial infarction or unstable angina. Circulation 1986; 73:286–293.
26. Ellis S, Alderman EL, Cain K, et al. Morphology of left anterior descending coronary territory lesions as a predictor of anterior myocardial infarction: A CASS registry study. J Am Coll Cardiol 1989; 13:1481–1491.
27. Ellis SG, Vandowmael MG, Cowley MJ, et al. Coronary morphologic and clinical determinants of procedural outcome with angioplasty for multivessel coronary disease. Circulation 1990; 82:1193–1202.
28. Myler RK, Shaw R, Stertzer SH, et al. Lesion morphology and coronary angioplasty: Current experience and analysis. J Am Coll Cardiol 1992; 19: 1641–1652.
29. Umans VAWM, Beatt KJ, Rensing BJWM, Hermans WRM, deFeyter PJ, Serruys PW. Comparative quantitative angiographic analysis of directional coronary atherectomy and balloon coronary angioplasty. Am J Cardiol 1991; 68:1556–1563.
30. Kalbfleisch SJ, McGillem MJ, Simon SB, et al. Automated quantitation of indexes of coronary lesion complexity: Comparison between patients with stable and unstable angina. Circulation 1990; 82:439–447.
31. Taeymans Y, Theroux P, Lesperance J, Waters D. Quantitative angiographic morphology of the coronary artery lesions at risk of thrombotic occlusion. Circulation 1992; 85:78–85.
32. Gould KL, Ornish D, Kirkeeide R, et al. Improved stenosis geometry by quantitative coronary arteriography after vigorous risk factor modification. Am J Cardiol 1992; 69:845–853.
33. Fischell TA, Bausback KN. Effects of luminal eccentricity on spontaneous coronary vasoconstriction after successful percutaneous transluminal coronary angioplasty. Am J Cardiol 1991; 68:530–534.

6

Angioscopy:

Clinical Correlation with Complex Lesion Morphology

Christopher J. White, MD,
Stephen R. Ramee, MD

Introduction

Coronary angioplasty, first performed in 1977,[1] has become established as a technique for coronary artery revascularization. As experience with angioplasty was gained, it became apparent that atherosclerotic coronary lesion morphology was a major determinant of a successful procedural outcome.[2–14]

The gold standard for imaging coronary artery lesion morphology is selective coronary angiography. Angiographic morphology studies of coronary arteries in patients with atherosclerotic coronary artery disease have allowed us to stratify patients with high-risk lesions.[15–17] These studies have been limited by the documented insensitivity of angiography for detecting subtle changes in coronary artery surface morphology, such as plaque fractures, dissections, intracoronary thrombi, and the assessment of residual stenosis, following angioplasty.[18–32]

Rapid advancements in angioplasty catheter design have led to the development of many new technologies for both therapeutic and

From: Ambrose JA (ed): *Complex Coronary Lesions in Acute Coronary Syndromes*.

diagnostic applications. One of these new devices is the angioscope.[33–63] The angioscope is a percutaneous catheter-based system designed to allow direct visual inspection of the endoluminal surface of the coronary arteries. The promise of the angioscope is that direct visual examination of the surface morphology of a diseased coronary artery will provide more specific, more sensitive, and more accurate information than angiography for identifying details of atherosclerotic plaque morphology.

Angioscope Equipment and Procedure

The imaging system is made up of components including illumination fibers, imaging fibers, a video camera and monitor, and a videotape recorder. The angioscope (Figure 1) (Imagecath, Baxter Edwards, Irvine, CA) contains 3,000 image fibers and is designed as a rapid ex-

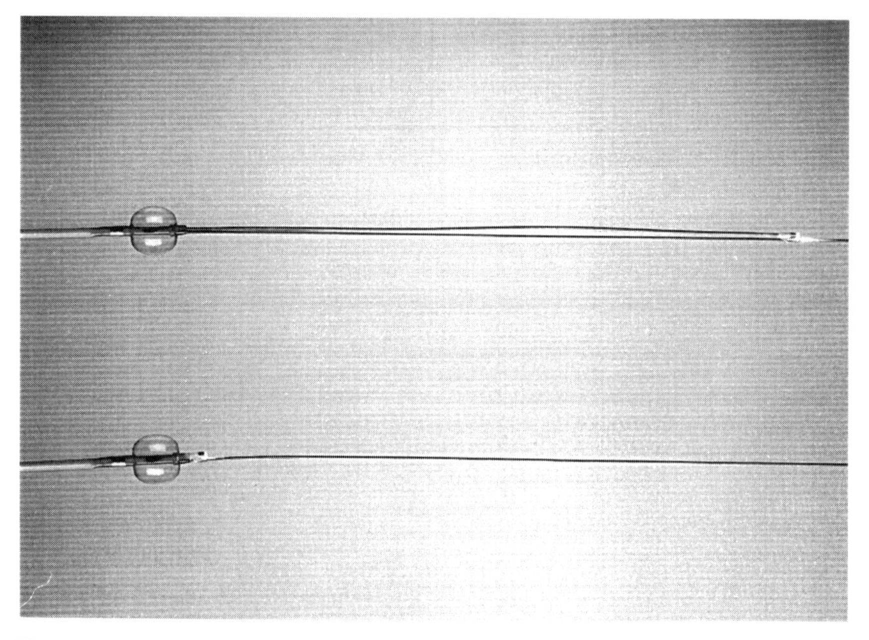

Figure 1: Photograph of the angioscope with the occlusion balloon inflated and inner image bundle extended (top) and retracted (bottom).

change catheter using a 0.014" angioplasty guidewire. The angioscope measures 4.5-French in diameter and has a lumen for inflating and deflating the occlusion balloon at its distal tip. The occlusion balloon is very compliant and achieves a variable final diameter up to a maximum diameter of 5.0 mm. An optically clear flush solution is infused through the angioscope's distal lumen to clear the field of view during inflation of the occlusion balloon. The image bundle may be advanced or withdrawn independently of the outer catheter a distance of approximately 5 cm, allowing examination of a large segment of the artery or lesion of interest.

An 8-French conventional angioplasty guiding catheter is placed in the coronary ostium of interest, and 10,000 units of heparin are administered. A 0.014" angioplasty guidewire is advanced across the "target lesion" and into the distal segment of the vessel. The angioscope has three umbilical connections for the light source, the video camera, and the flush lumen which are connected when the scope is outside of the body. The scope is "white balanced," focused, and flushed before introduction into the guiding catheter.

The angioscope is then advanced over the guidewire and positioned proximal to the region to be examined. Optically clear flush solution (warmed Ringer's lactate) is infused through the distal lumen of the scope with a power injector at a rate 0.5 cc to 1.0 cc per second. The occlusion balloon is hand-inflated with a 1-cc syringe filled with a 50:50 mixture of saline and radiographic contrast. Special care is taken not to overinflate the balloon which may damage the vessel. The imaging bundle is then advanced over the guidewire to view the intraluminal surface of the vessel. Each imaging sequence lasts approximately 30 to 45 seconds after which the occlusion balloon is deflated and antegrade blood flow restored. These steps can be repeated several times until the region of interest has been adequately investigated.

Complex Lesion Morphology

Saphenous Vein Bypass Grafts

The angiographic appearance of "friable" or loosely adherent plaque lining saphenous vein coronary bypass grafts has been suggested by some investigators to be a relative contraindication to balloon angioplasty due to the increased risk of distal embolization of atherosclerotic material.[64–66] Histological studies of saphenous vein bypass graft stenoses demonstrate the progression from fibrointimal proliferation in early graft lesions (less than 1 year old) to the development of typical atherosclerotic plaque in grafts more than 3 years old.[67–69] These plaques differ very little in their composition from native coronary artery atherosclerotic lesions with the exception that the plaques may be larger in ectatic saphenous vein grafts, and because of their bulk they may be more likely to cause clinically significant embolization during angioplasty.[67] There are reports that angioplasty of saphenous vein bypass grafts more than 3 years old (atherosclerotic versus fibrotic lesions) have been associated with increased risk of distal embolization.[64,66,67,70] However, other investigators have not confirmed the increased association of angioplasty complications with any specific angiographic lesion morphology in bypass grafts or that older vein grafts are associated with an increased risk of procedural complications.[71–75]

We compared angiographic and angioscopic lesion morphology in 21 saphenous vein bypass grafts.[60] All but one of the patients had unstable angina. The mean age of the saphenous vein coronary bypass grafts was 10.1 ± 2.4 years (range 5 to 15 years). Restenosis, at a prior angioplasty site, was present in seven patients.

Combining before and after angioplasty data, angioscopy demonstrated the presence of intravascular thrombi in 15 (71%) of 21 grafts in contrast to only four (19%) detected by angiography ($P<0.001$) (Figure 2). The incidence of intracoronary thrombi detected by angioscopy was not different between the restenosis graft lesions 71% (5/7) and the de novo graft lesions 71% (10/14). There was no correlation between the age of a bypass graft and the presence of thrombus.

Dissection was seen either before or after PTCA in 14 (66%) grafts by angioscopy versus two (9.5%) grafts by angiography ($P<0.01$). No patients had angiographic evidence of dissection prior to PTCA, whereas seven patients had intimal tears seen with angioscopy before angioplasty. Following PTCA there were two (9.5%) angiographic dissections versus 11 (52.3%) which were seen with the angioscope. The presence of dissection did not correlate with the age of the bypass graft.

Graft friability was detected before PTCA by angioscopy in 11 (52.3%) versus only four (19%) grafts by angiography ($P<0.05$) (Figure 3, see color plate on page 108A). Graft age did not correlate with the presence of friable plaque. Angioscopy confirmed the presence of a friable plaque in 3/4 grafts identified by angiography. The vein graft incorrectly identified as friable by angiography had a lesion with a white fibrotic-appearing nonshaggy intimal lining by angioscopy.

These data demonstrate the ability of angioscopy to detect features of lesion morphology that are frequently not seen by angiography in

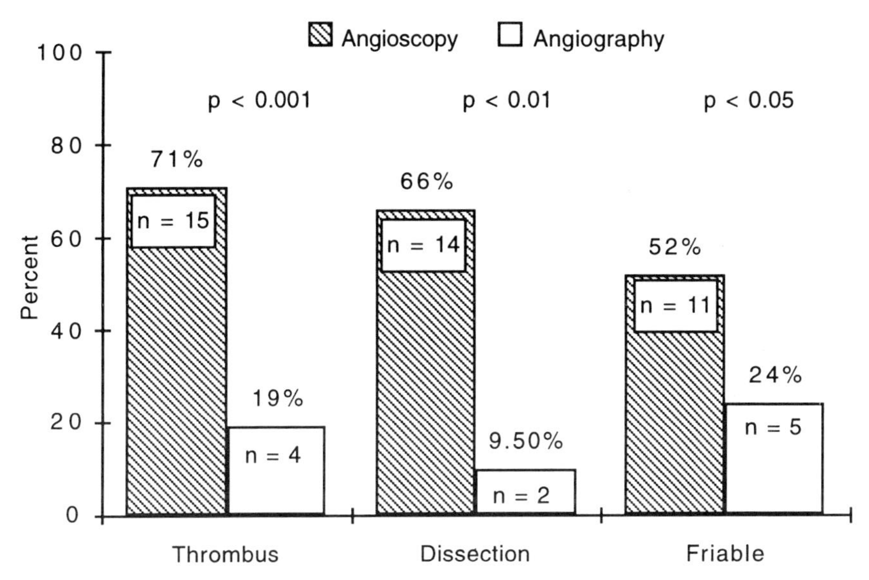

Figure 2: Bar graph comparing the angioscopic and angiographic findings in saphenous vein grafts undergoing angioplasty.

saphenous vein coronary bypass grafts. This uncertainty regarding the risk of embolization and the questionable ability of angiography to identify a high-risk subgroup for bypass graft angioplasty may be related to the insensitivity of angiography for detecting friable lesions as we have shown. None of our patients experienced embolization associated with angioplasty of these older vein grafts including the 11 patients with demonstrable friability of the luminal surface by angioscopy. Furthermore, we could not demonstrate that the presence of a friable appearance of the plaque surface correlated with the age of the bypass graft.

Angioscopic identification of friable plaque does not preclude an uncomplicated angioplasty procedure. In these older grafts, there is no correlation between their absolute age and the presence of friable or loosely adherent plaque. Whether the angioscopic appearance of plaque can predict in which grafts atheroembolism is more likely to occur will require a larger number patients to be studied.

Abrupt Occlusion after Angioplasty

Abrupt occlusion, the sudden closure of a coronary artery or saphenous vein graft after attempted angioplasty, is the major cause of in-hospital morbidity and mortality associated with percutaneous angioplasty. Prompt restoration of blood flow is essential to avoid myocardial infarction. Available therapies include repeat (long) balloon dilation, intracoronary thrombolysis, directional atherectomy, stent implantation, emergency coronary bypass surgery, and administration of intracoronary nitroglycerin. Treatment of abrupt occlusion may either be empirically determined or guided by the angiographic appearance of the lesion.

The speed and efficiency of restoring patency in a failed angioplasty vessel may be improved if specific information regarding the causes of the occlusion is known to the operator. For example, thrombolytic therapy would be expected to be much more effective in recanalizing a thrombosed vessel, but would be ineffective in re-establishing patency in a vessel occluded with tissue fragments or by dissection.

Percutaneous coronary angioscopy was performed in 10 patients following abrupt occlusion after balloon angioplasty. Intravascular thrombi were observed at the site of the abrupt occlusion in nine of 10 (90%) patients and were occlusive in two (20%) patients (Figure 4, see color plate on page 108A). Fragmented plaque and tissue flaps secondary to dissection of the artery wall were seen in all 10 patients and were occlusive in eight patients (80%) (Figure 5, see color plate on page 108B).*

Angioscopy revealed the cause of abrupt occlusion in each case by allowing direct visual inspection at the site of occlusion. Angioscopy may be useful in selecting the specific therapy for abrupt occlusion (thrombolysis for thrombus, or long balloon inflations, atherectomy, or stents for dissection).

The endovascular morphology we observed in these patients clearly demonstrated the primary cause of the vascular obstruction. It is interesting to note that although the majority of the patients had unstable angina, a condition that has been associated with a high incidence of intracoronary thrombi,[43,55] the majority of occlusions after PTCA were due to dissection and obstructive tissue flaps, not red thrombi.

We were able to determine a "primary cause" of the abrupt occlusion with the angioscope when both thrombi and dissections were present. Angioscopic information was used in these patients to select specific treatment modalities directed at the underlying cause of the failed

Editor's note: These observations have been published recently in a full article: White, et al. JACC 1995; 25:1681. Angioscopy was preformed in 17 vessels after post PTCA acute closure. Dissection was the primary cause in 14 (82%).

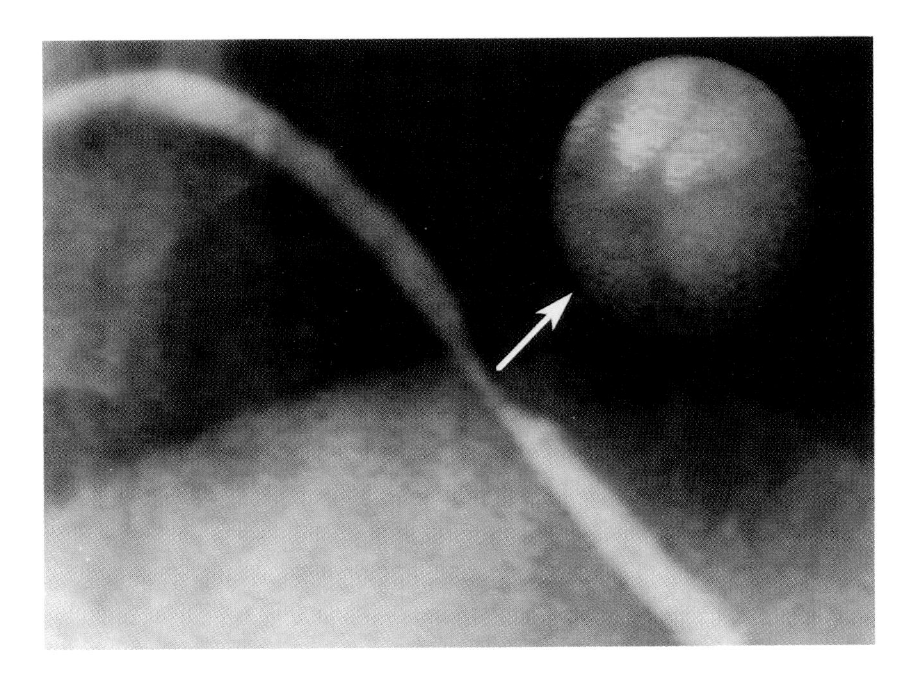

Figure 3: Angiography and angioscopy of a "friable" lesion in the mid-body of a saphenous vein graft. In the angioscopic photography, note yellow lobes of plaque loosely attached to the vessel wall.

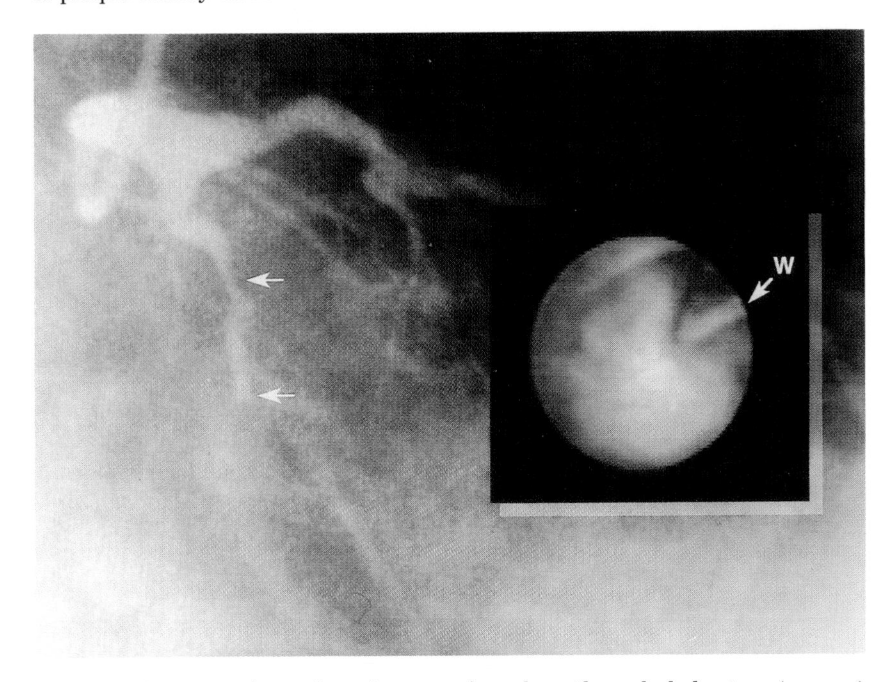

Figure 4: Angiography and angioscopy of an abruptly occluded artery (arrows) following PTCA, with the occlusion due to plaque in the lumen of vessel. Note the absence of red thrombus. (W = guidewire).

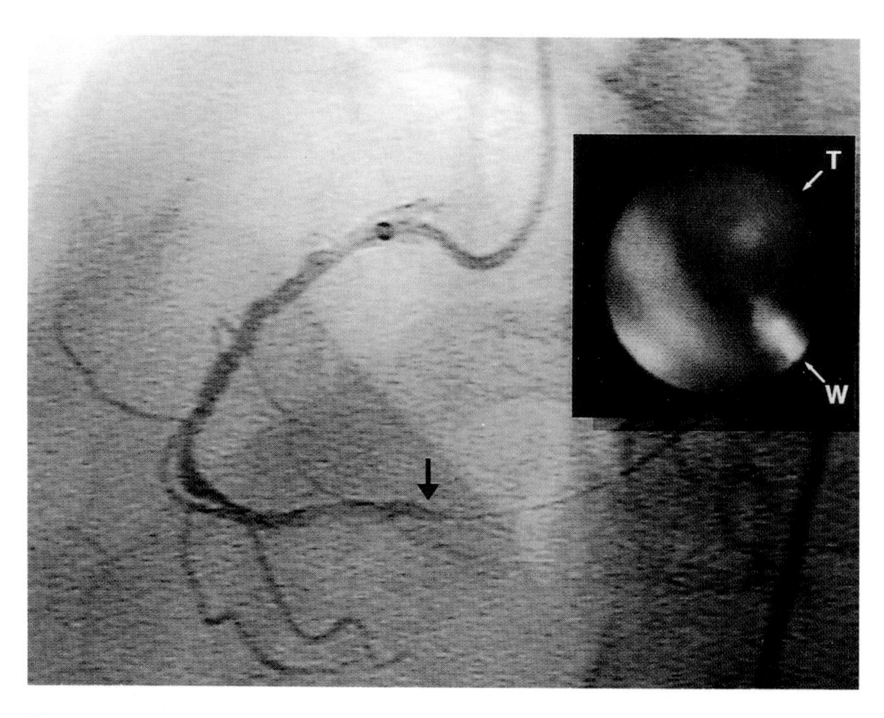

Figure 5: Angiography and angioscopy of abrupt occlusion (arrow) due to thrombus. (T = thrombus, W = guidewire).

angioplasty attempt, i.e., thrombolytic therapy for thrombus and repeat balloon dilation, directional atherectomy, or stent placement for occlusive dissections (tissue flaps).

We believe that specific information regarding the causes of the occlusion allows the operator to more efficiently select an appropriate treatment strategy. This knowledge, if it can be gained rapidly and safely, should expedite the re-establishment of coronary flow and avoid inappropriate (thrombolysis for tissue obstruction) or unattractive (stents in thrombus-filled arteries) therapies.*

Coronary Thrombi and PTCA Outcomes

There are conflicting reports in the literature regarding the significance of intracoronary thrombus as a harbinger of potential complications associated with coronary angioplasty.[2–12] The presence of intracoronary thrombus might be expected to predispose a traumatized endovascular surface to thrombotic occlusion. The inability of angiography to convincingly demonstrate a relationship between intracoronary thrombi and angioplasty complications may be related to angiography's documented insensitivity for coronary thrombus.[43,55,60,62]

Angioscopy was far more sensitive for intracoronary thrombus than was angiography detecting coronary thrombi in 74/122 (61%) vessels by angioscopy versus 24/122 (20%) patients by angiography ($P<0.001$). Angioscopic thrombus was visualized in 70/95 (74%) of the unstable angina patients compared to 4/27 (15%) of the stable angina patients ($P<0.001$). In the 24 vessels with angiographic evidence of thrombus, angioscopy confirmed the presence of intracoronary thrombus in 20 (83%). The sensitivity of angiography for intracoronary thrombi was 27% and the specificity was 92% when compared to angioscopy.

In-hospital complications (death, myocardial infarction, recurrent ischemia, or emergency coronary bypass surgery) were more likely to occur in patients with angioscopic thrombus, 24 of 74 (32.4%) than in those without thrombus, 5 of 48 (10.4%) ($P = 0.01$). The relative risk, or odds ratio, of a complication occurring with angioscopic thrombus was 3.11, (95% CI 1.28–7.60, $P = 0.01$) versus 0.85 (95% CI 0.36–2.00, $P = 0.91$) for angiographic thrombus. Multivariate analysis of clinical

* Editor's note: The results of the EPIC Trial reported in the NEJM in 1994 indicated that a bolus of $c7E_3$ plus a 12-hour infusion significantly reduced the need for emergent reintervention versus placebo. Thus, inhibiting thrombus may significantly reduce acute closure in spite of the presence of dissection.

Table 1
Multivariate Analysis of Variables Associated with In-hospital Complications following PTCA

	Coefficient	*P Value*
Scope thrombus	0.214	0.012
Angio thrombus	−0.126	0.22
Type A lesion	$-2.15e^{-3}$	0.99
Type B lesion	0.069	0.58
Type B1 lesion	0.027	0.85
Type B2 lesion	0.083	0.51
Type C lesion	0.209	0.24
Sex (M/F)	0.063	0.56
Angina (UA/SA)	$8.10e^{-3}$	0.94

M = male; F = female; UA = unstable angina; SA = stable angina.

(age, sex, unstable/stable angina), angiographic (AHA/ACC lesion type, minimal lumen diameter before or after PTCA, and thrombus) and angioscopic thrombus demonstrated that only angioscopic thrombus was significantly related to any in-hospital complication (Table 1).

The specificity of angiography for detecting intracoronary thrombi is also weakened when one realizes that not all angiographic filling defects are thrombi. Angioscopy, by depicting both color and texture, can readily distinguish white or yellow plaque fragments protruding into the vessel lumen from red thrombus. However, one limitation of angioscopy is the difficulty in differentiating "white" thrombus from white tissue elements that may be present in the vessel lumen. The angioscopic distinguishing feature of these white intraluminal masses is their shape and texture. Tissue fragments or dissection flaps usually demonstrate sharp, angular margins analogous to tattered white bed sheets on a clothesline blowing in the wind, whereas white thrombi (platelet aggregates and fibrin strands) are globular masses with fuzzy indistinct borders.

Patients with unstable angina had a significantly increased incidence of intracoronary thrombi compared to stable angina patients which is in agreement with prior angioscopic studies.[43,55] Intracoronary thrombus was also more commonly associated with the more complex AHA/ACC types B and C lesions compared to the less complex type A lesions. Univariate analysis of these angiographic lesion morphologies did not demonstrate a significant association with in-hospital complications.

Prior studies have demonstrated an increased incidence of angioplasty complications associated with unstable angina and complex coronary lesion morphology.[2,4,5,8,11,12,76,77] Some studies have also demonstrated an association of angiographic intracoronary thrombi with angioplasty complications[4–7] while others have not.[2,3,8] It appears that thrombi detected by angioscopy, but too small to be identified by angiography, may have clinical significance and be related to adverse outcomes following angioplasty. Multivariate analysis demonstrated that when compared to clinical variables (age, sex, unstable angina, and stable angina) or angiographic morphology (thrombus or lesion complexity), angioscopic intracoronary thrombus was most strongly associated with in-hospital adverse events following PTCA.

Conclusion

Angioscopic lesion morphology has definite clinical utility in guiding interventional therapy in selected patients. The angioscope may be useful to identify vein grafts with friable plaque likely to embolize with intervention, to select a treatment strategy for an abruptly occluded artery after angioplasty, or to visualize and identify an angiographic filling defect to determine if it is thrombus or a tissue flap protruding into the lumen.

The greatest potential impact for angioscopy appears to be in stratifying risk in patients at high risk for having coronary thrombus in association with a coronary lesion, such as those with unstable angina or complex AHA/ACC type B or type C lesions. Although the risk of a complication appears to be strongly related to the presence of intracoronary thrombus, we have yet to demonstrate a cause-and-effect relationship between the intracoronary thrombi visualized by angioscopy and the occurrence of an angioplasty complication. Thrombus may occur in association with lesions more likely to fail angioplasty rather than directly contributing to the failure. Alternatively, a small amount of red thrombus may serve as a nidus for subsequent growth of a thrombus directly contributing to vessel closure or recurrent ischemia. Resolution of this question will require us to demonstrate that angioscopically directed therapy to resolve the red thrombus can reduce the incidence of in-hospital complications compared to a control population.

References

1. Grüntzig AR, Senning A, Siegenthaler WE. Nonoperative dilatation of coronary artery stenosis. Percutaneous transluminal coronary angioplasty. N Engl J Med 1979; 301:61–68.

2. de Feyter PJ, van den Brand M, Jaarman G, van Domburg R, Serruys PW, Suryapranata H. Acute coronary occlusion during and after percutaneous transluminal coronary angioplasty. Frequency, prediction, clinical course, management, and follow-up. Circulation 1991; 83:927–936.
3. Simpfendorfer C, Belardi J, Bellamy G, Galan K, Franco I, Hollman J. Frequency, management and follow-up of patients with acute coronary occlusions after percutaneous transluminal coronary angioplasty. Am J Cardiol 1987; 59:267–269.
4. Ellis SG, Roubin GS, King SB III, Douglas JS, Weintraub WS, Thomas RG, Cox WR. Angiographic and clinical predictors of acute closure after native vessel coronary angioplasty. Circulation 1988; 77:372–379.
5. Detre KM, Holmes DR Jr., Holubkov R, Cowley MJ, Bourassa MG, Faxon DP, Dorros GR, Bentivoglio LG, Kent KM, Myler RK and coinvestigators of the National Heart, Lung, and Blood Institute's Percutaneous Transluminal Coronary Angioplasty Registry. Incidence and consequences of periprocedural occlusion. The 1985–1986 National Heart Lung and Blood Institute Percutaneous Transluminal Coronary Angioplasty Registry. Circulation 1990; 82:739–750.
6. Sugrue DD, Holmes DR Jr, Smith HC, Reeder GS, Lane GE, Vlietstra RE, Bresnahan JF, Hammes LN, Piehler JM. Coronary artery thrombus as a risk factor for acute vessel occlusion during percutaneous transluminal coronary angioplasty: improving results. Br Heart J 1986; 56:62–66.
7. Mabin TA, Homes DR, Smith HC, Vlietstra RE, Bove AA, Reeder GS, Chesebro JH, Bresnahan JF, Orszulak TA. Intracoronary thrombus: role in coronary occlusion complicating percutaneous transluminal coronary angioplasty. J Am Coll Cardiol 1985; 5:198–202.
8. de Feyter PJ, Suryapranata H, Serruys PW, Beatt K, van Domburg R, van den Brand M, Tijssen JJ, Azar AJ, Hugenholtz PG. Coronary angioplasty for unstable angina: Immediate and late results in 200 consecutive patients with identification of risk factors for unfavorable early and late outcome. J Am Coll Cardiol 1988; 12:324–333.
9. Sinclair IN, McCabe CH, Sipperly ME, Baim DS. Predictors, therapeutic options and long-term outcome of abrupt reclosure. Am J Cardiol 1988; 61:61G-66G.
10. Bredlau CE, Roubin GS, Leimbruber PP, Douglas JS, King SB III, Gruentzig AR. In-hospital morbidity and mortality in patients undergoing elective coronary angioplasty. Circulation 1985; 72:1044–1052.
11. Ellis SG, Roubin GS, King SB III, Douglas JS, Shaw RE, Stertzer SH, Myler RK. In-hospital cardiac mortality after acute closure after coronary angioplasty: analysis of risk factors from 8,207 procedures. J Am Coll Cardiol 1988; 11:211–216.
12. de Feyter PJ, de Jaegere PPT, Murphy ES, Serruys PW. Abrupt coronary artery occlusion during percutaneous coronary angioplasty. Am Heart J 1992; 123:1634–1642.
13. Breshnahan DR, Davis JL, Holmes DR, Smith HC. Angiographic occurrence and clinical correlates of intraluminal coronary artery thrombus: Role of unstable angina. J Am Coll Cardiol 1985; 6:285–289.
14. Ambrose JA, Hjemdahl-Monsen CE, Borrico S, Gorlin R, Fuster V. Angio-

graphic demonstration of a common link between unstable angina pectoris and non-Q wave myocardial infarction. Am J Cardiol 1988; 61:244–247.
15. Ambrose JA, Winters SL, Stern A. Angiographic morphology and the pathogenesis of unstable angina pectoris. J Am Coll Cardiol 1985; 5:609–616.
16. Rehr R, Disciascio G, Vetrovec G, Cowley M. Angiographic morphology of coronary artery stenoses in prolonged rest angina: Evidence of intracoronary thrombosis. J Am Coll Cardiol 1989; 14:1429–1437.
17. Levin DC, Fallon JT. Significance of the angiographic morphology of localized coronary stenoses: Histopathologic correlations. Circulation 1982; 66: 316–320.
18. Vlodaver Z, Frech R, Van Tassel RA, Edwards JE. Correlations of the antemortem coronary arteriogram and the postmortem specimen. Circulation 1973; 47:162–169.
19. Grondin CM, Dyrda I, Pasternac A, Campeau L, Bourassa MG, Lesperance J. Discrepancies between cineangiographic and postmortem findings in patients with coronary artery disease and recent myocardial revascularization. Circulation 1974; 49:703–708.
20. Pepine CJ, Feldman RL, Nichols WW, Conti CR. Coronary arteriography: Potentially serious sources of error in interpretation. Cardiovasc Med 1977; 2:747–752.
21. Arnett EN, Isner JM, Redwood DR, et al. Coronary artery narrowing in coronary heart disease: Comparison of cineangiographic and necropsy findings. Ann Int Med 1979; 91:350–356.
22. Isner JM, Kishel J, Kent KM, Ronan JA, Ross AM, Roberts WC. Accuracy of angiographic determination of left main coronary arterial narrowing: Angiographic-histologic correlative analysis in 28 patients. Circulation 1981; 63:1056–1064.
23. Spears JR, Sandor T, Baim DS, Paulin S. The minimum error in estimating coronary luminal cross-sectional area from cineangiographic diameter measurements. Cathet Cardiovasc Diag 1983; 9:119–128.
24. White CW, Wright CB, Doty DB, et al. Does visual interpretation of the coronary arteriogram predict the physiologic importance of a coronary stenosis? N Engl J Med 1984; 310:819–824.
25. Isner JM, Donaldson RF. Coronary angiographic and morphologic correlation. Cardiol Clin 1984; 2:571–592.
26. Gould KL. Quantification of coronary artery stenosis in vivo. Circ Res 1985; 57:341–353.
27. Zijlstra F, van Ommeren J, Reiber HC, Surruys PW. Does the quantitative assessment of coronary artery dimensions predict the physiologic significance of a coronary stenosis? Circulation 1987; 75:1154–1161.
28. Marcus ML, Skorton DJ, Johnson MR, Collins SM, Harrison DG, Kerber RE. Visual estimates of percent diameter coronary stenosis: "A battered gold standard" (editorial). J Am Coll Cardiol 1988; 11:882–885.
29. Katritsis D, Webb-Peploe M. Limitations of coronary angiography: An underestimated problem? Clin Cardiol 1991; 14:20–24.
30. Block PC, Myler RK, Stertzer S, Fallon JT. Morphology after transluminal angioplasty in human beings. N Engl J Med 1981; 305:382–385.
31. Duber C, Jungbluth A, Rumpelt HJ, Erbel R, Meyer J, Thoenes W. Morphology of the coronary arteries after combined thrombolysis and percuta-

neous transluminal coronary angioplasty for acute myocardial infarction. Am J Cardiol 1986; 58:698–703.
32. Essed CE, Van Den Brand M, Becker AE. Transluminal coronary angioplasty and early restenosis: Fibrocellular occlusion after wall laceration. Br Heart J 1983; 49:393–396.
33. Mizuno K, Kurita A, Imazeki N. Pathological findings after percutaneous transluminal coronary angioplasty. Br Heart J 1984; 52:588–590.
34. Cutler EC, Levine, Beck CS. The surgical treatment of mitral stenosis: Experimental and clinical studies. Arch Surg 1924; 9:689–821.
35. Harken DE, Glidden EM. Experiments in intracardiac surgery. II. Intracardiac visualization. J Thorac Surg 1943; 12:566–572.
36. Bolton HE, Bailey CP, Costas-Durieux J, Gemeinhardt W. Cardioscopy: simple and practical. J Thorac Surg 1954; 27:323–329.
37. Sakakibara S, Ilkawa T, Hattori J, Inomata K. Direct visual operation for aortic stenosis: Cardioscopic studies. J Int Coll Surg 1958; 29:548–562.
38. Litvack F, Grundfest WS, Lee ME, Carroll RM, Foran R, Chaux A, Berci G, Rose HB, Matloff JM, Forrester JS. Angioscopic visualization of blood vessel interior in animals and humans. Clin Cardiol 1985; 8:65–70.
39. Grundfest WS, Litvack F, Sherman T, Carroll RM, Lee M, Chaux A, Kass R, Matloff J, Berci G, Swan HJC, Morgenstern L, Forrester J. Delineation of peripheral and coronary detail by intraoperative angioscopy. Ann Surg 1985; 202:394–400.
40. Sanborn TA, Rygaard JA, Westbrook BM, Lazar HL, McCormick JR, Roberts AJ. Intraoperative angioscopy of saphenous vein and coronary arteries. J Thorac Cardiovasc Surg 1986; 91:339–343.
41. Lee G, Garcia JM, Corso PJ, Chan MC, Rink JL, Pichard A, Lee KK, Reis RL, Mason DT. Correlation of coronary angioscopic to angiographic findings in coronary artery disease. Am J Cardiol 1986; 58:238–241.
42. Grundfest WS, Litvack F, Glick D, et al. Intraoperative decisions based on angioscopy in peripheral vascular surgery. Circulation 1988; 78(Suppl I):l-13-I-17.
43. Sherman CT, Litvack F, Grundfest W, Lee M, Hickey A, Chaux A, Kass R, Blanche C, Matloff J, Morgenstern L, Ganz W, Swan HJC, Forrester J. Coronary angioscopy in patients with unstable angina pectoris. N Engl J Med 1986; 315:913–919.
44. Spears JR, Spokojny AM, Marais HJ. Coronary angioscopy during cardiac catheterization. J Am Coll Cardiol 1985; 6:93–97.
45. Susawa T, Yui Y, Hattori R, Takatsu Y, Yui N, Takahashi M, Aoyama T, Murohara Y, Shirotani M, Kawai C. Direct observation of coronary thrombus using a newly developed ultrathin (1.2 mm) flexible angioscope (abstract). J Am Coll Cardiol 1987; 9(Suppl A):197A.
46. Takahashi M, Yui Y, Susawa T, Hattori R, Takatsu Y, Yui N, Aoyama T, Murohara Y, Shirotani M, Yasumoto H, Morishita H, Kadota K, Kawai C. Evaluation of coronary thrombus by a newly developed ultrathin (0.75 mm) flexible quartz microfiber angioscope (abstract). Circulation 1987; 76(Suppl IV):lV-282.
47. Uchida Y, Furuse A, Hasegawa K. Percutaneous coronary angioscopy using a novel balloon guiding catheter in patients with ischemic heart diseases (abstract). Circulation 1987; 76(Suppl IV):lV-185.

48. Uchida Y. Tomaru T, Nakamura F, Furuse A, Fujimori Y, Hasegawa K. Percutaneous coronary angioscopy in patients with ischemic heart disease. Am Heart J 1987; 114:1216–1222.
49. Inoue K, Kuwaki K, Ueda K, Shirai T. Angioscopy guided coronary thrombolysis (abstract). J Am Coll Cardiol 1987; 9(Suppl A):62A.
50. Morice M-C, Marco J, Fajadet J, Castillo-Fenoy A. Percutaneous coronary angioscopy before and after angioplasty in acute myocardial infarction: Preliminary results (abstract). Circulation 1987; 76(Suppl IV):lV-282.
51. Inoue K, Kuwaki K, Ueda K, Takano E. Angioscopic macropathology of coronary atherosclerosis in unstable angina and acute myocardial infarction (abstract). J Am Coll Cardiol 1988; 11(Suppl A):65A.
52. Kuwaki K, Inoue K, Ueda K, Shirai T, Ochiai H. Percutaneous transluminal coronary angioscopy during cardiac catheterization: The results of experiences in the first 30 patients (abstract). Circulation 1987; 76(Suppl IV):lV-186.
53. Uchida Y, Hasegawa K, Kawamura K, Shibuya I. Angioscopic observation of the coronary luminal changes induced by percutaneous transluminal angioplasty. Am Heart J 1989; 117:769–776.
54. Uchida Y. Percutaneous coronary angioscopy by means of a fiberscope with a steerable guidewire. Am Heart J 1989; 117:1153–1155.
55. Ramee SR, White CJ, Collins TJ, Mesa JE, Murgo JP. Percutaneous angioscopy during coronary angioplasty using a steerable microangioscope. J Am Coll Cardiol 1991; 17:100–105.
56. White CJ, Ramee SR. Percutaneous coronary angioscopy: Methods, findings, and therapeutic implications. Echocardiography 1990; 7:485–494.
57. Mizuno K, Arai T, Satomura K, et al. New percutaneous transluminal coronary angioscope. J Am Coll Cardiol 1989; 13:363–368.
58. Ventura H0, White CJ, Ramee SR, et al. Percutaneous coronary angioscopy findings in patients with cardiac transplantation (abstract). J Am Coll Cardiol 1991; 17:273A.
59. Ventura H0, White CJ, Ramee SR, Collins TJ, Mesa JE, Jain A. Coronary angioscopy in the diagnosis of graft coronary artery disease in heart transplant recipients (letter). J Heart Lung Transplant 1991; 10:488.
60. White CJ, Ramee SR, Collins TJ, Mesa JE, Jain A. Percutaneous angioscopy of saphenous vein coronary bypass grafts. J Am Coll Cardiol 1993; 21:1181–1185.
61. White CJ, Ramee SR, Collins RJ, Jain A, Mesa JE, Ventura HO. Percutaneous coronary angioscopy: Applications in interventional cardiology. J Interven Cardiol 1993; 6:61–67.
62. White CJ, Ramee SR, Mesa J, Collins TJ. Percutaneous coronary angioscopy in patients with restenosis after coronary angioplasty. J Am Coll Cardiol 1991; 17(Suppl B):46B-49B.
63. Mizuno K, Satomura K, Miyamoto A, Arakawa K, Shibuya T, Arai T, Kurita A, Nakamura H, Ambrose JA. Angioscopic evaluation of coronary-artery thrombi in acute coronary syndromes. N Engl J Med 1992; 326: 287–291.
64. Reeves F, Bonan R, Cote G, Crepeau J, deGuise P, Gosselin G, Campeau L, Lesperance J. Long-term angiographic follow-up after angioplasty of venous coronary bypass grafts. Am Heart J 1991; 122:620–627.

65. Cote G, Myler RK, Stertzer SH, Clark DA, Rosen JF, Murphy M, Shaw RE. Percutaneous transluminal angioplasty of stenotic coronary artery bypass grafts: 5 years' experience. J Am Coll Cardiol 1987; 9:8–17.
66. Block PC, Cowley MJ, Kaltenbach M, Kent KM, Simpson J. Percutaneous angioplasty of bypass grafts or of bypass graft anastomotic sites. Am J Cardiol 1984; 53:666–668.
67. Saber RS, Edwards WD, Holmes DR, Vlietstra RE, Reeder GS. Balloon angioplasty of aortocoronary saphenous vein bypass grafts: A histopathologic study of six grafts from five patients, with emphasis on restenosis and embolic complications. J Am Coll Cardiol 1988; 12:1501–1509.
68. Waller BF, Rothbaum DA, Gorfinkel JH, Ulbright TM, Linnemeier TJ, Berger SM. Morphologic observations after percutaneous transluminal balloon angioplasty of early and late aortocoronary saphenous vein bypass grafts. J Am Coll Cardiol 1984; 4:784–792.
69. Garratt KN, Edwards WD, Kaufmann UP, Vlietstra RE, Holmes DR. Differential histopathology of primary atherosclerotic and restenotic lesions in coronary arteries and saphenous vein bypass grafts: Analysis of tissue obtained from 73 patients by directional atherectomy. J Am Coll Cardiol 1991; 17:442–448.
70. Platko WP, Hollman J, Whitlow PL, Franco I: Percutaneous transluminal angioplasty of saphenous vein graft stenosis: Long-term follow-up. J Am Coll Cardiol 1989; 14:1645–1650.
71. Dorros G, Lewin RF, Mathiak LM, Johnson WD, Brenowitz J, Schmahl T, Tector A. Percutaneous transluminal coronary angioplasty in patients with two or more previous coronary artery bypass grafting operations. Am J Cardiol 1988; 61:1243–1247.
72. Marquis JF, Schwartz L, Brown R, Matushinsky E, Mickleborough L, Aldridge H, Henderson M. Percutaneous transluminal angioplasty of coronary saphenous vein bypass grafts. Can J Surg 1985; 28:335–337.
73. Jost S, Gulba D, Daniel WG, Amende I, Rudiger S, Eckert S, Lichtlen PR. Percutaneous transluminal angioplasty of aortocoronary venous bypass grafts and effect of the caliber of the grafted coronary artery on graft stenosis. Am J Cardiol 1991; 68:27–30.
74. Reeder GS, Bresnahan JF, Holmes DR Jr, Mock MB, Orszulak TA Smith HC, Vlietstra R. Angioplasty for aortocoronary bypass graft stenosis. Mayo Clin Proc 1986; 61:14–19.
75. Ernst SM, van der Felts TA, Ascoop CA, Bal ET, Vermeulen FE, Knaepen PJ, van Bogerijen L, van den Berg EJ, Plokker HW. Percutaneous transluminal coronary angioplasty in patients with prior coronary artery bypass grafting: Long-term results. J Thorac Cardiovasc Surg 1987; 93:268–275.
76. Ellis SG, Vandormael MG, Cowley MJ, DiSciascio G, Delingonul U, Topol EJ, Bulle TM, and the Multivessel Angioplasty Prognosis Study Group. Coronary morphologic and clinical determinants of procedural outcome with angioplasty for multivessel coronary disease: implications for patient selection. Circulation 1990; 82:1193–1202.
77. de Feyter PJ. Coronary angioplasty for unstable angina. Am Heart J 1989; 118:860–868.

7

Biochemical Markers and Complex Lesion Morphology

Jonathan D. Marmur, MD, John Venditto, MD

Introduction

Advanced atherosclerotic plaques are focal intimal lesions that develop in areas of low or oscillatory shear stress. They are composed mainly of smooth muscle cells, an extracellular matrix rich in glycosaminoglycans, collagen, elastin, and lipid. Lipid may be contained in foam cells or located extracellularly in the form of cholesterol or cholesterol ester. The lipid-rich core of the plaque is separated from the lumen by a fibromuscular cap. When thrombus forms on an atherosclerotic plaque, a tear in the fibromuscular cap with a thrombus anchored to the subintimal surface will be present in 75% of cases. In the remaining 25%, a superficial ulceration of the intimal surface will be present.

Exposure of the highly thrombogenic substrate of the plaque to blood leads to platelet deposition upon the subintimal components of the vessel wall. Activation of coagulation by tissue factor and other substances leads to thrombin generation and fibrin formation. The extent of thrombus formation is a complex process depending in part on the degree of plaque disruption, the plaque contents, the degree of plasma hypercoagulability, and hemodynamic factors that promote hemostasis and vasoconstriction. The thrombus that forms at the site of

From: Ambrose JA (ed): *Complex Coronary Lesions in Acute Coronary Syndromes*. © Futura Publishing Co., Inc., Armonk, NY, 1996.

plaque disruption is usually platelet-rich while the distal tail is usually fibrin-rich and if large enough may be occlusive.

Reliable markers of this process in vivo could be clinically useful given the significance of intracoronary thrombus formation in the acute coronary syndromes. Biochemical markers of thrombin generation and platelet activation have been studied extensively in patients with stable and unstable coronary artery disease. There are, however, limited data available correlating markers of thrombus formation directly with complex coronary lesion morphology. The following is a review of this literature.

The rapid conversion of blood from a fluid to a solid involves a cascade of reactions in which inactive circulating zymogens (enzyme precursors) are converted to active serine proteases that ultimately result in the generation of fibrin. Each step of the coagulation cascade is characterized by the formation of a complex comprised of a substrate (a zymogen or fibrinogen), a converting enzyme (e.g., factor Xa, thrombin), and a co-factor (e.g., factors V and VIII).[1] These complexes form on natural surfaces (such as membrane derived from platelets, leukocytes, or vascular cells) that help to both accelerate and localize the clotting process to areas of vascular injury. Dissemination of coagulation beyond the site of injury is also limited by endogenous circulating anticoagulants that inhibit the cascade at several steps (e.g., C1-inhibitor, tissue factor pathway inhibitor, antithrombin III).

In patients with primary hemorrhagic or thrombotic diatheses, measurement of the plasma level of zymogens, co-factors, inhibitors, or substrates may provide important diagnostic information. However, in the majority of atherosclerotic patients presenting with acute arterial thrombosis, these molecules are present in large excess, and only small fractions of the zymogens are converted to their active form. Thus, in the setting of acute coronary syndromes, plasma levels of circulating zymogens are unable to provide an assessment of the degree to which the coagulation cascade has been activated.

The enzymes generated during clotting in vivo have not been amenable to direct quantification in plasma because these activated molecules bind to the surfaces upon which they are generated. Furthermore, active enzymes that enter the circulation are rapidly neutralized by endogenous protease inhibitors. For example, whereas prothrombin has a half-life of 48–72 hours, free thrombin circulates for only seconds.[2] For these reasons, investigators interested in monitoring the activity of the coagulation cascade have focused efforts on assaying peptides that are released upon cleavage of zymogens to their active forms. Unlike active enzymes, these biologically inactive peptides are released into the circulation and possess circulatory half-lives that permit accurate determination of their plasma concentration. Because these peptides are released during activation of the blood coagulation system, they have been termed "activation peptides," and have been used as biochemical markers of thrombosis.[1]

The activation peptides that have been most extensively studied in patients presenting with acute coronary syndromes[3] include fibrinopeptide A (FPA)[4,5] and the prothrombin fragment F_{1+2}.[6,7] FPA is a small 16-amino acid peptide that is released from the a-chain of fibrinogen when thrombin converts fibrinogen to fibrin, and is therefore an indicator of thrombin activity. F_{1+2} is a 31-kD polypeptide that is released from the amino terminal portion of prothrombin when it is converted to thrombin by factor Xa and is therefore an indicator of thrombin generation of factor Xa activity (Figure 1). Once generated, thrombin may be inhibited by the endogenous heparin sulfate-antithrombin III mechanism to form stable thrombin-antithrombin (TAT) complexes. Immunoassays have been developed for the detection of TAT,[8,9] which can also be used as an index of thrombin generation in vivo.

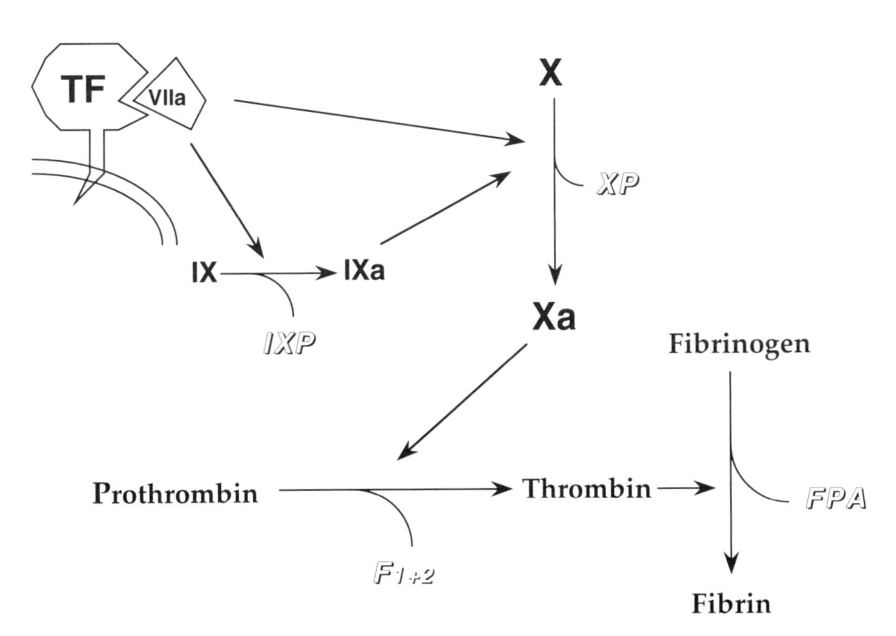

Figure 1: Schematic of tissue factor (TF) pathway leading to thrombin generation and fibrin formation. IX P = factor IX activation peptide; X P = factor X activation peptide; F_{1+2} = the peptide fragment cleaved when prothrombin is converted to thrombin; FPA = fibrinopeptide A.

The Tissue Factor Pathway of Blood Coagulation

In addition to its ability to cleave fibrinogen, thrombin activates platelets and exerts a variety of regulatory effects on vascular cells.[10] The generation of thrombin, as indicated by increased levels of F_{1+2}, is therefore a central event in hemostasis and the vascular response to injury. The coagulation cascade that leads to thrombin generation has been traditionally divided into intrinsic and extrinsic pathways that converge at the level of factor X activation.[11,12] All of the clotting factors involved in the intrinsic pathway of blood coagulation circulate within, and therefore are intrinsic to, the vasculature. In contrast, the extrinsic pathway of blood coagulation involves both intravascular clotting factors as well as an extravascular, tissue-bound clotting co-factor, known as tissue factor.

Over the last several years, many investigators have pointed to the extrinsic, or tissue factor (TF), pathway of blood coagulation as the predominant mechanism of clotting in vivo.[13–15] TF is a noncirculating glycoprotein that is tightly bound to the plasma membrane of a variety of tissues.[16] It possesses a large extracellular domain that serves as the catalytic site, and a single transmembrane domain that serves to anchor the molecule to the cell membrane. Upon contact with blood, the extracellular domain of TF binds to circulating factor VII/VIIa, and the resulting complex converts factors IX and X to IXa and Xa, respectively, triggering the clotting cascade (Figure 1).

TF is expressed on the cell surface in its fully functional form. There are therefore no biochemical markers of TF activation. However, the expression of TF protein and mRNA within vascular tissue can be studied using immunohistochemistry, procoagulant activity assays, and in situ hybridization. Wilcox et al.[17] have shown that TF is not expressed at significant levels in the intima or media of normal adult artery. This presumably protects the organism from unnecessary intravascular clotting.[18] In contrast, the outermost layer of the vessel wall, comprised mainly of adventitial fibroblasts, demonstrates intense TF immunostaining and mRNA hybridization. In atherosclerotic plaques from carotid endarterectomy specimens, TF mRNA and protein have been shown in smooth muscle-like intimal cells as well as in foam cells, and in the extracellular matrix.[17]

The expression of TF within atherosclerotic plaque may play an important role in the thrombotic events associated with plaque disruption. In its chronic stable state, the plaque is covered by a smooth, endothelialized fibrous cap which provides a relatively nonthrombogenic surface. Rupture of the atherosclerotic plaque, either spontaneously or during percutaneous coronary angioplasty, results in exposure of circulating blood to procoagulant elements within the plaque that were previously sequestered from the circulation, including collagen type 1[19] and TF. The extent to which each of these procoagulant elements is responsible for the thrombogenicity of the atherosclerotic plaque has not been defined.

The excision and retrieval of atherosclerotic plaque during directional coronary atherectomy (DCA) affords investigators the opportunity to study the expression of TF in patients presenting with angiographically significant coronary artery disease. Using a monoclonal anti-human TF antibody, Marmur et al.[20] have identified TF antigen within human coronary atherectomy specimens in 8 of 24 (33%) lesions examined. In this preliminary study, lesions in which TF was detected had a higher incidence of complex angiographic morphology (ulceration, irregular borders, or filling defects) versus lesions in which TF was not detected (6/8 versus 4/16, $p = 0.03$).

In addition to TF antigen, procoagulant TF activity has been detected in human coronary atheroma.[21] Plaques placed in an assay mix consisting of factor VIIa, factor X, and calcium will generate factor Xa if TF is present and available for binding to VIIa. The amount of Xa generated can be measured by adding a Xa-sensitive colorometric substrate (pNA) whose product is detectable by optical densitometry. Using this TF-specific functional colorometric assay, TF activity has been detected in 13 of 15 (87%) coronary atherectomy specimens.[21] The amount of TF activity detected varied markedly between patients, raising the possibility that variations in plaque TF content and bioavailability may account for the variable thrombotic tendency of atherosclerotic lesions that are disrupted spontaneously or iatrogenically during percutaneous interventions. Marked variations in total procoagulant activity (i.e., TF- and non-TF-mediated) have also been demonstrated by measuring the generation of FPA by plaques incubated with recalcified plasma in vitro.[22] Nine of 11 plaques examined (82%) demonstrated procoagulant activity. Specimens derived from complex, Ambrose type II lesions[23] were associated with marked procoagulant activity and organizing thrombus. These preliminary data support the notion that the expression and activity of lesion-bound coagulation factors, as well as the behavior of circulating clotting factors, play an important role in the pathogenesis of thrombosis associated with complex lesions.

Markers of Thrombin Generation and Activity in Coronary Artery Disease

The atherosclerotic plaque disruption that underlies acute coronary syndromes is presumed to result in the activation of the intrinsic or extrinsic pathways of coagulation. At each step of the coagulation cascade, a plasma zymogen is converted to its active form through limited proteolysis, and a marker peptide is released (Figure 1). By measuring the plasma level of these peptides in patients presenting with acute coronary arterial insufficiency, investigators have sought to gain insight into the activity of the coagulation cascade following the occurrence of a presumed plaque disruption.

FPA, an indicator of thrombin activity, was one of the first coagulation marker peptides to be measured in clinical blood samples.[4] Early studies established an association between the presence of coronary atherosclerosis and elevated plasma FPA levels, but were unable to detect differences in levels between patients presenting with myocardial infarction, unstable angina, or chronic exertional angina.[24–26] In light of the observation that acute myocardial infarction is associated with occlusive coronary thrombosis,[27] it was anticipated that particularly high plasma levels of FPA would be seen in this clinical syndrome. To test the hypothesis that peak plasma FPA levels occur early in patients with acute myocardial infarction, Eisenberg et al. compared levels in patients presenting early (<10 hr) and late (>10 hr) after the onset of symptoms.[28] FPA levels were found to be elevated to a significantly greater degree in the early patients, demonstrating that the timing of blood withdrawal in clinical investigations of coronary thrombosis is important.

By performing serial blood withdrawal from the same patients, the changes in plasma FPA levels over time have been investigated for both myocardial infarction and unstable angina. Plasma FPA levels have been shown to decrease to near normal levels within 24 hours of transmural infarction,[28] and within 6 days of an episode of unstable angina.[29] Decreases in plasma FPA may be accelerated by the administration of intravenous heparin. In patients with acute myocardial infraction, significant decreases in FPA have been demonstrated within 20 minutes of heparinization.[30] A more chronic time course of FPA and F_{1+2} levels in acute coronary syndromes has recently been reported by Merlini et al.[31] The plasma concentration of these peptides was measured in consecutive patients presenting with unstable angina (n = 80) or acute myocardial infarction (n = 32). At 6 months, plasma determinations were repeated in patients who had experienced an uneventful clinical course. Patients presenting with unstable angina or myocardial infarction had high levels of plasma FPA and F_{1+2} in comparison to patients with stable angina or healthy individuals. At 6 months, FPA levels were significantly reduced to near normal levels in both unstable angina and myocardial infarction patients. In contrast, plasma F_{1+2} levels, which reflect thrombin generation, remained elevated at 6 months for both groups of patients. Chronic elevations in plasma F_{1+2} have been documented in patients with thrombotic disorders, such as inherited antithrombin and protein C deficiency.[2] The persistence of elevated plasma F_{1+2} levels in patients presenting with acute coronary syndromes suggests that acute coronary thrombosis may be occurring on the background of a chronic hypercoagulable state. Thus, activation of the coagulation cascade in clinical syndromes associated with complex coronary lesions[23] may represent not only an effect of plaque disruption, but a cause of thrombosis as well.

The association between plasma FPA and complex angiographic coronary lesion morphology has been reported in a study of 29 unstable angina patients.[32] Of the 11 patients in whom a complex lesion was noted on the angiogram, plasma FPA levels were elevated in seven (64%), all of whom had exhibited reversible ST segment shifts on admission. In addition to monitoring thrombin generation and activity with plasma levels of F_{1+2} and FPA, respectively, it is possible to assess the rate of thrombin neutralization by assaying plasma levels of thrombin-antithrombin III (TAT) complexes.[7] Like F_{1+2}, plasma levels of TAT have been found to be elevated in unstable angina and in non-Q-wave and Q-wave myocardial infarction.[33]

Thrombin Generation and Activity in Percutaneous Transluminal Coronary Angioplasty

Percutaneous transluminal coronary angioplasty (PTCA) results in plaque fracturing and dissection,[34] and therefore provides a model to study the events associated with coronary plaque rupture under controlled conditions. To investigate the relationship between coronary atherosclerotic plaque injury and activation of the coagulation cascade, we have measured F_{1+2} and FPA coronary blood levels before, during, and immediately following PTCA.[35] After demonstrating that blood withdrawal through a PTCA catheter does not artifactually elevate the plasma levels of these markers in heparinized patients, coronary

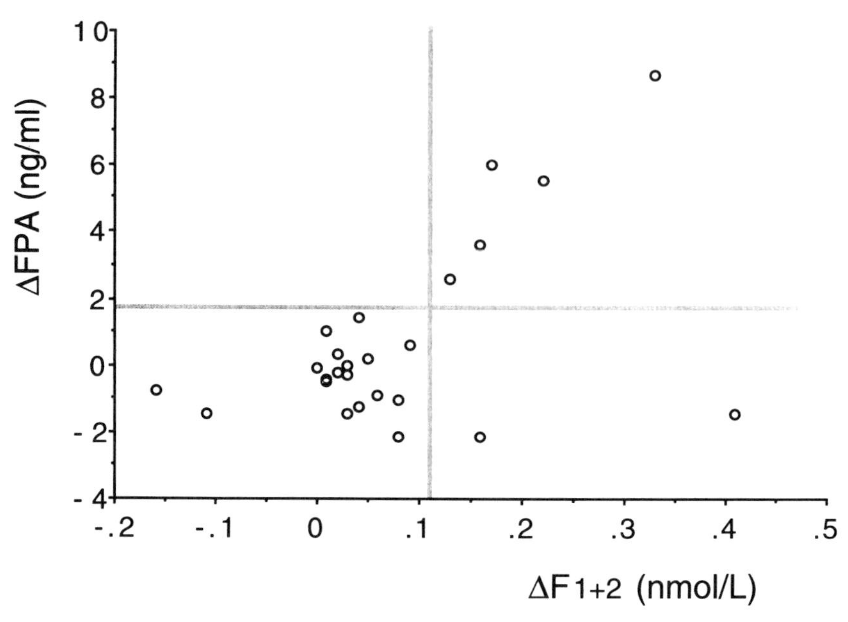

Figure 2: Changes in FPA (Δ FPA) and F_{1+2}) (Δ F_{1+2}) from pre-PCTA proximal to the lesion to post-PCYA distal to the lesion.

arterial samples were collected proximal and distal to the lesion prior to balloon inflation, and distal to the lesion after balloon inflation. For the total study population (n = 26) plasma levels of F_{1+2}, but not of FPA, rose significantly following PTCA. After defining a normal range of interassay variability based on plasma levels measured in blood collected prior to balloon inflation, seven patients (27%) were judged to have experienced a significant rise in F_{1+2} plasma levels post PTCA distal to the lesion. A significant rise in plasma FPA occurred in five of these seven patients post PTCA (Figure 2). These data, which were derived from systemically heparinized patients, suggest that balloon-mediated plaque disruption triggers an increase in thrombin generation and activity within the coronary artery.

Angiographically Complex Lesions Are Associated with Increased Levels of Thrombin Generation and Activity Following PTCA

Angiographically complex coronary lesions (irregular borders, overhanging edges, or filling defects) are associated with unstable coro-

Table 1
Plasma FPA and F_{1+2} Levels [median (95% confidence intervals)] in 50 Patients Treated with PTCA

Coagulation Marker	*Lesion Morphology*	*Pre PTCA*	*10 Min Post PTCA*
FPA ng/mL	Complex n = 24	2.1 (1.6–3.5)‡	3.3 (2.6–5.8) ‡‡
	Simple n = 26	1.9 (1.3–3.9)	2.1 (1.5–9.8)
F_{1+2} nmol/L	Complex n = 24	0.65 (0.54–1.04)*	0.76 (0.64–1.03)**
	Simple n = 26	0.64 (0.53–0.77)	0.61 (0.48–1.08)

$p < 0.02$: ‡ vs ‡‡ $p < 0.03$: * vs **

nary syndromes and an increased incidence of thrombosis following coronary angioplasty (PTCA). To study the relationship between angiographic lesion morphology and activation of the coagulation cascade, we measured coronary plasma levels of FPA and F_{1+2} in an additional series of 50 patients undergoing PTCA.[36] Pre-PTCA samples were withdrawn through a catheter placed proximal to the lesion prior to PTCA and post-PTCA samples were collected 10 minutes after the final balloon inflation with the catheter positioned distal to the lesion. Angiographic interpretations of lesion complexity were made without knowledge of the plasma FPA and F_{1+2} levels.

As shown in Table 1, pre-PTCA FPA and F_{1+2} values were similar for simple and complex lesions. After PTCA, FPA, and F_{1+2} values increased in arterial blood while FPA decreased in venous blood and F_{1+2} remained the same (Table 2). Thus, PTCA appears to increase

Table 2
Plasma FPA and F_{1+2} Levels (mean ± SD) Drawn from a Peripheral Vein (venous sheath) and a Coronary Artery (PTCA catheter) before and after PTCA (n = 50 patients)

Site	*Timing*	*FPA (ng/mL)*		*F_{1+2} (nmol/L)*	
Venous sheath	pre-PTCA	5.77 ± 3.42	$p < 0.001$	0.72 ± 0.35	p = NS
Venous sheath	post-PTCA	3.41 ± 2.49		0.71 ± 0.36	
PTCA catheter	pre-PTCA	3.06 ± 2.44	$p < 0.02$	0.75 ± 0.36	$p < 0.05$
PTCA catheter	post-PTCA	4.94 ± 4.73		0.82 ± 0.54	

thrombin activity and generation locally at the site of balloon injury, despite the systemic effects of heparin. These data suggest that peripheral venous sampling is inadequate for the monitoring of coagulation cascade activity during PTCA.

Markers of Platelet Activation

The discovery of a highly sensitive and specific marker of in vivo platelet activation that would be able to detect dynamic changes in underlying platelet physiology has been described as one of the "holy grails" in the field of hemostasis and thrombosis.[37] There have been numerous investigations of platelet activation in coronary artery disease (Figure 3). The methods employed have assessed platelet activation indirectly by studying in vitro platelet responsiveness, or directly by either measuring substances that are released from activated platelets into plasma or by the direct detection of activation-dependent changes on the platelet surface. Only the more clinically useful methods of detecting in vivo platelet activation including measures of platelet aggregation, thromboxane metabolites, secreted platelet proteins, and activation-dependent changes in platelet membrane proteins will be discussed.

Commonly used markers for studying platelet activation:

I. Platelet aggregation:
   A. Spontaneous platelet aggregation
   B. Agonist induced platelet aggregation

II. Thromboxane metabolites

III. Secreted platelet proteins:
   A. B-thromboglobulin (BTG)
   B. Platelet factor 4 (PF4)

IV. Activation dependent changes in platelet membrane proteins using flow cytometry:
   A. Activation-dependent membrane receptor changes
   B. Surface exposure of platelet membrane proteins

Figure 3: Commonly used markers for studying platelet activation.

Platelet Aggregation

Several authors have suggested that measures of ex vivo platelet reactivity, the tendency to form aggregates either spontaneously or in response to platelet agonists, may serve as an indirect marker of platelet activation in patients with coronary artery disease.[38] Such platelet hyperreactivity might also identify patients at increased risk for coronary thrombosis.

Several studies have measured spontaneous platelet aggregation (SPA) as an indirect marker of increased in vivo platelet activity. To determine SPA, a platelet-rich solution is stirred and the formation of platelet aggregates over time is measured. Normal platelets do not aggregate or do so only minimally after several minutes. Trip et al. detected abnormal spontaneous platelet aggregation (SPA) in 36% of patients surviving a myocardial infarction.[38] Wu and Hoak found SPA in 7 of 10 (70%) patients with an acute myocardial infarction, 6 of 32 (19%) patients with chronic stable angina, and in 0 of 22 (0%) healthy controls.[39] Trip et al. also sought to determine the prognostic significance of increased platelet aggregability as measured by SPA in 149 patients with recent myocardial infarction.[38] Platelet aggregation was tested 3 months after a myocardial infarction and at 6-month intervals for up to 5 years. SPA was graded as either positive (<10 min), intermediate (10–20 min) or negative. The 5–year mortality in the SPA-negative group was 6.4% (6 of 94), 10.3% (3 of 29) in the intermediate group, and 34.6% (9 of 26) in the SPA-positive group. The SPA-positive group had a relative risk of death of 5.4, and a relative risk of a recurrent cardiac event of 3.1 compared to the SPA-negative group. Nearly 50% of SPA-positive patients later experienced cardiac death or another nonfatal infarction.

Several studies employing ex vivo platelet aggregation as an indirect marker of in vivo platelet activity have demonstrated that an increased sensitivity to aggregating agents is associated with acute cardiac events in patients with coronary artery disease. For example, there is a clear circadian variation in the onset of myocardial infarction and sudden death with a peak incidence occurring between 6 AM and noon.[40] Furthermore, platelet hyperreactivity over 24 hours in normal subjects has been found to coincide with a peak in ADP-induced platelet aggregation occurring between 6 AM and 9 AM.[41] In the Physicians Health Study, Ridker et al. showed that the circadian variation seen in the incidence of myocardial infarction in the placebo group was abolished in the group receiving aspirin.[42] These data suggest that platelet hyperreactivity may be the trigger for myocardial infarction, aspirin may decrease platelet reactivity, and platelet aggregation may be a clinically useful indirect marker of underlying platelet activation.

However, there have been inconsistencies in the results of aggregation studies that may be related to methodological limitations and differences in study design. For example, Elwood et al. reported an association between ADP-induced but not collagen-induced platelet aggregation and the presence of ischemic heart disease.[43] Thaulow et al. found an association between enhanced ADP-induced but not collagen or thrombin-induced platelet aggregation and cardiovascular death.[44] Yet Lam et al. found that enhanced thrombin-induced but not ADP, collagen, epinephrine, or platelet activating factor-induced aggregation was associated with progression of coronary atherosclerosis and subsequent coronary events in patients with angiographically documented coronary artery disease.[45] Theroux et al. failed to demonstrate any association between platelet aggregation and cardiac events in patients with unstable angina and myocardial infarction.[29] Zahavi et al. demonstrated an inverse relation between platelet activity and unstable coronary artery disease.[47] They showed that in comparison to patients with stable angina, patients with unstable angina have decreased platelet aggregation.[46]

The conflicting data from the above studies suggest that ex vivo platelet aggregation may not accurately reflect platelet physiology in vivo. Other markers to assess platelet activity include thromboxane metabolism, secreted platelet proteins, and activation dependent changes in platelet membrane proteins.

Thromboxane Metabolism

Platelet activation results in the conversion of arachidonic acid to thromboxane A_2. The detection of thromboxane A_2 metabolites in plasma and urine has been used as a marker of in vivo platelet activation. Radioimmunoassay studies have demonstrated elevated levels of thromboxane metabolites in plasma and in urine in patients with coronary artery disease.[47–51] Fitzgerald et al. found increases in thromboxane activity in the urine in patients with unstable angina compared to those with stable angina.[51] Elevated metabolites of thromboxane in plasma in patients with unstable angina and concurrent rest pain have also been detected.[52] Hamm et al. have also confirmed transient increases in thromboxane B_2 related to episodes of ischemia in patients with unstable angina.[54] However, results have varied greatly and some studies have failed to detect any alteration in thromboxane activity in patients with coronary artery disease. Theroux et al., for example, measured thromboxane B_2 production in patients with coronary artery disease found no difference between patients with rest angina and those with stable angina.[29]

The sensitivity of measuring peripheral thromboxane metabolites in plasma may be limited by dilution factors. To avoid the dilutional effects of peripheral venous sampling, Hirsch et al. measured transcardiac gradients of thromboxane A_2 and demonstrated a temporal relation between clinical ischemia in patients with unstable angina and increases in this metabolite.[48] Though peripheral dilution is to a large extent eliminated, catheter sampling from the aortic root and coronary sinus is more invasive and introduces the possibility of catheter-induced platelet activation.

Thromboxane metabolites accumulate in plasma and in urine over time with half-lives of several hours. Measures of thromboxane activity in plasma and urine are a reflection of cumulative platelet activation over several hours and may be insensitive to transient episodes of platelet activation. There has been no study to date correlating thromboxane metabolites with specific lesion morphologies in patients with unstable angina.

Secreted Platelet Proteins

One of the most frequently used methods to detect in vivo platelet activation in patients with coronary artery disease is the measurement of secreted platelet proteins in plasma. Two proteins that may be measured by commercially available kits are B-thromboglobulin (BTG) and platelet factor 4 (PF4). These proteins are contained within the platelet alpha-granules and are secreted from these granules when platelets are activated. Therefore, plasma levels may reflect in vivo platelet activation.

Levels of BTG and PF4 have been studied extensively in patients with coronary artery disease, often with inconsistent results. For example, elevated levels of BTG and PF4 in patients with stable angina have been reported in several studies.[53–61] Whereas other papers have reported normal levels in patients with stable angina,[62,63] Smitherman et al. detected elevated levels of BTG in patients with unstable angina.[64] Others have reported elevated BTG and PF4 levels in patients with unstable angina only when samples were obtained within 4 hours of ischemic chest pain.[65] However, Schmitz-Huebner et al. reported normal levels of BTG and PF4 in 105 patients with stable angina and in 120 with unstable angina.[66]

Several other studies have failed to detect elevated levels of BTG and PF4 in patients with unstable angina.[29,49,66–68] Similar inconsistencies have been reported in patients with acute myocardial infarction.[69–71]

Based on these data, BTG and PF4 do not appear to be very useful markers of in vivo platelet activation. This may in part be due to the fact that these proteins are released in vitro after phlebotomy.[72] Kaplan et al. have shown that secretion from as little as 10^6 platelets/mL would be sufficient to double normal levels of these proteins.[73] Because BTG and PF4 are secreted in similar amounts in vitro but have significantly different rates of clearance in vivo, PF4 clearance is more rapid, and expressing the data as a ratio of BTG/PF4 has been used to control for artifactual release. A low BTG/PF4 ratio, for example, would suggest in vitro artifact. This ratio may be influenced by a variety of factors including renal insufficiency and hyperlipoproteinemia, which increase BTG, and heparin, which increases PF4. Although a ratio of 5:1–10:1 is thought to reflect in vivo platelet activation, normal and abnormal ranges for BTG and PF4 values have not been well defined. As in the case with thromboxane metabolites, again the relatively long half-lives of these platelet proteins in plasma may preclude the detection of transient episodes of platelet activation.

Activation-Dependent Changes in Platelet Membrane Proteins

Perhaps the most promising method for studying in vivo platelet activation involves the direct detection of activated platelets in whole blood by flow cytometry. Platelet activation results in significant changes in platelet membrane proteins. For example, platelet activation exposes the ligand binding site within the GP IIb/IIIa molecule for several ligands, including fibrinogen. A fluorescence-labeled monoclonal antibody (PAC1) bound specifically to the activated IIb/IIIa molecule can be detected on the platelet surface by fluorescence-activated flow cytometry. The proportion of platelets with bound activation-specific antibody can be accurately measured in a sample population of cells. The limit of detection for this method is approximately 1% activated platelets.[73] Surface markers of platelet secretion and activation-dependent ligand binding have also been used to detect platelet activation. A frequently used marker of alpha-granule release is P-selectin, (CD62), which is an integral alpha-granule membrane protein that becomes expressed on the outer surface of activated platelets (Figure 4).[74]

There have been only a few studies using fluorescence-activated flow cytometry to investigate platelet activation in patients with coronary artery disease and most of these are only preliminary reports. Palabrica et al. measured platelet P-selectin expression in 20 patients with stable angina and in six with unstable angina or myocardial infarction.[75] Samples were drawn from a peripheral vein and from the coronary sinus. P-selectin expression was detected in 6% of circulating platelets in patients with stable angina, and in 25% in patients with unstable angina. Measures made in the coronary and systemic venous circulation were the same. Becker et al. measured P-selectin expression in 22 patients with unstable angina enrolled in the TIMI IIIB study who had received aspirin, heparin, and either t-PA or placebo.[76] P-selectin expression prior to treatment and over a 96-hour period after therapy was increased in patients with unstable angina compared to healthy controls.

Fluorescence-activated flow cytometry has also been used to detect platelet activation in patients undergoing coronary angioplasty. Palabrica et al. measured pre-PTCA and post-PTCA coronary sinus platelet P-selectin expression in 19 patients.[77] There was a significant increase in P-selectin expression within the coronary sinus following PTCA. P-selectin expression appeared to be most elevated in four patients

Commonly used markers of platelet activation by flow cytometry:

Platelet receptor and membrane changes	Monoclonal antibodies	Activation-specific binding sites
GP IIb-IIIa: Activation-dependent conformational changes in receptor	PAC1	ligand binding site of GP IIb-IIIa receptor
Alpha-granule platelet membrane proteins	S12 and AC 1.2	P-Selectin (GMP-140)

Figure 4: Commonly used markers of platelet activation by flow cytometry.

who experienced vessel closure and/or infarction within 24 hours of the procedure. Tschoepe et al. measured platelet P-selectin, GP 53, a lysosomal membrane protein, and thrombospondin expression in 102 patients prior to elective PTCA.[78] The prevalence of acute ischemic events over a 24-hour period following PTCA was related to pre-PTCA platelet activation. Scharf et al. measured platelet activation using a panel of activation-specific monoclonal antibodies in five patients undergoing PTCA.[79] Platelet activation was measured in whole blood samples drawn continuously from a heparin-bonded catheter in the coronary sinus before, during, and for 30 minutes following PTCA. Patients undergoing angiography without PTCA were used as controls. Binding of antibodies specific for the activated GP IIb/IIIa complex were significantly elevated during and for 30 minutes following PTCA in four of five patients. P-selectin expression was detected in one of five patients. No significant expression of these markers was noted in eight patients undergoing angiography without PTCA. Activation markers were not detected in samples drawn from the peripheral venous circulation in this study.

Unlike any other method of detecting in vivo platelet activation, fluorescence-activated flow cytometry can directly identify subpopulations of activated platelets within the circulation. The data suggest that in vivo platelet activation in patients with coronary artery disease can be detected by measuring the expression of activation-specific changes on the platelet surface by fluorescence-activated flow cytometry. Because the analysis is performed on fixed whole blood samples and therefore involves very little ex vivo manipulation, there is less chance for spurious activation. There has been some variation between studies regarding normal and abnormal ranges of platelet activation using fluorescence-activated flow cytometry. Scharf et al. failed to detect activation in peripheral samples following PTCA though other studies have shown significantly increased expression of activation markers.[77,79] Differences in fixation techniques, platelet inhibitors, buffers, antibodies, and flow cytometry parameters may explain these inconsistences. Although this method appears to be highly sensitive and specific, there have been relatively few studies reported thus far and the clinical usefulness of flow cytometry as a marker of platelet activation remains to be determined. In addition, platelet activation by flow cytometry has been correlated only with the clinical presentation of unstable angina. There have been no studies demonstrating the prognostic significance of these findings. There also have been no studies to date correlating coronary lesion morphology with these markers of platelet activation.

Thrombosis and Leukocyte Activation

Rupture of a lipid-rich plaque and subsequent intracoronary thrombosis is thought to underlie in most cases the pathophysiology of acute coronary syndromes. There is, however, recent evidence suggesting that an acute inflammatory cell reaction may also play a role in the pathogenesis of unstable angina and myocardial infarction. Activation of monocytes and neutrophils in patients with unstable angina may induce coronary vasospasm,[79] platelet activation,[80] and may increase thrombin generation.[81–84]

Several studies have reported evidence of increased leukocyte activation in patients with unstable angina.[84–88] Dinerman et al. for example, found marked increases in plasma levels of neutrophil elastase in patients with unstable angina versus controls.[85] Berk et al. detected increased levels of C-reactive protein in patients with unstable angina.[86] These findings were reconfirmed by Liuzzo et al. who noted increases in C-reactive protein (>0.3 mg/dL) in a subgroup of patients with unstable angina and no evidence of myocardial necrosis. Patients with a high C-reactive protein had a worse in-hospital prognosis than those with normal levels (<0.3 mg/dL).[87] Mazzone et al. also found significantly increased monocyte and neutrophil expression of CD11b/CD18 adhesion receptors in blood drawn from the coronary sinus in patients with unstable angina versus those with chronic stable angina.[88]

Histopathological studies have demonstrated an inflammatory response in patients with acute coronary syndromes. Ruptured plaques are usually associated with inflammatory cells that accumulate at the site of disrupture.[89] Moreno et al. detected macrophage-rich sclerotic tissue and macrophage-rich atherosclerotic material more often in atherectomy specimens from patients with unstable angina and non-Q-wave myocardial infarction than in patients with stable angina.[90]

There are other potential sites for inflammatory infiltrates in acute syndromes. Following ischemia for as little as 3 hours in an experimental model, there is accumulation of leukocytes in the microcirculation which is potentiated by reperfusion.[91] Thus, prolonged ischemia in unstable angina even without evidence of myocardial necrosis might lead to inflammatory infiltrates in the microcirculation. Platelet deposition on vascular surfaces in experimental models is accompanied by leukocyte adhesion as well. This leukocyte adhesion may be platelet-dependent.[83] A proposed model of the interrelationship between inflammation and thrombosis is shown in Figure 5. More information on this subject should be available in the near future.

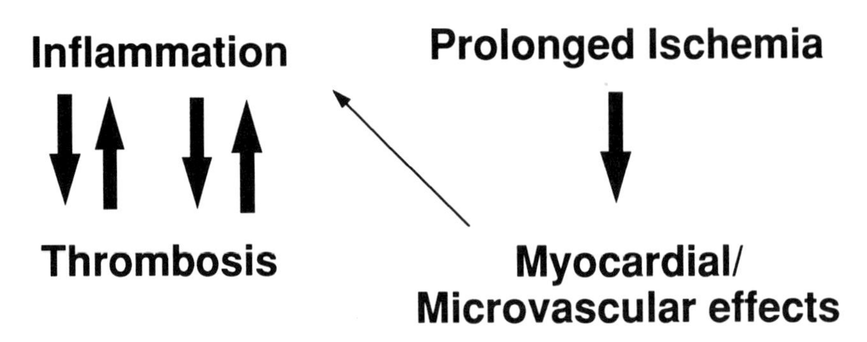

Figure 5: Proposed mechanisms of inflammation and thrombosis in unstable angina.

References

1. Seligsohn U, Kasper CK, Osterud B, Rapaport SI. Activated factor VII: Presence in factor IX concentrates and persistence in the circulation after infusion. Blood 1979; 53:828.
2. Bauer KA, Rosenberg RD. The pathophysiology of the prethrombotic state in humans: insights gained from studies using markers of hemostatic system activation. Blood 1987; 70:343–350.
3. Fuster V, Badimon L, Badimon JJ, Chesebro JH. The pathogenesis of coronary artery disease and the acute coronary syndromes. N Engl J Med 1992; 326:242–250.
4. Nossel HL, Yudelman I, Canfield RE, et al. Measurement of fibrinopeptide A in human blood. J Clin Invest 1974; 54:43–53.
5. Nossel HL, Ti M, Kaplan KL, Spanondis K, Soland T, Butler VP Jr. The generation of fibrinopeptide A in clinical blood samples. Evidence for thrombin activity. J Clin Invest 1976; 58:1136–1144.
6. Lau HK, Rosenberg JS, Beeler DL, Rosenberg RD. The isolation and characterization of a specific antibody population directed against the prothrombin activation fragments F_2 and F_{1+2}. J Biol Chem 1979; 254: 8751–8761.
7. Teitel JM, Bauer KA, Lau HK, Rosenberg RD. Studies of the prothrombin activation pathway utilizing radioimmunoassays for the F_2/F_{1+2} fragment and thrombin-antithrombin complex. Blood 1982; 59:1086–1097.
8. Lau HK, Rosenberg RD. The isolation and characterization of a specific antibody population directed against the thrombin-antithrombin complex, J Biol Chem 1980; 255:5885–5893.
9. Pelzer H, Schwarz A, Heimburger N. Determination of human thrombin-antithrombin III complex in plasma with an enzyme-linked immunosorbent assay. Thromb Haemost 1988; 59:101–106.
10. Walz D, Fenton JW II, Shuman M. Bioregulatory functions of thrombin. Ann NY Acad Sci 1986; 485:14–49.

11. MacFarlane RG. An enzyme cascade in the blood clotting mechanism, and its function as a biochemical amplifier. Nature 1964; 202:498–499.
12. Davie EW, Ratnoff OD. Waterfall sequence for intrinsic blood clotting. Science 1964; 145:1310–1312.
13. Nemerson Y. Tissue factor and hemostasis. Blood 1988; 71:1–8.
14. Bauer KA, Kass BL, ten Cate H, Hawiger JJ, Rosenberg RD. Factor IX is activated in vivo by the tissue factor mechanism. Blood 1990; 76:731–736.
15. ten Cate H, Bauer KA, Levi M, et al. The activation of factor X and prothrombin by recombinant factor VIIa in vivo is mediated by tissue factor. J Clin Invest 1993; 92:1207–1212.
16. Edgington TS, Mackman N, Brand K, Ruf W. The structural biology of expression and function of tissue factor. Thromb Haemost 1991; 66:67–79.
17. Wilcox JN, Smith KM, Schwartz SM, Gordon D. Localization of tissue factor in the normal vessel wall and in the atherosclerotic plaque. Proc Natl Acad Sci USA 1989; 86:2839–2843.
18. Drake TA, Morrissey JH, Edgington TS. Selective cellular expression of tissue factor in human tissues. Am J Pathol 1989; 134:1087–1097.
19. Badimon L, Badimon JJ, Turitto VT, Vallabhajosula S, Fuster V. Platelet thrombus formation on collagen type 1. A model of deep vessel injury influence on blood rheology, von Willebrand factor and blood coagulation. Circulation 1988; 78:1431–1442.
20. Marmur JD, Fyfe B, Sharma SK, Ambrose JA, et al. Immunohistochemical detection of tissue factor in human coronary atheroma (abstract). J Am Coll Cardiol 1994; (Feb Suppl):64A.
21. Marmur JD, Singanallore TV, Sharma SK, et al. Detection and quantification of tissue factor activity in coronary atherectomy specimens (abstract). J Am Coll Cardiol 1994; (Feb Suppl):65A.
22. Lucore CL, Winters KJ, Eisenberg PR. Procoagulant activity of coronary atherosclerotic plaques (abstract). Circulation 1992; 86:1–20.
23. Ambrose JA, Winters SL, Stern A, et al. Angiographic morphology and the pathogenesis of unstable angina pectoris. J Am Coll Cardiol 1985; 5: 609–616.
24. Neri Serneri GG, Gensini GF, Abbate R, et al. Increased fibrinopeptide A formation and thromboxane A_2 production in patients with ischemic heart disease: Relationships to coronary pathoanatomy, risk factors, and clinical manifestations. Am Heart J 1981; 101:185–194.
25. Nichols AB, Owen J, Kaplan KL, et al. Fibrinopeptide A, platelet factor 4, and B-thromboglobulin levels in coronary heart disease. Blood 1982; 60: 650–654.
26. Douglas JT, Lowe GDO, Forbes CD, Prentice RM. Plasma fibrinopeptide A and beta-thromboglobulin in patients with chest pain. Thromb Haemost 1983; 50:541–542.
27. DeWood MA, Spores J, Notske R, et al. Prevalence of total coronary occlusion during the early hours of transmural myocardial infarction. N Engl J Med 1980; 303:897–902.
28. Eisenberg PR, Sherman LA, Schectman K, et al. Fibrinopeptide A: a marker of acute coronary thrombosis. Circulation 1985; 71:912–918.
29. Theroux P, Latour J-G, Leger-Gauthier C, De Lara J. Fibrinopeptide A

and platelet factor levels in unstable angina pectoris. Circulation 1987; 75:156–162.
30. Mombelli G, Im Hof V, Haeberli A, Straub PW. Effect of heparin on plasma fibrinopeptide A in patients with acute myocardial infarction. Circulation 1984; 69:684–689.
31. Merlini PA, Bauer KA, Oltrona L, et al. Persistent activation of coagulation mechanism in unstable angina and myocardial infarction. Circulation 1994; 90:61–68.
32. Eisenberg PR, Kenzora JL, Sobel BE, Ludbrook PA, Jaffe AS. Relation between ST segment shifts during ischemia and thrombin activity in patients with unstbale angina. J Am Coll Cardiol 1991; 18:898–903.
33. Merlini PA, Bauer KA, Mannucci PM, et al. Biochemical markers of activation of the coagulation cascade in acute ischemic syndromes (abstract). Circulation 1992; 86 (Suppl 1):1–802.
34. Losordo DW, Rosenfield K, Pieczek A, et al. How does angioplasty work? serial analysis of human iliac arteries using intravascular ultrasound. Circulation 1992; 86:1845–1858.
35. Marmur JD, Merlini PA, Sharma SK, et al. Thrombin generation in human coronary arteries after percutaneous transluminal balloon angioplasty. J Am Coll Cardiol 1994; 24:1484–1491.
36. Marmur JD, Sharma SK, Kantrowitz NE, et al. Angiographically complex lesions are associated with increased levels of thrombin generation and activity following PTCA (abstract). J Am Coll Cardiol (in press).
37. Abrams C, Shatil S. Immunological detection of activated platelets in clinical disorders. Thromb Haemost 1991; 65(5):467–473.
38. Trip MD, Manger Cats V, van Capelle F. Platelet hyperreactivity and prognosis in survivors of myocardial infarction. N Engl J Med 1990; 322: 1549–1554.
39. Wu KK, and Hoak JC. Spontaneous platelet aggregation in arterial insufficiency: Mechanisms and implications. Thromb Haemost 1976; 35:702.
40. Muller JE, Stone PH, Turi ZG, et al. Circadian variation in the frequency of onset of acute myocardial infarction. N Engl J Med 1985; 313:1315.
41. Tofler GH, Brezinski D, Schafer AI, et al. Concurrent morning increase in platelet aggregability and the risk of myocardial infarction and sudden cardiac death. N Engl J Med 1987; 316:1514–1518.
42. Ridker PM, Manson JAE, Buring JE, et al. Circadian variation of acute myocardial infarction and the effect of low-dose aspirin in a randomized trial of physicians. Circulation 1990; 82:897–902.
43. Elwood PC, Renaud S, Sharp DS, et al. Ischemic heart disease and platelet aggregation. The Caerphilly Collaborative Heart Disease Study. Circulation 1991; 83:38–44.
44. Thaulow E, Erikssen J, Sandvik L, et al. Blood platelet count and function are related to total cardiovascular death in apparently healthy men. Circulation 1991; 84:613–617.
45. Lam JYT, Latour J, Lesperance J, et al. Platelet aggregation, coronary artery disease progression and future coronary events. Am J Cardiol 1994; 73:333–338.
46. Theroux P, Latour J, Leger-Gauthier C, et al. Fibrinopeptide A and platelet factor levels in unstable angina pectoris. Circulation 1987; 75:156.

47. Zahavi M, Zahavi J, Schafer R, et al. Abnormal pattern of platelet function and thromboxane generation in unstable angina. Thromb Haemost 1989; 62:840.
48. Rubenstein MD, Wall RT, Baim DS, et al. Platelet activation in clinical coronary artery disease and spasm. Am Heart J 1981; 102:363–367.
49. Hirsh PD, Hillis LD, Campbell WB, et al. Release of prostaglandins and thromboxane into the coronary circulation in patients with ischemic heart disease. N Engl J Med 1981; 304:685–691.
50. deBoer AC, Turpie AG, Butt RW, et al. Platelet release and thromboxane synthesis in symptomatic coronary artery disease. Circulation 1982; 66: 327–333.
51. Fitzgerald DJ, Roy L, Catella F, et al. Platelet activation in unstable coronary disease. N Engl J Med 1986; 315:989–993.
52. Mehta J, Mehta P, Feldman RL, et al. Thromboxane release in coronary artery disease: Spontaneous versus pacing induced angina. Am Heart J 1984; 107:286–292.
53. Grande P, Grauholt A, Madsen JK. Platelet behavior and prognosis in progressive angina and intermediate coronary syndrome. Circulation 1990; 81(1):I-16-I-19.
54. Hamm CW, Lorenz RL, Bleifield W, et al. Biochemical evidence of platelet activation in patient with persistent unstable angina. J Am Coll Cardiol 1987; 10:998–1004.
55. Doyle DJ, Chesterman CN, Cade JF, et al. Plasma concentrations of platelet specific proteins correlated with platelet survival. Blood 1980; 55:82.
56. Files JC, Malpass T, Yee EK, et al. Studies of human platelet alpha-granule release in vivo. Blood 1981; 58:607.
57. Levine SP, Lindenfeld J, Ellis B, et al. Increased plasma concentrations of platelet factor four in coronary artery disease. A measure of in vivo platelet activation and secretion. Circulation 1981; 64:626.
58. White GC, Marouf AA. Platelet factor IV levels in patients with coronary artery disease. J Lab Clin Med 1981; 97:369.
59. Pumphery CW, Dawes J. Plasma beta-thromboglobulin as a measure of platelet activity. Effect of risk factors and findings in ischemic heart disease after myocaridal infarction. Am J Cardiol 1982; 50:1258.
60. deBoer AC, Han P, Turpie AG, et al. Platelet tests and antiplatelet drugs in coronary artery disease. Circulation 1983; 76:500.
61. van Hulsteijn H, Kolff J, Briet E, et al. Fibrinopeptide A and beta-thromboglobulin in patients with angina pectoris and myocardial infarction. Am Heart J 1984; 107:39
62. Nichols AB, Owen J, Kaplan KL, et al. Fibrinopeptide A, platelet factor 4, and beta-thromboglobulin levels in coronary heart disease. Blood 1982; 60:650.
63. Cella G, Colby SI, Taylor AD, et al. Platelet factor 4 and heparin-releasable platelet factor 4 patients with cardiovascular disorders. Thromb Res 1983; 29:499.
64. Smitherman TC, Milam M, Woo J, et al. Elevated beta-thromboglobulin in peripheral venous blood of patients with acute myocardial ischemia: Direct evidence for enhanced platelet reactivity in vivo. Am J Cardiol 1981; 48:395.

65. Sobel M, Salzman EW, Davies GC, et al. Circulating platelet products in unstable angina pectoris. Circulation 1981; 63:300.
66. Schmitz-Huebner U, Thompson SG, Balleisen L, et al. Lack of association between hemostatic variables and the presence and extent of coronary atherosclerosis. Br Heart J 1988; 59:287.
67. Douglas JT, Lowe GD, Forbes CD, et al. Plasma fibrinopeptide A and beta-thromboglobulin in patients with chest pain. Thromb Haemost 1983; 50: 541.
68. Swahn E, Wallentin L. Platelet reactivity in unstable coronary artery disease. Thromb Haemost 1987; 57:302.
69. De Caterina R, Gazzetti P, Mazzone A, et al. Platelet activation in angina at rest. Evidence by paired measurement of plasma beta-thromboglobulin and platelet factor 4. Eur Heart J 1988; 9:913.
70. Kutti J, Wadenvik H, Johnson S, et al. The relation between platelet reactivity and coronary angiographic findings in young female survivors of acute myocardial infarction. Thromb Haemost 1986; 56:207.
71. Ring ME, Feinberg WM, Bruck DC, et al. Platelet activity during acute myocardial infarction treated with tissue plasminogen activator. Thromb Res 1988; 51:331.
72. Rapold HJ, Haeberli A, Kuemmerli H, et al. Fibrin formation and platelet activation in patients with myocardial infarction and normal coronary arteries. Eur Heart J 1989; 10:323.
73. Kaplan KL, Owen J. Plasma levels of beta-thromboglobulin and platelet factor 4 as indices of platelet activation in vivo. Blood 1981; 57:199.
74. Shattil SJ, Cunningham M, Hoxie JA. Detection of activated platelets in whole blood using activation-dependent monoclonal antibodies and flow cytometry. Blood 1987; 70:307–315.
75. Palabrica T, Smith J, Aronovitz M, et al. Platelet PADGEM expression in the coronary and systemic circulation in stable and unstable angina. Circulation 1990; 82(4):(Suppl)III-277.
76. Becker R, Tracy R, Bovill E, et al. Platelet activation persists among patients with unstable angina and non-Q wave myocardial infarction. Circulation 1993; 88(4):(Suppl)I-609.
77. Palabrica T, Smith J, Aronovitz M, et al. Flow cytometric analysis of platelet PADGEM expression during PTCA. Circulation 1990; 80(4):III-655.
78. Tschoepe MD, Schultheib HP, Kolarov MD, et al. Platelet membrane activation markers are predictive for increased risk of acute ischemic events after PTCA. Circulation 1993; 88:37–42.
79. Scharf RE, Tomer A, Marzec UM, et al. Activation of platelets in blood perfusing angioplasty-damaged coronary arteries: Flow cytometric detection. Arterioscler Thromb 1992; 12:1475–1487.
80. Harlan J. Leukocyte-endothlial interactions. Blood 1985; 65:513–523.
81. Faint RW. Platelet-neutrophil interactions: their significance. Blood Rev 1992; 6:83–91.
82. Yasuda M, Takeuchi K, Hiruma M, et al. The complement system in ischemic heart disease. Circulation 1990; 81:156–163.
83. Palabrica T, Lobb R, Furie B, et al. Leukocyte accumulation promoting fibrin deposition is mediated in vivo by P-selectin on adherent platelets. Nature 1992; 359:848–851.

84. Neri Serneri G, Abbate R, Gori AM, et al. Transient intermittent lymphocyte activation is responsible for the instability of angina. Circulation 1992; 86:790–797.
85. Dinerman J, Mehta J, Saldeen T, et al. Increased neutrophil elastase in unstable angina and acute myocardial infarction. Am J Cardiol 1990; 15: 1559–1563.
86. Berk B, Weintraub W, Alexander R. Elevation of C-reactive protein in "active" coronary artery disease. Am J Cardiol 1990; 65:168–172.
87. Liuzzo A, Biasucci LM, Gallimore JR, et al. The prognostic value of C-reactive protein and serum amyloid 'a' protein in severe unstable angina. N Engl J Med 1994; 331(7):417–424.
88. Mazzone A, De Servi S, Ricevuti G, et al. Increased expression of neutrophil and monocyte adhesion molecules in unstable coronary artery disease. Circulation 1993; 22:358–363.
89. van der Wal A, Becker A, van der Loos, et al. Site of intimal rupture or erosion of thrombosed coronary atherosclerotic plaques is characterized by an inflammatory process irrespective of the dominant plaque morphology. Circulation 1994; 89:36–44.
90. Moreno PR, Falk E, Palacios IF, et al. Macrophage infiltration in acute coronary syndromes: Implications for plaque rupture. Circulation 1994; 90:775–778.
91. Engler RL, Dahlgren MD, Peterson MA, et al. Accumulation of polymorphonuclear leukocytes during 3-h experimental myocardial ischemia. Am J Physiol 1986; 251:H93-H100.

II

Prognosis and Therapy

8

Prognostic Implications of Lesion Morphology

Raffaele Bugiardini, MD, Alberico Borghi, MD

Introduction

Unstable angina is a broad clinical diagnosis that includes patients at different levels of risk for an unfavorable outcome. Although, as in other categories of coronary artery disease, the state of left ventricular function and the extent of coronary artery disease will determine long-term prognosis, recognition of clinical markers of an early unfavorable outcome may be of value in defining management strategies. This report focuses on the relevance of noninvasive data and lesion morphology in assessing the prognosis of patients with unstable angina.

Angiography, Lesion Morphology, and Prognosis

The quantitative and qualitative appearance of coronary artery lesions in unstable angina have been reported by several investigators. A number of studies[1,2] reported that the site of occlusive thrombosis causing infarction cannot be predicted by preinfarction angiograms, since thrombosis may occur at the site of mild stenosis whereas severe stenosis remains unchanged. Ambrose et al.[3] reported type II eccentric lesions (irregular eccentric stenoses or eccentric lesions with a narrow

From: Ambrose JA (ed): *Complex Coronary Lesions in Acute Coronary Syndromes*.

neck) to be common in unstable angina (54%) as compared with stable angina (4%). Type II lesions are frequently associated with intracoronary thrombus. The angiographic evidence of type II lesions with or without intracoronary thrombus is commonly defined as complex coronary morphology.[4] Angioscopic and postmortem studies established that these lesions represent atherosclerotic plaque disruption and/or fissuring.[5,6]*

Freeman et al.[7] found complex angiographic lesions in 29/78 unstable angina patients. Of these 29 patients, 55% had cardiac events (death, myocardial infarction, or emergency revascularization), the remainder having a good clinical outcome. These authors reported evidence of a coronary thrombus (intracoronary filling defects) in 32/78 patients. Of these 32 patients, 72% showed subsequent coronary events, the remainder having a favorable outcome. They concluded that cardiac events were more frequent in patients with coronary thrombus and/or complex coronary morphology.

Our findings add a piece of information relative to the coronary vascular disorder seen in unstable angina.[8] We found a high incidence of complex lesions and/or coronary thrombi in 66% (58/88 patients) of unstable angina. Of the 58 patients with complex morphology, 32 (55%) had an unfavorable clinical outcome. A similar outcome, however, occurred in only two of the 30 (7%) patients without complex coronary morphology (Figure 1). These data therefore indicate that:

1. Unstable angina frequently has a dynamic component of coronary thrombosis that is often superimposed onto irregular stenosis (complex morphology).
2. The unfavorable evolution of unstable angina is almost invariably associated with the evidence of irregular stenosis at angiography.
3. Irregular stenosis is necessary but not sufficient to activate the dynamic process leading to coronary artery occlusion and related consequences; some patients with complex coronary morphology may live for years, although others may die quickly.

Since prognostic statements for any one patient cannot be made with certainty by using angiography alone, an understanding of the underlying probability of death or myocardial infarction as assessed by clinical indices and noninvasive techniques is essential for a correct definition of risk. This approach may identify functional prognostic factors, quantify their strength, and assess their possible interplay with concurrent angiographic information.

* Editor's note: See Chapter 3.

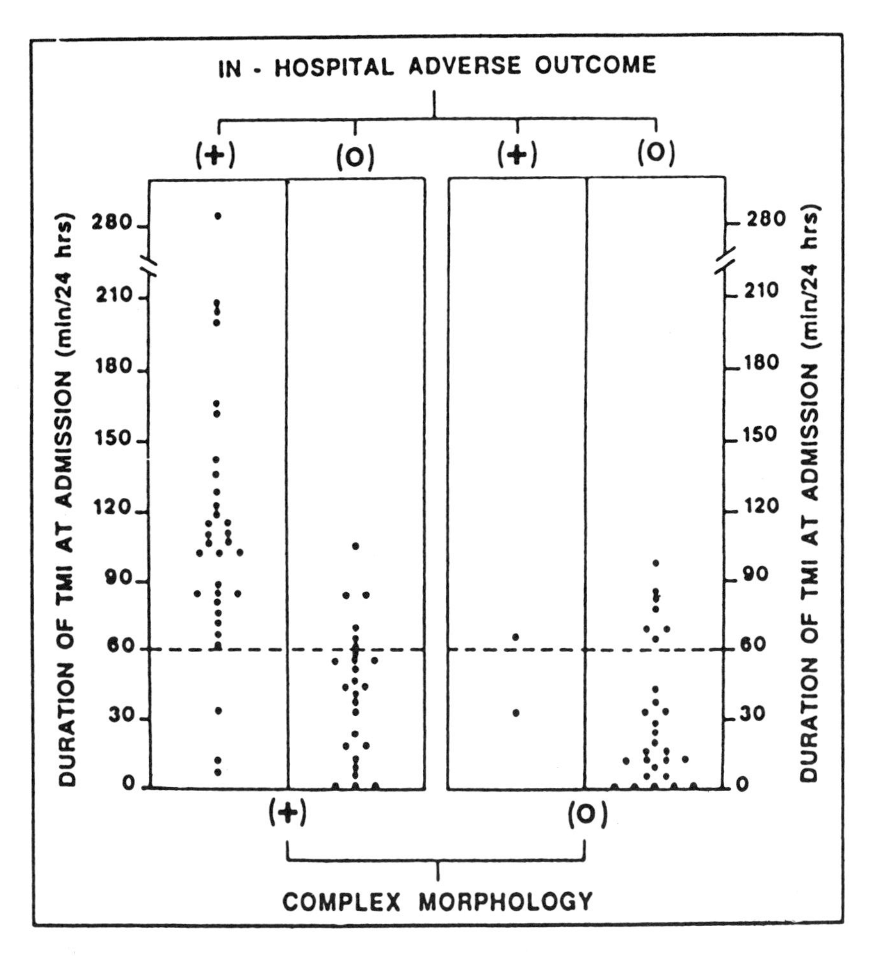

Figure 1: Relationship among complex stenosis morphology, transient myocardial ischemia (TMI), and in-hospital outcome in patients with unstable angina. Association of complex morphology with TMI ≥60 minutes per 24 hours is highly predictive of in-hospital adverse clinical outcome. (Reproduced with permission of The American Journal of Cardiology.[8])

Severity of Symptoms, Lesion Morphology, and Prognosis

Chest pain has been used traditionally to guide management and therapy of unstable angina.[9–11] Patients without recurrent chest pain had a lower event rate than those with pain.[11] Recurrence of chest pain within 48 hours after admittance has been shown to carry a reduction in likelihood of survival at 1 year of about 20% in patients with progressive or prolonged angina.[9,12] Symptoms, however, do not help to predict early (in-hospital) complications. Recurrent angina, i.e., the occurrence of one or more anginal episodes during hospitalization, was observed in the majority of patients admitted to the Coronary Care Unit regardless of their early prognosis.[1]

Efforts were therefore directed to assess the quality and/or severity of angina and not simply its presence or absence. Murphy et al.[13] studied 141 patients and demonstrated that the event-free probability was similar in different subgroups of patients, as defined by their presenting clinical features, i.e., angina of recent onset, of increasing severity, and at rest. Ahmed et al.[14] reported that patients with early postinfarction angina, patients with primary unstable angina and a history (within 1 month) of pain at rest, and patients with unstable angina secondary to a non cardiac condition but with recent (≤48 hours) episodes of pain at rest, all had high probability of discovering intracoronary thrombus and lesion complexity during angiography. One hundred four unstable patients were examined in a concomitant study.[15] Exclusion criteria included age ≥75 years and severe heart failure. Forty-eight hour monitoring was performed shortly after admission and coronary angiography within 1 week. Unfavorable outcomes were cardiac death (5 patients), myocardial infarction (14 patients), or need for urgent revascularization (22 patients), the latter based on angina not controlled with medical therapy and the presence of a 70% or greater coronary stenosis. Severity of angina was numerically scored; scores were based on frequency and persistence of pain, duration of each single episode of angina and length of pain-free intervals. It was found that the length of the pain-free intervals (<1 hour) and the duration (>15 minutes) of episodes of angina both correlated with a higher incidence of coronary lesion complexity, and subsequent in-hospital coronary events (Figures 2 and 3).

Based on this estimation, however, 19% of patients were grouped as "high risk" and 81% as "low risk," whereas many more patients (39%) actually developed an unfavorable clinical course and far less (61%) had a good outcome. *It follows that symptoms are specific (92%) but not sensitive (32%) enough for identifying the majority of patients with oncoming events.* The prognostic significance of chest pain in patients with unstable angina is further limited by two important considerations: (1) quantitative evaluation of symptoms has a subjective component that may cause uncertainty as to how to establish risk

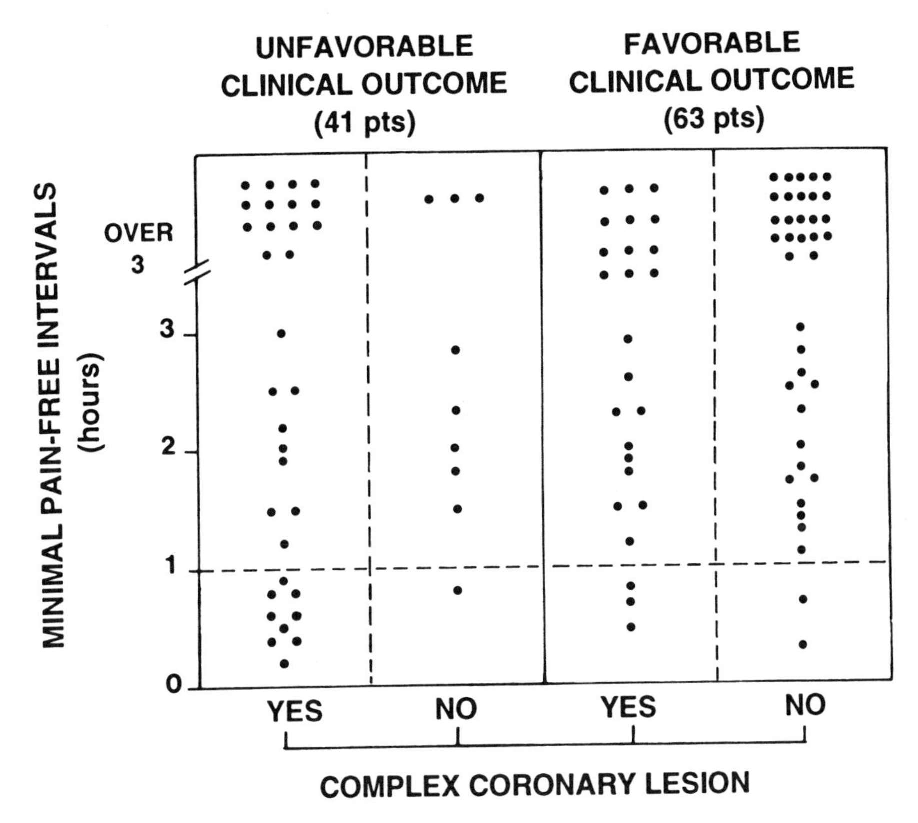

Figure 2: Relationship among prognosis, duration of minimal pain-free intervals, and angiographic coronary morphology in patients with unstable angina. A minimal pain-free interval <1 hour is correlated with the presence of a complex coronary stenosis. The association of both findings shows a low sensitivity, but a high specificity in predicting subsequent early adverse outcome.

adequately in each individual patient. In practice it appears to be extremely difficult to find clear-cut categories. For example, prolonged episodes (>15 minutes) of angina generally occur in association with symptoms not controlled by medical therapy, and usually are analyzed in this fashion; (2) since persistence of symptoms is commonly used to determine the need for revascularization, it would be expected that such symptoms would be specific for an unfavorable outcome. Indeed, the statistical power for detecting a prognostic factor is determined chiefly by the quality and the number of adverse events. Thus, an analysis such as that we reported, of 41 events consisting of five deaths, 14 nonfatal myocardial infarctions, and 22 surgical procedures could have primarily identified the factors used to select patients for inter-

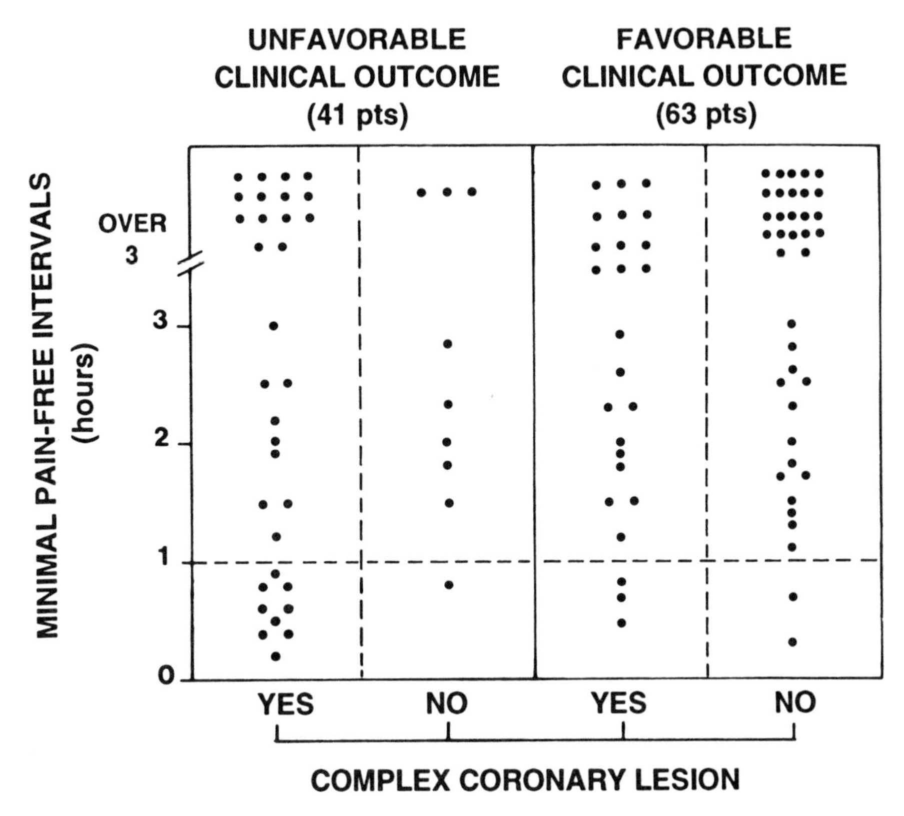

Figure 3: Relationship among prognosis, maximal duration of anginal episodes, and angiographic coronary morphology in patients with unstable angina. Prolonged (>15 minutes) anginal episodes are often associated with a complex coronary stenosis. Again, combination of these findings is poorly sensitive, even though highly specific, in predicting an adverse in-hospital prognosis.

vention, not the determinants of the "natural history" of the disease. In other words, the effects of angina on outcome may be overestimated.

Transient Myocardial Ischemia, Lesion Morphology, and Prognosis

The role of ECG changes in either symptomatic or asymptomatic patients has been widely investigated. Cohen et al.[16] found ST changes on the emergency room electrocardiogram to be a reliable predictor of adverse in-hospital clinical outcome (recurrent ischemia, infarction, or need for revascularization). Also, the cumulative duration of transient ST changes on Holter monitoring has been shown to be an important predictor of subsequent late and early events. Gottlieb et al.[17] reported that patients presenting with more than 60 minutes of ischemia in 24 hours had a higher in-hospital event rate (48%) than did those with less than 60 minutes of ischemia (20%). Other studies reported similar findings in patients followed-up for 6 to 72 months.[18,19] Langer et al. showed that the duration of ischemia was greater in patients with an unfavorable outcome, multivessel disease, and left main artery stenosis.[20] We reported that the duration of transient myocardial ischemia correlates with the underlying angiographic anatomy, i.e., is a complex coronary morphology, and may thus help in making decisions regarding diagnostic and interventional procedures.[8,21] Most of these studies analyzed the strength of a continuous prognostic factor, i.e., the duration of transient myocardial ischemia, by setting an arbitrary "cut-point" and dividing the patients into subgroups with values above and below the cut-point. Although this technique is useful in facilitating the drawing of survival curves, it discards additional prognostic information of this variable. Ischemia is described as being above or below 60 minutes/24 hours. Dividing patients in this fashion implicitly assumes that a duration of ischemia of 59 minutes has the same prognostic impact as a duration of 1 minute, which may be a risky statement.

Further studies were then performed to clarify whether a different analysis of Holter recordings may give better prognostic information. Pozzati et al.[22] confirmed the relation of transient myocardial ischemia to unstable plaque and to certain morphological features. The importance of this study lies in the demonstration that the electrocardiographic correlates of the unstable plaque decrease or disappear with time, which may provide prognostic information. Patients showing more than 60 minutes per 24 hours of transient myocardial ischemia on the first day of monitoring had a poor prognosis with a 70% risk of subsequent coronary events. Three days of full medical treatment resulted in a significant decrease in the daily duration of ischemia in all subgroups of patients. In this setting, "residual" myocardial ischemia (>0 minutes per 24 hours) occurred in 85% of patients later having a major coronary event and was related to the in-hospital and 1-year clinical outcome. This finding may have several explanations. Response of unstable angina to treatment depends on its pathological substrate.[23] Conventional intensive medical treatment (including aspirin and 12,500 IU/day subcutaneous calcium-heparin) should reduce myocardial oxygen consumption, coronary vasoconstriction and platelet aggregation, which have all been suggested to play a role in precipitating acute myocardial ischemia.[24] Transient myocardial ischemia may be, therefore, significantly reduced in all subsets of patients by full medical treatment. The degree of benefit, however, varies among patients. Patients with complex lesions are likely to show residual ischemia at a mean interval of 3 days after admission. This suggests that treatment has little effect when applied to intracoronary thrombus formation or growth, which is the dynamic process superimposed on an injured atherosclerotic plaque.[25] It also seems conceivable that ischemia persisting despite medical treatment, rather than the amount of ischemia observed at admission,[22] could better correlate with the angiographic finding of complex coronary lesions, hence with the early clinical outcome of those patients having unstable angina due to plaque disruption (Figure 4).

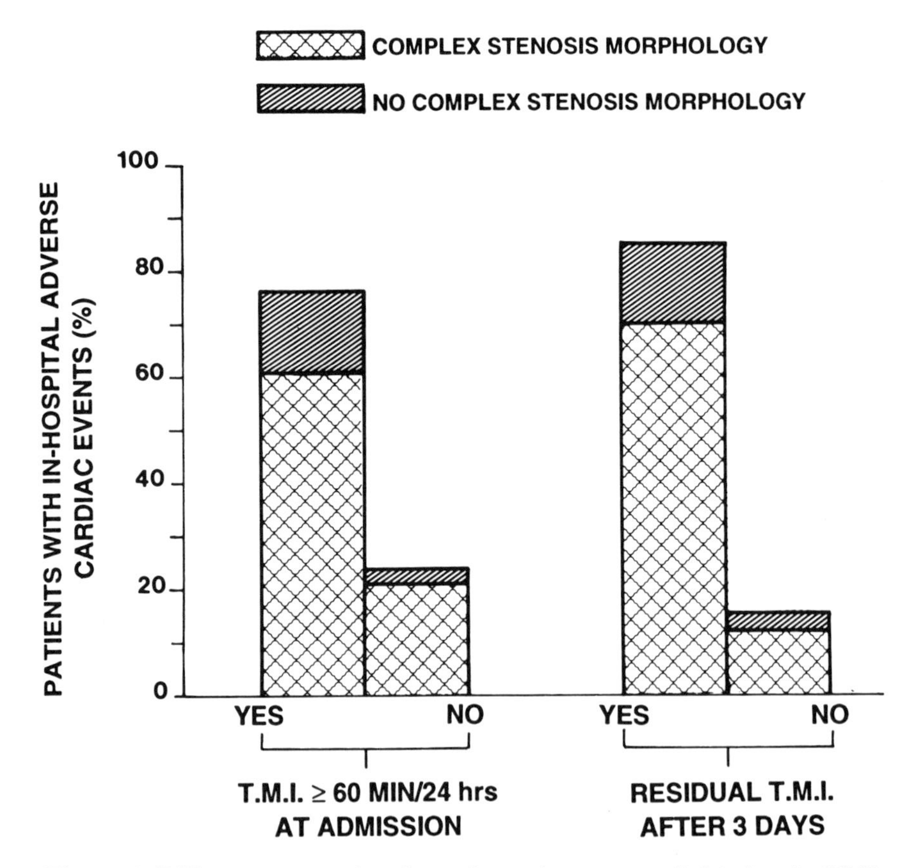

Figure 4: Different prognostic values of transient myocardial ischemia (TMI) detected at admission or following 3 days of full medical treatment in a group of patients with unstable angina. Residual TMI seems to better correlate with the presence of complicated coronary stenosis and unfavorable in-hospital prognosis than duration of TMI detected at admission.

Estimation of Prognosis by Using Combined Angiographic and Noninvasive Findings

Prognosis in unstable angina is presumably affected by a large number of factors including the patient's age, gender, extent of coronary artery disease, morphological coronary findings, and coexisting medical disorders. Regression modeling techniques for prognostic analysis can be enhanced by the use of several clinical variables measuring different aspects of the same underlying pathophysiological phenomenon. For instance, the presence of prolonged episodes of angina, short pain-free intervals, prolonged duration of transient myocardial ischemia at admission, residual transient myocardial ischemia despite 3 days of full medical treatment, and complex coronary morphology with or without angiographically detectable thrombus all measure different aspects of the underlying pathophysiological substrate, i.e., the atherosclerotic plaque and its degree of instability. A clinical index that combines the information provided from the above related variables could be a more powerful prognostic factor than any individual variable. The observation of complex coronary morphology in patients exhibiting angina with pain-free intervals <1 hour or prolonged episodes of chest pain (>15 minutes) is highly specific (97%) but is not sensitive (34%) for predicting subsequent coronary events.[15] Detection of complex coronary morphology in patients with ischemia ≥ 60 minutes per 24 hours or in those having "residual" ischemia despite full medical treatment is both specific and sensitive in identifying acute coronary syndromes evolving toward myocardial infarction.[8,22] Urgent definition of coronary anatomy and left ventricular global function seems therefore necessary in patients with specific symptoms and/or persisting ischemia on Holter monitoring.

From Angiography to Revascularization

These studies have emphasized the relation of acute myocardial infarction to unstable plaque and to certain clinical and electrocardiographic features. Exactly how this translates in terms of early revascularization remains to be determined. Early intervention is associated with a threefold increase in mortality,[26] thus the preferred strategy is deferring revascularization after plaque stabilization, i.e., 2 to 4 weeks later.[27] However, it should not be assumed that this strategy must be applied to all patients. In most studies, the majority (65%–80%) of patients who suffered fatal or nonfatal myocardial infarction, did so 2 to 6 days after admission.[8,17] If these high-risk patients could have been simply identified, they would have been able to undergo coronary revascularization early enough to prevent myocardial infarction. Lesion irregularity itself cannot be considered crucial in clinical decision making because it can be found in a substantial portion (40%) of patients having good short-term clinical outcome. This means that immediate coronary revascularization in all subjects exhibiting critical coronary stenosis as well as complex coronary morphology may expose many of these patients to the risks of an unnecessary procedure.

It is important to recognize that the most powerful detectable clinical predictors of the evolution toward infarction are the persistence and duration of ischemic episodes, despite full medical therapy. If, despite an intensive pharmacological approach, patients continue to have angina with pain-free intervals <1 hour or prolonged episodes of chest pain (>15 minutes) or persistence (more than 3 days) of transient myocardial ischemia, treatment may be regarded as being ineffective, thus they should undergo immediate catheterization to determine the type of coronary lesion representing the underlying cause of ischemia. In the presence of significant left main disease or complex coronary morphology, an attempt at myocardial revascularization should be instituted without delay because progression to myocardial infarction usually occurs soon after hospitalization.*

References

1. Little WC, Costantinescu M, Applegate RJ, et al. Can coronary arteriography predict the site of a subsequent myocardial infarction in patients with mild-to-moderate coronary artery disease? Circulation 1988; 78: 1157–1166.
2. Hackett D, Davies G, Maseri A. Pre-existing coronary stenosis in patients with first myocardial infarction are not necessarily severe. Eur Heart J 1988; 9:1317–1323.
3. Ambrose JA, Winters SL, Stern A, et al. Angiographic morphology and the pathogenesis of unstable angina pectoris. J Am Coll Cardiol 1985; 5: 609–616.
4. Ambrose JA, Winters SL, Arora RR, et al. Coronary angiographic morphol-

* Editor's note: Complex stenoses that stabilize clinically tend to progress angiographically on follow-up. Chen, et al. Circulation 1995; 91:2319.

ogy in myocardial infarction: A link between the pathogenesis of unstable angina and myocardial infarction. J Am Coll Cardiol 1985; 6:1233–1238.
5. Sherman CT, Litvack F, Grundfest W, et al. Coronary angioscopy in patients with unstable angina pectoris. N Engl J Med 1986; 315:913–919.
6. Davies MJ, Thomas AC. Plaque fissuring-the cause of acute myocardial infarction, sudden ischemic death and crescendo angina. Br Heart J 1985; 53:363–373.
7. Freeman MR, Williams AE, Chrisholm RT, Armstrong PW. Intracoronary thrombus and complex morphology in unstable angina: Relation to timing of angiography and in-hospital cardiac events. Circulation 1989; 80:17–23.
8. Bugiardini R, Pozzati A, Borghi A, et al. Angiographic morphology in unstable angina and its relation to transient myocardial ischemia and hospital outcome. Am J Cardiol 1991; 67:460–464.
9. Mulcahy R, Daly L, Graham I, et al. Unstable angina: natural history and determinants of prognosis. Am J Cardiol 1981; 48:525–528.
10. Report of HINT (Holland Interuniversity Nifedipine Trial) Research Group. Early treatment of unstable angina in the coronary care unit: a randomized, double blind, placebo controlled comparison of recurrent ischaemia in patients treated with nifedipine or metoprolol or both. Br Heart J 1986; 56:400–413.
11. Wilcox I, Freedman SB, Kelly DT, et al. Clinical significance of silent ischemia in patients with suspected unstable angina pectoris. Am J Cardiol 1990; 65:1313–1316.
12. Gazes PC, Mobley EM Jr, Faris HM Jr, et al. Preinfarctional (unstable) angina: a prospective study. Ten-year follow-up: prognostic significance of electrocardiographic changes. Circulation 1973; 48:331–337.
13. Murphy JJ, Connell PA, Hampton JR. Predictors of risk in patients with unstable angina admitted to a district general hospital. Br Heart J 1992; 67:395–401.
14. Ahmed WH, Bittl JA, Braunwald E. Relation between clinical presentation and angiographic findings in unstable angina pectoris, and comparison with that in stable angina. Am J Cardiol 1993; 72:544–550.
15. Bugiardini R, Borghi A, Pozzati A, et al. Is chest pain a reliable predictor of subsequent coronary events in unstable angina? Eur Heart J 1992; 13: 205 (abstract).
16. Cohen M, Hawkins L, Greenberg S, Fuster V. Usefulness of ST-segment changes in ≥2 leads on the emergency room electrocardiogram in either unstable angina pectoris or non-Q-wave myocardial infarction in predicting outcome. Am J Cardiol 1991; 67:1368–1373.
17. Gottlieb SO, Weisfeldt ML, Ouyang P, et al. Silent ischemia as a marker for early unfavorable outcomes in patients with unstable angina. N Engl J Med 1986; 314:1214–1219.
18. Nademanee K, Intrachot V, Josephson MA, et al. Prognostic significance of silent myocardial ischemia in patients with unstable angina. J Am Coll Cardiol 1987; 10:1–7.
19. Romeo F, Rosano GMC, Martuscelli E, et al. Unstable angina: role of silent ischemia and total ischemic time (silent plus painful ischemia): a 6-year follow-up. J Am Coll Cardiol 1992; 19:1173–1179.
20. Langer A, Freeman MR, Armstrong PW. ST segment shift in unstable

angina: pathophysiology and association with coronary anatomy and hospital outcome. J Am Coll Cardiol 1989; 13:1495–1502.
21. Bugiardini R, Borghi A, Sassone B, et al. Prognostic significance of silent myocardial ischemia in variant angina pectoris. Am J Cardiol 1991; 68: 1581–1586.
22. Pozzati A, Bugiardini R, Borghi A, et al. Transient ischaemia refractory to conventional medical treatment in unstable angina: angiographic correlates and prognostic implications. Eur Heart J 1992; 13:360–365.
23. Epstein SE, Palmeri ST. Mechanisms contributing to precipitation of unstable angina and acute myocardial infarction: implication regarding therapy. Am J Cardiol 1984; 54:1245–1252.
24. Fuster V, Badimon L, Cohen M, et al. Insights into the pathogenesis of acute ischemic syndromes. Circulation 1988; 77:1213–1220.
25. Falk E. Unstable angina with fatal outcome: dynamic coronary thrombosis leading to infarction and/or sudden death. Circulation 1985; 71:699–708.
26. Kamp O, Beatt KJ, De Feyter PJ, et al. Short-, medium-, and long-term follow-up after percutaneous transluminal coronary angioplasty for stable and unstable angina pectoris. Am Heart J 1989; 117:991–997.
27. De Feyter PJ. Coronary angioplasty for unstable angina. Am Heart J 1989; 118:860–868.

9

Unstable Angina/Complex Lesions and the Response to Conventional Antithrombotic Therapy

Marc Cohen MD, Philip C. Adams MD

Introduction

Patients with unstable angina pectoris represent a broad spectrum, ranging from progressive or accelerating angina to the higher risk subset of rest angina with reversible electrocardiographic changes.[1] Large scale randomized, placebo-controlled, therapeutic trials have established a beneficial role for antithrombotic therapy with aspirin alone, or with heparin or warfarin alone, in progressive unstable angina.[2–6] Clinical trials have also demonstrated a beneficial effect of antithrombotic therapy in the higher risk patients with rest angina[5–8] or non-Q-wave myocardial infarction[6,9,10] who usually have complex coronary lesions. Therefore, antithrombotic therapy with either antiplatelet agents alone, or anticoagulants alone, are of proven benefit in patients with complex lesions presenting with the acute coronary syndromes of unstable angina and/or non-Q-wave infarction.

Pathoanatomic observations implicate acute plaque rupture and overlying thrombosis as the usual triggering mechanism for these

From: Ambrose JA (ed): *Complex Coronary Lesions in Acute Coronary Syndromes.*

acute coronary syndromes.[11–13] In addition, prior studies have shown that failure of medical therapy in these syndromes most often occurs within the first few days after admission.[14] Therefore, in view of the dynamic intra-arterial processes precipitating unstable angina and non-Q-wave infarction, more aggressive antithrombotic therapy with platelet inhibition *plus* anticoagulation may offer more benefit than either agent alone. Based on the trend to lower mortality and morbidity with combination therapy in the RISC[6] study and in the small pilot study of Cohen et al.,[14] a larger multicenter, binational study was undertaken of combination antithrombotic therapy in unstable angina and non-Q-wave infarction. The therapy tested in this trial utilized low doses of aspirin with or without anticoagulation for 12 weeks. The study population was prospectively stratified into patients without or with prior aspirin use (Figure 1). The main end-points were recurrent ischemia with electrocardiographic changes, progression to infarction, death, and/or major bleeding, assessed during hospitalization and over a 12-week follow-up period.

Patients with *no prior aspirin* (ASA) use were randomized into one of two limbs: (1) ASA alone, or (2) ASA + heparin/warfarin. The hypothesis tested in this subgroup was whether combination anti-

NO PRIOR ASA USE: TRIAL A

Group 1	**Group 2**
At randomization: ASA 162.5 mg po	At randomization: ASA 162.5 mg po plus, loading heparin 100u/kg iv push
Maintainance: ASA 162.5 mg/day for 12 weeks	Maintainance: ASA 162.5 mg/day plus, heparin drip (PTT 2X control for 3 days) then warfarin (PT 1.3-1.5X control (INR 2-3) for 12 weeks

PRIOR ASA USE: TRIAL B

Group 1	**Group 2**
At randomization: CR-ASA 75 mg po plus, loading heparin 100 u/kg iv push	At randomization: Conventional ASA 75 mg po plus, loading heparin 100 u/kg iv push
Maintainance: CR-ASA 75 mg/day plus, heparin drip (PTT 2X control for 3 days) then warfarin (PT 1.3-1.5X control (INR 2-3) for 12 weeks	Maintainance: Conventional ASA 75 mg/day plus heparin drip (PTT 2X control for 3 days then warfarin (PT 1.3-1.5X control (INR 2-3) for 12 weeks.

Figure 1: Protocol for antithrombotic trial therapy for non-prior aspirin versus prior aspirin users.

thrombotic therapy with an antiplatelet and an anticoagulant reduced morbidity and mortality compared to an antiplatelet agent alone.

Patients with *prior* ASA use were randomized into one of the following two limbs: (1) controlled release aspirin (CR-ASA[15]) + heparin/warfarin, or (2) conventional ASA + heparin/warfarin. Controlled release aspirin (recently tested in normal volunteers[15]), acetylates platelets in the enterohepatic circulation but doesn't reach the systemic circulation thereby preserving endothelial prostacyclin synthesis. Patients experiencing unstable angina, in spite of conventional aspirin therapy, probably have a strong thrombotic stimulus that may be aggravated by the loss of local prostacyclin-mediated vasodilation. The hypothesis tested in this subgroup was whether addition of a prostacyclin-sparing formulation of ASA to heparin/warfarin was more beneficial than conventional ASA plus heparin/warfarin in patients who have failed conventional ASA and need maximal antithrombotic therapy.

Methods

The study was a prospective, partially blinded, randomized, multicenter study of antithrombotic therapy in the treatment of men and women (over age 21) with acute chest pain due to rest unstable angina or non-Q-wave myocardial infarction admitted to the hospital. To select a high-risk population, patients with chest pain had to have definite evidence of ischemic heart disease, but no evidence of evolving Q-wave infarction. Three hundred fifty-eight patients gave informed consent and were randomized.

Selection of Patients; Inclusion/Exclusion Criteria

The details of the inclusion and exclusion criteria have been described in prior publications.[10,16,17] All patients enrolled in the study presented to the hospital within 48 hours of ischemic pain caused by either rest unstable angina or non-Q-wave infarction. In addition, there must have been prior evidence of underlying ischemic heart disease, e.g., electrocardiographic (ECG) changes during chest pain or a previous coronary angiography showing a 50% or greater luminal narrowing in a coronary artery. If ST segment elevation was present, it must have resolved within 30 minutes of relief of pain post nitroglycerin. Patients with persistent ST elevation were not randomized.

There were several exclusion criteria including ischemic pain due to evolving Q-wave myocardial infarction, angina precipitated by congestive heart failure, tachyarrhythmia, or hypertension, and contraindications to anticoagulation.

Study Design

The study design is outlined in Figure 1. Once consent was obtained, patients were prospectively stratified into either the non-prior aspirin use group (Trial A), or prior ASA use (Trial B), and randomized accordingly. Prior aspirin use was defined as ingestion of greater than or equal to 150 mg of ASA within 3 days of randomization. Separate randomization schemes were provided for Trial A and Trial B. All trial therapy was instituted immediately upon randomization in the emergency room. Therapy was not withheld until enzymatic analysis excluded evolving transmural infarction. Trial therapy was continued for 12 weeks. After 12 weeks, continued administration of ASA or anticoagulation was left to the discretion of the private physician.

Treatment Protocol: Trial Antithrombotic Therapy

TRIAL A: Patients with No Prior Aspirin Use

These patients were randomized to receive one of two treatments:

1. *ASA Alone*—Upon randomization ASA 162.5 mg p.o. as a loading dose, followed by ASA 162.5 mg daily.

2. *ASA + Anticoagulation*—Upon randomization ASA 162.5 mg p.o. and a loading dose of heparin 100 units/kg intravenous bolus. This was followed by ASA 162.5 mg daily, plus a continuous heparin infusion to maintain the activated partial thromboplastin time (PTT) at 2.0 X control for 3–4 days. Partial thromboplastin time tests were drawn 6 hours after the initial bolus and then once daily to maintain the PTT at 2.0 times control. Warfarin was to be started by the second or third day presuming that coronary arteriography did not appear imminent. When the prothrombin time (PT), reached 1.3 to 1.5 times control (INR of 2.0–3.0), heparin was discontinued. Aspirin and warfarin were continued for 12 weeks.

TRIAL B: Patients with Prior Aspirin Use

These patients were randomized to receive one of two treatments:

1. *Controlled Release Aspirin + Anticoagulation*—Upon randomization, controlled release aspirin 75 mg, (CR-ASA 75 mg), followed by CR-ASA 75 mg daily. In addition, a loading dose of heparin 100 units/kg intravenous bolus was given followed by a continuous infusion and initiation of warfarin as described above.
2. *Conventional Aspirin + Anticoagulation*—Upon randomization, conventional ASA 75 mg, followed by ASA 75 mg/day. In addition, a loading dose of heparin was given followed by a continuous infusion and initiation of warfarin as mentioned above.

In Trial B, the controlled release ASA appeared identical to the conventional ASA and both the patient and the physician were blinded with regard to the type of ASA given. Aspirin and warfarin were continued for 12 weeks.

Treatment Protocol: Standard Medical Therapy

In addition to trial antithrombotic therapy, anti-anginal therapy was administered to all patients according to the algorithm described by Cohen et al.[16] Doses of the three classes of oral anti-anginal drugs, beta adrenergic blockers, calcium channel blockers, and nitrates were maximized as tolerated within 48 hours of hospital admission in order to titrate the systolic blood pressure to $\leq$130 mm Hg, and the heart rate to $\leq$65 beats/minute. Aspirin-containing medication other than trial drugs were prohibited and a supply of acetaminophen was given. In the absence of any revascularization procedure, patients were discharged on the above standard medical regimen that was clinically effective, in addition to their trial antithrombotic therapy.

Primary End-Points

1. *Recurrent angina:* Defined as recurrent chest pain at rest *with* ischemic ECG ST-T wave changes occurring despite *full* medical therapy. Prolonged rest angina necessitating an urgent intervention, (intra-aortic balloon counterpulsation, coronary angioplasty, or bypass surgery) was considered an end-point. Chest pain without acute ECG changes, even if suggestive of ischemia, was not considered an end-point unless this pain prompted coronary revascularization.

2. *Myocardial infarction:* The presence of prolonged chest pain unrelieved by nitroglycerin, associated with new and persistent ST-T wave changes or Q-waves, *and* a rise in serum creatine kinase (CK) to two times above the upper limit of normal, or an increase of 50% or more in CK activity above the preceding sample but at least 1.5 times the upper limit of normal was required for the diagnosis of infarction. Perioperative myocardial infarction was identified by a combination of ECG criteria, *and* enzyme criteria. In this setting, the CK MB must have been greater than 50 mμ/mL when the normal reference was 15–16 mμ/mL.

3. *Total deaths:* All deaths regardless of etiology. Fatal myocardial infarction, or sudden death from which the patient was resuscitated, was counted as a death.

Protocol Deviations

Analysis of serial electrocardiograms and enzymes revealed that 19 patients had an evolving transmural myocardial infarction. One was anterior and the remaining 18 were true posterior wall infarctions. In 17 patients, trial therapy was discontinued prematurely by the personal physician who referred the patients to a revascularization procedure even though there had been no recurrent ischemia on trial therapy.

Statistics

Analyses of events were performed under the principle of intention to treat. In addition, a secondary analysis was performed censoring events at the time a patient withdrew from ATACS therapy (efficacy analysis). Comparison of time to event was displayed using Kaplan-Meier plots of percent free of event. Therapy groups were compared using a log rank statistic separately for patients who had not had aspirin prior to entry (Trial A), and patients who had used aspirin (Trial B). Comparison of baseline characteristics was performed using a chi square statistic or t-test as appropriate. A P value of less than 0.05 was considered significant.

Results

Three hundred fifty-eight patients were randomized; 214 had not been taking aspirin prior to admission (Trial A), and 144 had (Trial

B). Among the non-prior aspirin users, 109 were randomized to receive aspirin and 105 to receive a combination of aspirin plus anticoagulation (heparin followed by warfarin). Among prior aspirin users, 72 were randomized to receive controlled release aspirin plus anticoagulation, and 72 were randomized to receive conventional aspirin plus anticoagulation. The mean time from "qualifying pain" to randomization and treatment was 18.2 ± 19.8 hours.

Non-Prior Aspirin Users

Among non-prior aspirin users, baseline characteristics were similar between the two treatment groups with the exception of history of hypertension and diastolic blood pressure at entry (Table 1). More patients with a history of hypertension were assigned to aspirin alone than to aspirin plus anticoagulation (38% vs. 23%, P = .02), and they had a higher diastolic blood pressure (79 mm Hg vs. 75 mm Hg, P = .02). The mean age of the 214 non-prior aspirin users was 61 years. Sixty-seven percent were male. One hundred forty-seven were admitted for unstable angina, 46 with a non-Q-wave myocardial infarction, and 16 with an evolving Q-wave infarction. Five patients had no cardiac enzyme information.

Thirty-one patients (28%) assigned to aspirin alone experienced a primary event, compared to 20 patients (19%) assigned to aspirin plus anticoagulation; P = .10 by log rank statistic after adjusting for history of hypertension and diastolic blood pressure at entry (Table 2, Figure 2). When exposure was censored at the time that a patient discontinued trial therapy, 27 patients (25%) assigned to aspirin experienced a primary event compared to 14 patients (13%) assigned to aspirin plus anticoagulation; P = .03 by log rank statistic after adjusting for history of hypertension and diastolic blood pressure at entry. If the study had been designed as an acute phase trial limiting exposure to 14 days, analysis by intention to treat would have shown a significant benefit for combination therapy (Table 3); 27% of patients assigned to aspirin experienced a primary event versus 10% of patients assigned to combination therapy (P = .002 by log rank statistic, after adjusting for history of hypertension and diastolic blood pressure at entry).

Withdrawal from therapy or occurrence of a secondary end-point, occurred in 26% of patients assigned to aspirin alone and in 43% of patients assigned to combination therapy prior to the end of the 12 weeks of follow-up. The reasons for withdrawal of therapy varied (Table 4). Compliance to aspirin therapy was adequate; patients took their tablets, on average, 80% of the time.

Table 1
Characteristics of Patient Population (Trial A)

	ASA *N = 109*	*ASA +* *Hep/War* *N = 105*	*Signif*
Demographic Characteristics			
Male (%)	63	72	ns
Mean age (years)	63	60	.06
Ethnic group (%)			
White	91	95	
Black	2	3	
Other	7	2	ns
Current smoker (%)	36	34	ns
Baseline Clinical History			
Hx of hypertension (%)	38	23	.02
Hx of diabetes (%)	7	9	ns
Hx stroke or TIA (%)	0	3	.07
Family hx of heart disease (%)	45	45	ns
Angina prior to last 4 wks (%)	45	53	ns
Hx myocardial infarction (%)	24	32	ns
Prior coronary angiogram (%)	10	11	ns
Prior PTCA (%)	1	2	ns
Prior CABG (%)	4	2	ns
Prior positive ETT (%)	61	48	ns
Baseline Clinical Characteristics			
Mean systolic BP (mmHg)	133	130	ns
Mean diastolic BP (mmHg)	79	75	.02
Cardiomegaly (%)	11	14	ns
LV hypertrophy on ECG (%)	2	6	ns
RBBB (%)	2	5	ns
Admission diagnosis:			
Unstable angina (N)	76	71	ns
Non Q-wave MI (N)	22	24	
Evolving Q-wave MI (N)	10	6	
Not classified	3	2	
Antianginal Medications at Study Entry			
Beta blockers (%)	31	21	.08
Calcium channel blockers (%)	22	27	ns
Admission ECG Findings			
Ischemic ST-T wave changes (%)	64	61	ns
New ST or T wave changes that reversed with NTG (%)	22	25	ns

Hx = history; MI = myocardial infarction; BP = blood pressure; Hep = heparin; War = warfarin.

Table 2
Primary End-Points (Trial A)

	ASA N = 109		*ASA + Hep/War N = 105*		
	No.	*Pct*	*No.*	*Pct*	*Signif**
Primary End-Point					
No event	78	72	85	81	
Event	31	28	20	19	.09
Recurrent Angina with ECG Changes or Prompting Intervention					
No event	89	82	93	89	
Event	20	18	12	11	ns
Myocardial Infarction					
No event	100	92	99	94	
Event	9	8	6	6	ns
All Deaths					
No event	107	98	103	98	
Event	2	2	2	2	ns

* After adjustment for history of hypertension and diastolic blood pressure at entry.

Prior Aspirin Users

Baseline characteristics for prior aspirin users were similar between the two treatment groups with the exception of history of prior stroke or transient ischemic attack, and cardiomegaly on chest X-ray (Table 5). More patients assigned to controlled release aspirin plus anticoagulation had a history of either prior stroke or TIA (15% vs. 4% of patients assigned to conventional aspirin plus anticoagulation), or cardiomegaly (29% vs. 14% of patients assigned to conventional aspirin plus anticoagulation). The mean age of the 144 prior aspirin users was 63 years. Seventy-three percent were male. One hundred twenty-one were admitted with unstable angina, 16 with a non-Q-wave myocardial infarction and three with an evolving Q-wave infarction. Four patients had no cardiac enzyme information.

There was no difference in outcome between controlled release aspirin versus conventional aspirin in combination with anticoagulation in this population (Table 6, Figure 3). Adjustment for co-variates not balanced by randomization (prior stroke or TIA and cardiomegaly) did not change these results.

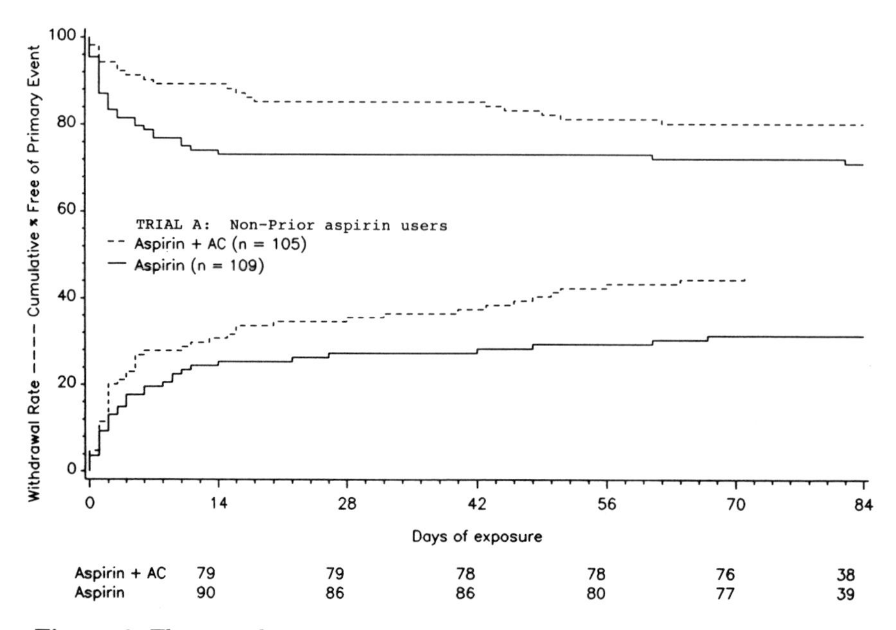

Figure 2: The cumulative percent of patients free of any primary end-point in non-prior aspirin users (Trial A). Also depicted in the bottom half of the panel is the withdrawal rate from trial therapy.

The rate of withdrawal from trial therapy was 26% in patients assigned to controlled release aspirin plus anticoagulation and 32% in patients assigned to conventional aspirin plus anticoagulation. The reasons for withdrawal varied (Table 7). Compliance to aspirin therapy was similar in this group compared to non-prior aspirin users with patients taking at least 80% of expected tablets.

Non-Q-Wave Myocardial Infarction

Based on an elevated admission serum creatine kinase, 62 patients were classified as having an admission non-Q-wave myocardial infarction. Forty-six patients entered Trial A and 16 entered Trial B. In specific, in Trial A, there were 22 patients assigned to aspirin alone and 24 assigned to aspirin plus anticoagulation. All of the events occurred in the first 14 days. The Kaplan-Meier estimate for percent free of primary events at 14 days for patients assigned to aspirin alone

Table 3
Primary End-Points Analysis and Time to Event (Trial A)

	ASA N = 109		*ASA + Hep/War N = 105*		
	No.	*Pct*	*No.*	*Pct*	*Signif**
Primary End-Point (12 weeks)					
Intention to Treat					
No event	78	72	85	81	
Event	31	28	20	19	.09
Primary End-Point (12 weeks)					
Efficacy					
No event	82	75	91	87	
Event	27	25	14	13	.06
Primary End-Point (14 day)					
Intention to Treat					
No event	80	73	94	90	
Event	29	27	11	11	.004
Primary End-Point (30 days)					
Intention to Treat					
No event	80	73	90	86	
Event	29	27	15	14	.03

* After adjustment for history of hypertension and diastolic blood pressure at entry.

was 68.2% (95% confidence interval 44.6–83.4), versus 83.3% (95% CI 61.5–93.4) in patients assigned to combination therapy. The number of non-Q-infarct patients in Trial B was too small for statistical comparison.

Monitoring the level of anticoagulation in patients assigned to warfarin (in both Trial A and Trial B), revealed a median International Normalized Ratio (INR) value of 2.2 over the 12-week period. Fifty percent of the INR values fell between 1.9 and 2.7, and 90% between 1.4 and 3.7. There were no spontaneous (unrelated to coronary revascularization) major bleeds in the Trial A patients assigned to aspirin alone therapy. In contrast, in the patients assigned to combination therapy the major bleeding rate was 2.9%. The major bleed rate in Trial B patients, all of whom received a combination antithrombotic therapy, averaged 3.0%. The frequency of minor bleeds or medication intolerance in the Trial A patients assigned to aspirin alone therapy was 2.8%. In contrast, the average frequency of minor bleeds or medica-

Table 4
Reasons for Withdrawal of Trial Therapy (Trial A)

	ASA N = 109		*ASA + Hep/War N = 105*	
	Number	*Pct*	*Number*	*Pct*
Withdrawal or Secondary End-Point				
No	81	74	62	59
Yes	28	26	43	41
Evolving Q wave Infarct	10	9.2	6	5.7
Major bleed	0	0	3	2.9
PTCA not prompted by recurrent pain	3	2.8	3	2.9
CABG not prompted by recurrent pain	4	3.7	1	1.0
Stroke	1	.9	0	0
Normal coronary arteries	2	1.8	4	3.8
Medication intolerance	3	2.8	7	6.7
Poor compliance	0	0	3	2.9
Patient request	0	0	4	3.8
Physician request	3	2.8	6	5.7
Other exclusions	2	1.8	6	5.7

tion intolerance for all patients assigned to combination therapy was 5.2%.

Discussion

In spite of several large scale, placebo-controlled trials in patients with the acute coronary syndromes of rest unstable angina or non-Q-wave myocardial infarction, several issues remain unresolved.

1. Is combination antithrombotic therapy with an antiplatelet agent and an anticoagulant better than the established benefit of either of these agents alone?

2. What is the impact of combination antithrombotic therapy on the ever-increasing proportion of patients, already taking aspirin, presenting with unstable angina or non-Q-wave infarction?

3. What is the impact of combination therapy on the acute coronary syndrome of non-Q-wave myocardial infarction?

4. If combination antithrombotic therapy is better, is it an effective

Table 5
Characteristics of Prior Aspirin Users (Trial B)

	CR-ASA + Hep/War N = 72	*Conv ASA + Hep/War N = 72*	*Signif*
Demographic Characteristics			
Male (%)	75	71	ns
Mean age (years)	63	62	ns
Ethnic Group			
White (%)	94	90	ns
Black	0	3	
Other	6	7	
Current smoker (%)	23	23	ns
Baseline Clinical History			
Hx of hypertension (%)	49	33	.05
Hx of diabetes (%)	6	11	ns
Hx stroke or TIA (%)	15	4	.03
Family hx of heart disease (%)	42	47	ns
Angina prior to last 4 wks (%)	75	74	ns
Hx Myocardial infarction (%)	49	54	ns
Prior Coronary angiogram (%)	32	37	ns
Prior PTCA (%)	4	6	ns
Prior CABG (%)	17	16	ns
Prior Positive ETT (%)	39	41	ns
Baseline Clinical Characteristics			
Mean Systolic BP (mm Hg)	129	130	ns
Mean Diastolic BP (mm Hg)	76	76	ns
Cardiomegaly (%)	29	14	.03
LV hypertrophy by ECG (%)	4	7	ns
RBBB (%)	1	7	ns
Admission diagnosis:			
Unstable angina (N)	64	57	ns
Non Q-wave MI (N)	7	9	
Evolving Q-wave MI (N)	1	2	
Not classified (N)	0	4	
Antianginal Medications at Study Entry			
Beta blockers (%)	44	60	.05
Calcium channel blockers (%)	48	39	ns
Admission ECG Findings:			
Ischemic ST-T wave changes (%)	59	57	ns
New ST or T wave changes that reversed with NTG (%)	23	24	ns

Hx = history; MI = myocardial in farction; BP = blood pressure; Hep = heparin; War = warfarin.

Table 6
Primary End-Points in Prior Aspirin Users (Trial B)

	CR ASA + Hep/War N = 72		*ASA + Hep/War N = 72*		
	No.	*Pct*	*No.*	*Pct*	*Signif*
Primary End-Points					
No event	51	71	51	71	1.0
Event	21	29	21	29	
Recurrent Angina with ECG Changes or Prompting Intervention					
No event	58	81	54	75	NS
Event	14	19	18	25	
Myocardial Infarction					
No event	70	97	69	96	
Event	2	3	3	4	NS
All Deaths					
No event	67	93	72	100.0%	
Event	5	7	0		NS

and safe "medical" regimen over the long term (post hospital discharge)?

Non-Prior Aspirin Users

The present study based on the investigations of the Antithrombotic Therapy in Acute Coronary Syndromes Research Group[16,17] is the first large-scale trial of patients with acute coronary syndromes to dichotomize patients into non-prior aspirin users versus conventional aspirin failures. In an earlier pilot trial conducted in the United States,[14] we observed a 31% rate of prior aspirin use in patients presenting with rest unstable angina. In the current trial which began in 1989, the rate increased to 40% (144/358).

In patients not already taking aspirin, our data suggest that combination antithrombotic therapy significantly reduces the incidence of primary ischemic events in the early phase (first 14 days). However, by 90 days, there is only a trend favoring combination therapy. If one censors the events that occurred after withdrawal from trial therapy, a significant benefit appears in favor of combination therapy at 90

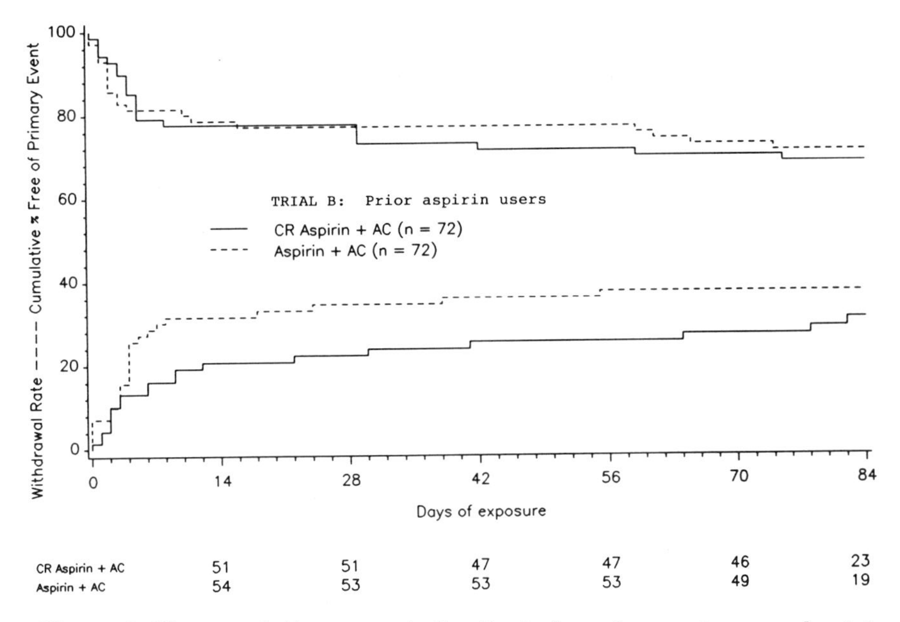

Figure 3: The cumulative percent of patients free of any primary end-point in prior aspirin users (Trial B). Also depicted in the bottom half of the panel is the withdrawal rate from trial therapy.

days. It is possible that the power to detect a significant difference at 90 days using an intention-to-treat analysis was too small given our sample size.

Combination therapy for unstable angina or non-Q-wave infarction has been prospectively evaluated in only three prior studies.[5,6,14] The trial by Theroux et al.[5] was the first randomized comparison of different antithrombotic regimens including combination therapy with aspirin plus heparin in patients with unstable angina. Trial therapy was terminated after a mean follow-up of 6 days. Combination therapy with aspirin plus heparin was significantly better than placebo; however, there were no statistically significant differences in recurrent ischemic events between the combination group versus the heparin alone or aspirin alone treatment limbs.[5] More recently, these investigators extended their studies in order to directly compare antithrombotic treatment with aspirin alone versus continuous intravenous heparin alone for 4 to 5 days.[8] They observed significantly fewer infarctions in the heparin-treated group compared to the aspirin-treated group.

The RISC study group[6,18] conducted a 90-day study of combination

Table 7
Reasons for Withdrawal of Trial Therapy in Prior Aspirin Users (Trial B)

	CR ASA + Hep/War N = 72		*ASA + Hep/War N = 72*	
	Number	*Pct*	*Number*	*Pct*
Withdrawal or Secondary End-Point				
No	53	74	49	68
Yes	19	26	23	32
Evolving Q-wave infarct	1	1.4	2	2.8
Major bleed	2	2.8	1	1.4
PTCA, no pain	0	0	1	1.4
CABG, no pain	2	2.8	3	4.2
Normal coronary arteries	2	2.8	1	1.4
Medication intolerance	4	5.6	2	2.8
Poor compliance	0	0	2	2.8
Patient request	2	2.8	2	2.8
Physician request	3	4.2	7	9.7
Other exclusions	3	4.2	2	2.8

low-dose aspirin (75 mg daily) and heparin, versus aspirin alone, or heparin alone in patients with either unstable angina or non-Q-wave infarction. The heparin in the combination group was continued for only 5 days. The combination of aspirin and short-term heparin resulted in the lowest rate of events at 5 days, but there were no significant differences in recurrent ischemic events between the combination group versus the aspirin alone treatment limbs.[6]

The three trials[5,6,16] using combination antithrombotic therapy versus aspirin alone demonstrated a similar relative risk reduction in infarction or death occurring within the first 5 days. The pooled estimate of the relative risk combining observed results from the three studies (calculated using the method of Mantel-Haenszel[19]) for infarction or death among patients treated with combination antithrombotic therapy compared to aspirin alone was 0.41 (95% confidence interval 0.20–0.99) (Table 8).

The higher ischemic event rate experienced in our study compared to the RISC study or those of Theroux et al. may be partially explained by the fact that randomization and treatment in our study occurred at the time of admission in the emergency room. In the RISC study[6]

Table 8
Pooled Analysis of Relative Risk of Combination Therapy Versus Aspirin Alone

	ATACS[16]		RISC[6]		Theroux et al.[5]		
	ASA n = 109	ASA + HEP n = 105	ASA n = 189	ASA + HEP n = 210	ASA n = 121	ASA + HEP n = 122	RR_{mh} (CI)
MI/Death	9 (8.3%)	4 (3.8%)	7 (3.7%)	3 (1.4%)	4 (3.3%)	2 (1.6%)	.44 (.21 – .93)

* CI = 95% confidence interval

randomization was allowed up to 72 hours after hospital admission. In the Theroux studies[5,8] only the events occurring within the first 5 days were counted and patients with non-Q-wave infarction were excluded. Our data indicate that recurrent ischemic events may occur within days of onset of pain. Therefore, any delay in randomization may overlook patients with early recurrent ischemia and artificially reduce the total number of events.

Prior Aspirin Users

The study of Cohen et al.[17] is the first blinded, prospective trial of antithrombotic therapy in patients with rest unstable angina who were aspirin users. Since these patients failed conventional aspirin, they provide a model to evaluate the impact of preserving prostacyclin synthesis during platelet inhibition. We observed no significant difference between the prostacyclin-sparing, combination antithrombotic regimen, versus the conventional combination regimen. It is possible that the endothelium around the plaque rupture site which triggered the acute coronary syndrome is too abnormal to benefit from any prostacyclin-sparing interventions. The primary event rate of 29% in the prior aspirin users was slightly higher than the overall rate of 24% for the non-prior users.

Combination antithrombotic therapy with prostacyclin-sparing controlled release aspirin plus anticoagulants was also evaluated by Meade and colleagues in a long-term primary prevention trial of ischemic heart disease.[20] Primary end-point analysis is not yet available but the withdrawal rate for medication intolerance, with or without frank bleeding—4.2%, experienced in the Thrombosis Prevention Trial[21] was similar to the study of Cohen.[17]

Non-Q-Wave Myocardial Infarction

The impact of combination therapy on the subset of patients with non-Q-wave infarction paralleled that for patients with rest unstable angina in that there appeared to be a trend (not significant) in favor of combination therapy in patients who were non-prior aspirin users. It has been suggested that the stimulus for clot propagation in these patients is greater than in patients with unstable angina.[22] This may explain why in spite of initiating trial antithrombotic therapy in the emergency room, even in combination, almost all recurrent ischemic events, in patients with non-Q-wave infarction occurred within the first 14 days.[10]

Clinical Implications

In summary, it is our belief that the dynamic complex arterial lesions precipitating the acute coronary syndromes necessitate prompt and aggressive antithrombotic therapy with both aspirin and an anticoagulant, especially in non-prior aspirin users. In the absence of trials showing that urgent revascularization with either PTCA[23,24] or urgent coronary bypass surgery[25,26] reduces acute morbidity or improves long-term survival compared to aggressive medical management, we feel that the combination antithrombotic regimen with anti-anginals should become the standard early phase "medical" regimen for these acute coronary syndromes. A more effective antithrombotic therapy needs to be identified for prior aspirin users, and for patients with non-Q-wave infarction.

Editor's Note

Since submission of this chapter, another randomized trial of aspirin versus aspirin and continuous intravenous heparin in unstable angina has been reported (Holbrook et al, JACC 1994: 24:39–45). This study did not show a benefit for the combination of aspirin and heparin over aspirin alone. However, the event rate (myocardial infarction and death) was extraordinarily high (27.3% in the H + ASA group, n = 154, vs. 30.5% in the ASA group, n = 131). This rate is up to 20 times higher than that reported in Table 8 of this chapter. The reasons for this descrepancy are unclear.

References

1. Farhi JI, Cohen M, Fuster V. The broad spectrum of unstable angina pectoris and its implications for future controlled trials. Am J Cardiol 1986; 58: 547–550.
2. Lewis HD Jr, Davis JW, Archibald DG, Steinke WE, Smitherman TC, Doherty JE III, Schnaper HW, LeWinter MM, Linares E, Pouget JM, Sabharwal SC, Chesler E, DeMots H. Protective effects of aspirin against acute myocardial infarction and death in men with unstable angina. N Engl J Med 1983; 309:396–403.
3. Cairns JA, Gent M, Singer J, Finnie KJ, Froggatt GM, Holder DA, Jablonsky G, Kostuk WJ, Melendez LJ, Myers MG, Sackett DL, Sealey BJ, Tanser PH. Aspirin, sulfinpyrazone or both in unstable angina: results of a Canadian multicenter trial. N Engl J Med 1985; 313:1369–1375.
4. Williams DO, Kirby MG, McPherson K. Anticoagulant treatment in unstable angina. Br J Clin Pract 1986; 40:114–116.
5. Theroux P, Quimet H, McCans J, Latour JG, Joly P, Levy G, Pelletier E, Juneau M, Stasiak J, deGuise P, Pelletier GB, Rinzler D, Waters DD. Aspirin, heparin, or both to treat acute unstable angina. N Engl J Med 1988; 319:1105–1111.
6. Wallentin L for the RISC Group. Risk of myocardial infarction and death during treatment with low dose aspirin and intravenous heparin in men with unstable coronary artery disease. Lancet 1990; 336:827–830.
7. Neri Serneri GG, Gensini GF, Poggesi L, Trotta F, Modesti PA, Boddi M, Ieri A, Margheri M, Casolo GC, Bini M, Rostagno C, Carnovali M, Abbate R. Effect of heparin, aspirin, or alteplase in reduction of myocardial ischemia in refractory unstable angina. Lancet 1990; 335:615–618.
8. Theroux P, Waters D, Qui S, McCans J, deGuise P, Juneau M. Aspirin versus heparin to prevent myocardial infarction during the acute phase of unstable angina. Circulation 1993; 88(Part 1):2045–2048.
9. Klimt CR, Knatterud GL, Stamler J, Meier P. Persantine-Aspirin Reinfarction Study. Part II. Secondary coronary prevention with persantine and aspirin. J Am Coll Cardiol 1986; 7:251–269.
10. Cohen M, Xiong J, Parry G, Adams PC, Chamberlain D, Wieczorek I, Fox KAA, McBride R, Chesebro J, Fuster V, and the Anti-thrombotic therapy in Acute Coronary Syndromes Research Group. Prospective comparison of unstable angina versus non-Q-wave myocardial infarction during antithrombotic therapy. J Am Coll Cardiol 1993; 22; 1338–1343.
11. Ambrose JA, Winters SL, Stern A, Eng A, Teichholz LE, Gorlin R, Fuster V. Angiographic morphology and the pathogenesis of unstable angina pectoris. J Am Coll Cardiol 1985; 5:609–616.
12. Willerson JT, Hillis LD, Winniford M, Buja LM. Speculation regarding mechanisms responsible for acute ischemic heart disease syndromes. J Am Coll Cardiol 1986; 8:245–250.
13. Fuster V, Badimon L, Cohen M, Ambrose J, Badimon JJ, Chesebro JH. Insights into the pathogenesis of acute coronary syndromes. Circulation 1988; 77:1213–1220.
14. Cohen M, Adams PC, Hawkins L, Bach M, Fuster V. Usefulness of anti-

thrombotic therapy in resting angina pectoris or non-Q-wave myocardial infarction (a pilot study from the Antithrombotic Therapy in Acute Coronary Syndromes Study Group). Am J Cardiol 1990; 66:1287–1292.
15. Clarke RJ, Mayo G, Price P, FitzGerald GA. Suppression of thromboxane A_2 but not of systemic prostacyclin by controlled-release aspirin. N Engl J Med 1991; 325:1137–1141.
16. Cohen M, Adams PC, Parry G, Xiong J, Chamberlain D, Wieczorek I, Fox KAA, Chesebro JH, Strain J, Keller C, Kelly A, Lancaster G, Ali J, Kronmal R, Fuster V, and the Antithrombotic Therapy in Acute Coronary Syndromes Research Group. Combination antithrombotic therapy in unstable rest angina and non-Q-wave infarction in nonprior aspirin users: Primary end-points analysis from the ATACS trial. Circulation 1994; 89:81–88.
17. Cohen M, Parry G, Xiong J, Adams P, Chamberlain D, Fox K, Wieczorek I, McBride R, Chesebro J, Strain J, Fuster V, for ATACS. Double blind randomized trial of a prostacyclin-sparing aspirin formulation in rest angina and non-Q-wave infarction. J Am Coll Cardiol 1993; 21(Suppl-A): 269A.
18. Wallentin LC and the Research Group on Instability in Coronary Artery Disease in Southeast Sweden. Aspirin (75 mg/day) after an episode of unstable coronary artery disease: Long-term effects on the risk for myocardial infarction, occurrence of severe angina and the need for revascularization. J Am Coll Cardiol 1991; 18:1587–1593
19. Mantel N, Haenszel W. Statistical aspects of the analysis of data from retrospective studies of disease. JNCI 1959; 22:719–748.
20. Meade TW. Low-dose warfarin and low-dose aspirin in the primary prevention of ischemic heart dissease. Am J Cardiol 1990; 65:7C-11C.
21. Meade TW, Roderick PJ, Brennan PJ, Wilkes HC, Kelleher CC. Extracranial bleeding and other symptoms due to low-dose aspirin and low intensity oral anticoagulation. Thromb Haemost 1992; 68:1–6.
22. Fuster V, Badimon L, Cohen M, Ambrose J, Badimon JJ, Chesebro JH. Insights into the pathogenesis of acute coronary syndromes. Circulation 1988; 77:1213–1220.
23. Seggewiss H, Fassbender D, Vogt J, Minami K, Schmidt HK, Baller D, Gleichmann U. PTCA in stable and unstable angina: Primary success and complications in 1329 patients. Eur Heart J 1992; 13:126.
24. van den Brand M, van Zijl A, Geuskens R, de Feyter PJ, Serruys PW, Simoons ML. Tissue plasminogen activator in refractory unstable angina. A randomized double-blind placebo-controlled trial in patients with refractory unstable angina and subsequent angioplasty. Eur Heart J 1991; 12: 1208–1214.
25. McCormick JR, Schick EC, McCabe CH, Kronmal RA, Ryan TJ. Determinants of operative mortality and long-term survival in patients with unstable angina: the CASS experience. J Thorac Cardiovasc Surg 1985; 89: 683–688.
26. Curtis JJ, Walls JT, Salam NH, Boley TM, Nawarawong W, Schmaltz RA, Landreneau RJ, Madsen R. Impact of unstable angina on operative mortality with coronary revascularization at varying time intervals after myocardial infarction. J Thorac Cardiovasc Surg 1991; 102:867–873.

10

Novel Strategies for Platelet Inhibition in Acute Coronary Syndromes

Ari Ezratty, MD, John A. Ambrose, MD

Introduction

Pathological, clinical, and angiographic studies have implicated platelets and thrombosis in the pathogenesis of unstable coronary syndromes. Coronary angiography in patients with unstable angina is more likely to demonstrate complex, irregular lesions consistent with thrombosis compared to patients with chronic stable angina. While conventional antiplatelet agents have been shown to be effective in both the primary and the secondary prevention of vascular events, the existing agents are both nonselective and relatively impotent. Thus, novel antiplatelet and antithrombotic agents have been developed that possess specific activity directed at virtually every step leading to platelet adhesion and aggregation. These include serotonin receptor antagonists, prostanoid derivatives and antagonists, fibrinogen receptor antagonists, von Willebrand factor receptor antagonists, and selective thrombin inhibitors. Although the clinical utility of most of these agents in acute coronary syndromes has yet to be determined, it is likely that several of these agents will have an important impact on the treatment of patients with unstable coronary syndromes in the future. After a brief review of the pathways leading to platelet aggrega-

From: Ambrose JA (ed): *Complex Coronary Lesions in Acute Coronary Syndromes*.

tion, this chapter will focus on the mechanisms of action of the various new classes of antiplatelet agents and, when available, discuss the results of representative in vivo studies in animals and in man.

Pathological and Clinical Studies

Pathological and clinical studies have established that platelets and thrombosis play a central role in the pathogenesis of unstable coronary syndromes. Necropsy studies by Davies and colleagues have revealed platelet aggregates in up to 50% of those suffering sudden ischemic death.[1,2] In these patients, platelet thrombi localized only to segments of myocardium downstream of an atheromatous plaque that had ruptured and were associated with the presence of multifocal myocardial necrosis. Further pathological studies demonstrated that patients with unstable angina were more likely to have intramyocardial platelet emboli compared to patients with stable angina.[2]

Clinical evidence confining these pathological findings has been derived from the cardiac catheterization laboratory. Coronary angiographic morphology indicating complex plaques, such as eccentric or concentric lesions with overhanging edges, irregular borders, ulcerations, abrupt shoulders, and/or filling defects proximal or distal to a significant stenosis, are found in the majority of "culprit" lesions in unstable angina and only in a minority of lesions in stable angina.[3] These findings have been subsequently corroborated by coronary angioscopic data which demonstrated intracoronary thrombus in patients with unstable coronary syndromes.[4]

In conjunction with the pathological and morphological evidence that has accumulated supporting the role of platelets in unstable coronary syndromes, there have been many randomized trials of antiplatelet agents in the primary and secondary prevention of coronary artery disease since the early 1970s. A recent meta-analysis of 25 randomized trials of various antiplatelet agents (aspirin, dipyridamole, sulfinpyrazone, suloctidil) that included 29,000 patients revealed a highly statistically significant decrease in nonfatal myocardial infarction, stroke, total cardiovascular death, and overall mortality in patients treated with antiplatelet agents compared with placebo.[5] Three major trials have examined the effects of aspirin therapy in unstable angina pectoris. The VA Cooperative Study[6] randomized 1,266 male patients with unstable angina to aspirin therapy or placebo. A 51% reduction in 12-week mortality was demonstrated in patients treated with aspirin. The McMaster study,[7] which randomized 555 patients with unstable angina to aspirin, sulfinpyrazone, both agents, or neither agent, demonstrated a 50% reduction in mortality in aspirin-treated groups at 18 months, and no added benefit for sulfinpyrazone. Finally, Theroux and colleagues randomized 479 patients with unstable angina to aspirin and heparin.[8] Both the aspirin- and the heparin-treated patients demonstrated a profound reduction in cardiac events compared to placebo though sample sizes were too small to differentiate between aspirin and heparin groups.

Thus, data have accumulated from diverse sources to establish the importance of platelets and thrombosis in the genesis of unstable coronary syndromes. This has provided the impetus to investigate novel strategies of platelet inhibition that may offer the potential for selectivity and increased potency. The classes of antiplatelet agents that will be reviewed after a review of the mechanisms of platelet aggregation include: serotonin receptor antagonists, prostanoid derivatives and antagonists, von Willebrand factor receptor antagonists, fibrinogen receptor antagonists, and selective thrombin inhibitors.

Mechanisms of Platelet Aggregation

The platelet surface membrane is composed of the glycocalyx, which contains glycoproteins that are available for binding to adhesive proteins, and a phospholipid bilayer. The sequence of platelet-dependent hemostasis consists of platelet adhesion (which requires the presence of multimers of von Willebrand factor) to exposed subendothelium in the injured vessel wall followed by platelet aggregation and the eventual formation of a stable platelet-fibrin thrombus. Phospholipase C is activated during platelet adhesion liberating diacylglycerol and inositol triphosphate. Diacyglycerol is involved in platelet granule secretion while inositol triphosphate is a platelet agonist and calcium ionophore. The increase in intracellular calcium activates phospholipase A_2 which releases arachidonic acid from membrane phospholipid pools. Arachidonic acid is oxidized by cyclo-oxygenase, yielding prostaglandin endoperoxides (platelet agonists), and ultimately thromboxane A_2, an agonist of platelet aggregation and vasoconstrictor.

During the course of platelet adhesion and aggregation, platelet granule contents are released from dense bodies and alpha granules. The contents of these granules include: ADP, serotonin, calcium, thrombospondin, platelet-derived growth factor, tissue growth factor beta, fibroblast growth factor, platelet factor 4, and beta-thromboglobulin. The aggregation of platelets requires a calcium-dependent conformational change in the glycoprotein IIb/IIIa complex that facilitates the binding of fibrinogen to this receptor. When exposed and activated, this receptor is capable of binding fibrinogen, fibronectin, von Willebrand factor, thrombospondin, and vitronectin. Interestingly, all of these proteins contain the tripeptide sequence arg-gly-asp (RGD) which represents a consensus sequence critical for ligand binding to the IIb/IIIa receptor. Thus, the formation of a stable platelet thrombus is quite complex but offers the opportunity for intervention at many steps along the cascade leading to platelet aggregation (Figures 1, 2).

Serotonin Receptor Antagonists

Serotonin is released from dense bodies in platelets during the course of platelet activation thereby enhancing the platelet aggregatory response at sites of vessel injury and inducing local vasoconstriction. These actions are mediated through specific serotonin receptors on the platelet surface.[9] Although numerous studies have demonstrated serotonin to be important in the induction of platelet aggregation responses in whole blood and in platelet-rich plasma,[10] data showing an independent effect of serotonin antagonists on in vitro platelet aggregation or on in vivo models of thrombosis are still scarce.

Willerson et al. evaluated the contribution of serotonin to cyclic flow variations, which are dependent on recurrent platelet thrombus formation in vivo.[11–14] The serotonin receptor antagonist, ketanserin, was compared to thromboxane receptor antagonists in a canine model of coronary thrombosis. Ketanserin abolished cyclic flow variations in 8 of 10 dogs while two different thromboxane receptor antagonists eliminated cyclic flow variations in 14 of 17 animals. Golino et al. studied the combined effects of serotonin and thromboxane receptor antagonists on the incidence of reocclusion after thrombolysis. Interestingly, the combination of ketanserin with SQ29548, a thromboxane A_2 receptor antagonist, was significantly more efficacious in the reduction of reocclusion and cyclic flow variations than any agent used alone.

Thus, serotonin may be an important mediator of platelet aggregation and thrombosis. However, the ubiquitous nature of serotonin, coupled with the fact that serotonin antagonists may have intolerable systemic side effects, argues for the use of more selective agents. Future trials will determine whether a combination of a serotonin receptor antagonist in a low dose with a thromboxane receptor antagonist will optimize platelet inhibition while limiting the systemic side effects.

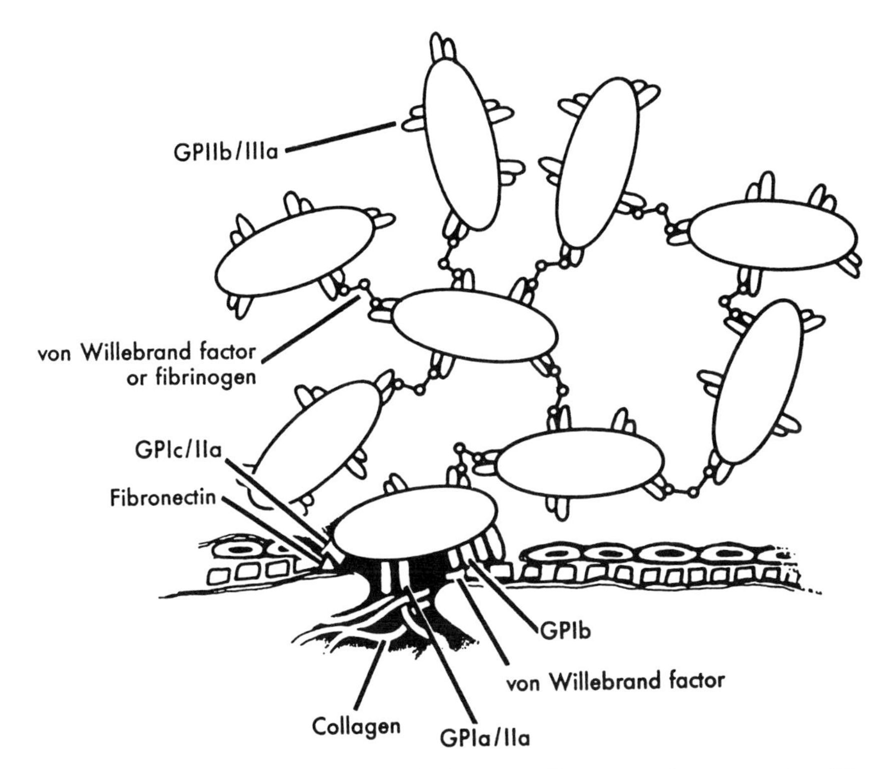

Figure 1: Schematic description of platelet adhesion and aggregation. The endothelium is a nonthrombogenic surface, but when it is damaged, adhesive glycoproteins such as collagen, von Willebrand factor, and fibrinonectin are exposed to the flowing blood. Platelets contain a number of different receptors on their surface that have a high affinity for the adhesive glycoproteins in the subendothelium, including GPIb, GPIa/IIa, and GPIc/IIa. After platelets adhere to the surface, their GPIIb/IIIa receptors undergo a transition that increases their affinity for several adhesive glycoproteins, with most evidence pointing to important roles for fibrinogen and von Willebrand factor, depending on the shear forces. In contrast to the multiplicity of receptors that may mediate platelet adhesion, at present it appears that all platelet aggregation is mediated by the GPIIb/IIIa receptor. (Used with permission from the author, Coller B, and Mosby Year Book Inc.)

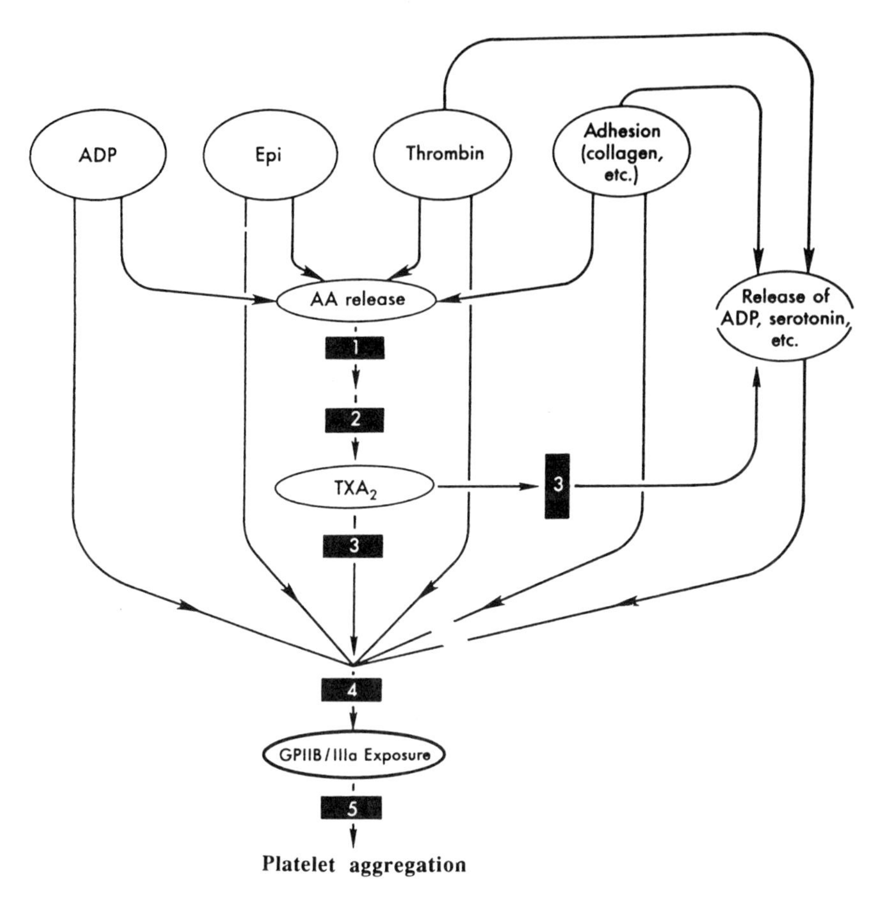

Figure 2: Platelet activation mechanisms leading to platelet aggregation. Several of the major agonists thought to operate in vivo are indicated, including adenosine diphosphate (ADP), epinephrine (Epi), and thrombin. In addition, platelet adhesion, whether mediated by collagen or other immobilized adhesive glycoproteins found in the subendothelium or in pathological lesions, is another potent stimulus for platelet activation. All of these agonists can cause arachidonic acid (AA) release, but even if the arachidonic pathway is blocked, they can all produce GPIIb/IIIa receptor exposure and platelet aggregation by bypass mechanisms. Arachidonic acid is metabolized to thromboxane A_2 (TXA_2) by the enzyme cyclo-oxgenase (box 1) and thromboxane synthase (box 2). Thromboxane A_2 can interact with its receptor (box 3) and produce the release of platelet agonists (e.g., ADP and serotonin) from specific platelet granules, which in turn augment aggregation. Two agonists, thrombin and collagen, can cause the release of the contents of platelet-storage granules even when the arachidonic acid pathway is blocked. The final pathway leading to the exposure of GPIIb/IIIa can be inhibited by increasing platelet cyclic AMP (box 4). Block-

Continued

Prostacyclin and Analogs

Endothelial cells produce prostacyclin from prostanoid endoperoxides generated from arachidonic acid through the action of several enzymes culminating in prostacyclin synthetase. Prostacyclin mediates vasodilation and platelet inhibition by increasing intracellular cyclic AMP and serves to counteract the vasoconstrictor and platelet aggregatory responses produced by thromboxane A_2. In in vitro models of ischemia, prostacyclin has been shown to reduce oxygen consumption and the release of lysosomal enzymes thereby limiting infarct size.[15–17]

Despite the early promise for prostacyclin, recent data gathered from in vivo trials have been less optimistic. Nicolini et al. examined the effects of the prostacyclin analog iloprost, on t-PA-induced thrombolysis in a canine model of thrombosis.[18] Similar reperfusion rates were achieved by the study group (t-PA plus iloprost) and the control group (t-PA alone). However, there was an increase in the time to reperfusion, a decrease in the duration of reperfusion, and increased reocclusion rates in all animals treated with iloprost. These findings were surprisingly associated with plasma levels of t-PA that were 30% lower in the iloprost group compared to the control group. Two mechanisms for this finding have been postulated: increased t-PA metabolism due to the increase in hepatic blood flow induced by iloprost, or alternatively, the induction of a coronary steal phenomenon whereby blood flow is increased preferentially to patent arteries thereby reducing the local concentration of t-PA at sites of thrombosis.[19]

The potential beneficial effects of prostacyclin in acute myocardial infarction[15–17] have been reported and are outweighed by the systemic side effects including hypotension and nausea, which have limited its widespread use. Likewise, iloprost, which has been shown to produce profound inhibition of ADP-induced platelet aggregation, has been

←

ade of the GPIIb/IIIa receptor can inhibit platelet aggregation by preventing the binding of fibrinogen or other adhesive glycoproteins. This inhibition of platelet aggregation can be achieved by blocking cyclo-oxygenase (e.g., with aspirin; box 1), blocking thromboxane synthase (box 2) with specific inhibitors, blocking the receptor that mediates the effect of thromboxane A_2 (box 3), increasing the production of intraplatelet cyclic AMP (e.g., with prostacyclin; box 4) or blocking the GPIIb/IIIa receptor (e.g., with monoclonal antibodies or peptides containing the recognition sequences found in the adhesive glycoproteins (box 5). (Used with permission from the author, Coller B, and the New England Journal of Medicine.)

troubled by the induction of nausea and systemic hypotension[20] in a trial in 14 patients with acute myocardial infarction. The use of prostaglandin E_1 (PGE_1), a cyclic AMP-dependent platelet inhibitor and vasodilator that stabilizes lysosomes and neutrophils, has been reported in 14 males with acute myocardial infarction in combination with intracoronary streptokinase.[21] The rates and times to lysis were improved in patients treated with the combination of agents compared with streptokinase alone. In addition, the does of streptokinase needed to produce reperfusion was lower in the PGE_1-treated patients than in the control group. Hypotension and systemic adverse effects were not a significant problem in this nonrandomized trial. Thus, the use of the available prostacyclin analogs, while theoretically promising, has not proven to be easily administered or clearly effective as antiplatelet agents in acute coronary syndromes. Given the early promise of PGE_1, further randomized studies are indicated to evaluate its efficacy in acute coronary syndromes.

Thromboxane A_2 Antagonists

Studies have demonstrated that in vivo thrombosis and platelet activation are associated with the release of thromboxane A_2 into the circulation. Thromboxane metabolites can be detected in the urine of patients with unstable angina.[22] In addition, it has recently been shown that thromboxane A_2 is released as a consequence of thrombolysis[23] due to platelet activation induced by plasmin, thrombin, or both. These data have provided the impetus to examine the effects of thromboxane A_2 antagonists on platelet aggregation and in in vivo models of thrombosis. Thromboxane synthetase inhibitors may offer an advantage over cyclo-oxygenase inhibitors by allowing the synthesis of prostacyclin to continue unabated in endothelial cells. Furthermore, the inhibition of thromboxane synthetase allows the intraplatelet pool of endoperoxidases to be shunted to the production of prostacyclin. Contrary to previous belief, low-dose aspirin will not selectively inhibit thromboxane synthesis and potentiate prostacyclin action. Therefore, this class of agents has the potential for increased vasodilatory platelet inhibitory effects compared with cyclo-oxygenase inhibitors.

A recent trial tested the thromboxane synthetase inhibitor sulatroban and its effects on t-PA-induced thrombolysis in a well-studied canine model of thrombosis.[24] Sulatroban inhibits thromboxane synthetase thereby reducing thromboxane A_2-mediated platelet aggregation and vasoconstrictor responses. Sulatroban produced a statistically significant, dose-related reduction in the time to lysis when compared with t-PA alone. In addition, reocclusion rates were decreased from 83% in the animals treated with t-PA alone to 11% in the animals treated with the combination of sulatroban plus t-PA. As mentioned previously, a recent trial that investigated the combination of a thromboxane A_2 receptor antagonist (SQ29548) with a serotonin receptor antagonist (ketanserin)[13] found that the combination of agents compared favorably with either agent alone in the prevention of reocclusion after t-PA in a dog model. Thus, combinations of specific antiplatelet agents may ultimately prove more beneficial than single agent therapy either by additive or frankly synergistic mechanisms.

Fibrinogen Receptor Antagonists

A-RGD Peptides

The binding of fibrinogen to the platelet glycoprotein IIb/IIIa receptor represents the final common pathway leading to platelet aggregation. The tripeptide sequence arg-gly-asp (RGD) is present in all ligands for this receptor including fibrinogen and mediates primary binding of the ligands to the platelet receptor. In order to produce an antagonist to glycoprotein IIb/IIIa there have been numerous attempts at synthesis of peptides, as well as isolation and purification of naturally occurring proteins containing this tripeptide sequence.

Bitistatin is derived from the venom of the viper *Bitis arietans* and is an 83-amino acid protein that contains the RGD sequence at residues 64–66. It is similar to two other compounds, trigramin and echistatin, also present in snake venoms.[25] In early experimental trials, bitistatin has shown very potent inhibition of fibrinogen binding to platelets similar to that observed with monoclonal antibodies directed at this receptor.[26] In addition, bitistatin inhibited platelet-dependent arterial cyclic flow variations ex vivo in a dose-dependent fashion. In contrast to monoclonal antibodies, the effects of bitistatin and other RGD peptides are reversible within 3 hours of cessation of the agent.

Bitistatin has been shown to influence the rate of t-PA-induced thrombolysis and reocclusion in a canine model[27] of coronary thrombosis. In this trial, five different treatment groups were investigated: (1) t-PA alone, (2) t-PA plus heparin, (3) t-PA plus heparin plus bitistatin, (4) t-PA plus bitistatin, and (5) no therapy. The combination of t-PA plus heparin plus bitistatin significantly increased the incidence of reperfusion, decreased the time to lysis, and decreased the rate of reocclusion compared to t-PA alone. These results were not observed in the groups treated with either heparin or bitistatin alone. The reocclusion rate observed in dogs treated with the combination of agents was reduced compared with t-PA alone, but still approached 20%. All groups treated with bitistatin demonstrated marked inhibition of platelet aggregation and three- to fourfold reversible prolongation of ternplate bleeding times. Schulman and co-workers recently reported that integrelin, another inhibitor of fibrinogen binding to glycoprotein IIb/IIIa, significantly reduced the number and duration of ischemic episodes in patients with unstable angina as evidenced by ST-segment changes on Holter monitoring.[28] Further evaluation of these agents is warranted in large-scale randomized trials of patients with unstable coronary syndromes.

Trigramin is a naturally occurring peptide of 72 amino acids purified from *Trimeresurus granieneus* which contains the RGD sequence and shares homologous sequences with von Willebrand factor, collagen, and laminin.[29] In in vitro experiments, trigramin has been shown to inhibit binding of human von Willebrand factor and fibrinogen to platelet glycoprotein IIb/IIIa in a dose-dependent manner.

In addition to the naturally occurring, purified, antithrombotic peptides that are under investigation, there are now several nonpeptide antagonists to platelet glycoprotein IIb/IIIa that are being evaluated for safety and efficacy in cohorts of patients with unstable coronary syndromes and those undergoing angioplasty.

B-Monoclonal Antibodies to Glycoprotein IIb/IIIa

Monoclonal antibodies to the glycoprotein IIb/IIIa receptor have recently been introduced into clinical trials. These agents similar to the RGD peptides compete with fibrinogen for binding to the fibrinogen receptor (glycoprotein IIb/IIIa) on platelets. However, unlike the RGD peptides, these antibodies bind with much greater affinity to the receptor. F(ab)'2 fragments are used in place of the intact antibody in order to prevent the removal of antibody-coated platelets by the spleen.[30,31] 7E3 and 10E5 (two different monoclonal antibodies to the IIb/IIIa receptor) abolished the periodic thrombus formation and platelet-dependent cyclic flow reductions in the Folt's model.[32] Treatment produced a dose-dependent inhibition of platelet aggregation to all agonists and caused a moderate increase in bleeding time.

The efficacy of 7E3 in combination with t-PA on the incidence of thrombolysis and reocclusion in a canine model of arterial thrombosis has been reported.[33] The combination of 7E3 (8 mg/kg) and a single bolus of t-PA (0.48 mg/kg) was associated with more rapid thrombolysis and no reocclusion when compared with t-PA alone. With this dose regimen, ADP-induced platelet aggregation was totally abolished and bleeding times were prolonged more than fourfold, persisting more than 30 minutes after infusion. Doses in the range of 0.1–0.4 mg/kg were not effective in the prevention of reocclusion, and bleeding time prolongation was much less marked. The effects of 7E3 on reocclusion rates after t-PA in a similar canine model of arterial thrombosis demonstrated that at an intravenous dose of 0.8 mg/kg, reocclusion was prevented in all dogs tested during a 2-hour observation period.[34] By contrast, treatment with aspirin, dipyridamole, or t-PA alone was associated with reocclusion in 5/7, 5/6, and 7/8 dogs, respectively.

The efficacy of 7E3 in 2,099 high-risk patients undergoing angioplasty has been investigated in the EPIC trial.[35] Patients were treated with aspirin and heparin and randomized to three treatment groups: (1) bolus 7E3 followed by 12-hour infusion, (2) bolus 7E3 followed by placebo infusion, and (3) placebo. There was a statistically significant improvement in the primary, combined end-point of death, myocardial infarction, stent implantation, urgent repeat angioplasty, or bypass surgery in the group treated with the bolus and infusion of 7E3 after a 30-day follow-up period. Specifically, the bolus and infusion resulted in a 35% reduction in the rate of primary end-points (12.8% vs. 8.3%) whereas the bolus alone resulted in a 10% reduction in the rate of primary end-point (12.8% vs. 11.5%). Thus, the EPIC trial has demonstrated that profound platelet inhibition with a glycoprotein IIb/IIIa antagonist can be given safely and prevents ischemic complications in high-risk patients undergoing angioplasty.*

Selective Thrombin Inhibitors

The generation of thrombin at sites of atherosclerotic plaque rupture catalyzes the conversion of fibrinogen to fibrin and is a potent mechanism by which platelets are activated in vivo. However, despite full-dose heparinization, reocclusion after thrombolysis or angioplasty occurs in up to 30% of patients.[36]** Alternative modes of thrombin inhibition[37–39] will be reviewed as they may be used in conjunction

*Editor's note: Other IIb/IIIa inhibitors are discussed in Chapter 12.
**Editor's note: This incidence of acute closure is obvioulsy extraordinarily high!

with standard platelet inhibitors and themselves serve as platelet inhibitors by impairing platelet aggregation induced by thrombin.

Argatroban is a synthetic, competitive thrombin inhibitor that has been shown to be more potent than heparin in the acceleration of thrombolysis and the prevention of reocclusion.[39] The effects of intravenous aspirin, argatroban, and 7E3 on thrombolysis, reocclusion, and bleeding after t-PA were compared in a canine model of arterial thrombosis.[40] Dogs treated with a combination of intravenous aspirin plus argatroban demonstrated decreased times to reflow and rates of reocclusion compared to animals treated with any single agent. Marked but reversible (within 1–3 hours) prolongation of bleeding time was noted in the group receiving the combination of aspirin plus argatroban which contrasted with the group receiving 7E3 in which the bleeding time abnormality was prolonged at 24 hours. D-phenylanalyl-L-prolyl-L-arginyl-chloromethyl-ketone (PPACK), an irreversible active site inhibitor of thrombin and other serine proteases, has been shown to decrease the deposition of fibrinogen and platelets in an animal model using arterial Dacron grafts.[41,42] However, the practical use of this agent may be limited by its relative lack of specificity.

The effect of recombinant hirudin, a specific thrombin inhibitor initially derived from the medicinal leech, has been examined in a porcine model of angioplasty.[43] Hirudin prevents thrombin-induced platelet aggregation, and inhibits the activation of factors V, VIII, and XIII thereby preventing fibrin formation and stabilization of fibrin-platelet thrombi. In the porcine in vivo model studied, hirudin reduced the deposition of platelets and fibrinogen at sites of deep arterial injury from carotid angioplasty, comparing favorably with high doses of heparin in the same model. A recent report by Abendschein and co-workers[44] investigated the efficacy of hirudin in a hypercholesterolemic swine carotid model of restenosis after balloon injury. Direct thrombin inhibition with hirudin was shown to be more effective in limiting luminal stenosis when compared with heparin despite equal, marked elevations of partial thromboplastin times in both groups. Meyer and co-workers[45] have recently demonstrated that thrombin inhibition with hirudin (but not heparin) significantly abolished thrombus progression on a pre-existing mural thrombus in a well-characterized porcine perfusion model of coronary stenosis.

Topol et al.[46] recently reported a pilot, multicenter, angiographic trial of recombinant hirudin in patients with unstable angina. Patients with unstable coronary syndromes and a baseline angiogram with evidence of intracoronary thrombus were randomized to either heparin or hirudin in a dose-escalating protocol. Patients treated with hirudin had significantly greater improvements in a cross-sectional area than those treated with heparin. The incidence of myocardial infarction in hirudin-treated patients (2.6%) compared favorably with that of patients treated with heparin (8%) although the sample size evaluated was too small to ascertain statistical significance.

Theroux et al.[47] characterized the antithrombotic effects of hirulog, a 20-amino acid synthetic thrombin inhibitor, in 40 patients with unstable angina. Hirulog predictably prolonged activated partial thromboplastin times and reduced fibrinopeptide A levels for the duration of the infusion. These findings were extended to the cohort of patients with acute myocardial infarction by Zeymer et al.[48] In the Thrombolysis and Myocardial Infarction (TIMI-7) study,[49] 410 patients with unstable angina were randomized to receive one of four doses of hirulog in combination with aspirin. The combined end-points of death, myocardial infarction, recurrent ischemia, or rapid clinical deterioration at 6 weeks' follow-up were significantly reduced in patients treated with higher doses (0.25–1.0 mg/kg/hr) of hirulog compared with those who received low doses (0.02 mg/kg/hr). Only one patient of the 410 patients enrolled experienced a major hemorrhagic episode. Whereas most previous reports have not been able to demonstrate additive effects of heparin when given with aspirin in patients with unstable angina, clinical outcomes at 6 weeks substantially improved in patients treated with the combination of aspirin and hirulog in higher doses. The results of the TIMI-5 trial which evaluated the efficacy of hirudin in conjunction with thrombolytic therapy and aspirin for acute myocardial infarction have been recently published.[50] Hirudin compared favorably to heparin as evidenced by improved infarct-related artery patency at 18–36 hours, a trend towards decreased reocclusion, and a reduction in in-hospital mortality and reinfarction without an increase in the incidence of hemorrhagic events. Thus, hirudin appears to be a promising adjunctive agent for the treatment of acute coronary syndromes. The TIMI-8 trial will investigate the efficacy of heparin versus hirulog in patients with unstable angina and non-Q-wave myocardial infarction.*

von Willebrand Factor Receptor Antatonists

Platelet aggregation induced by shear stress is dependent on large multimers of von Willebrand factor (vWF) and their binding to glyco-

*Editor's note: This trial has been canceled.

protein Ib (IX) and IIb/IIIa. Large vWF multimers originate from endothelial cells and are secreted in greater numbers from dysfunctional cells than from normal cells.[51,52] These findings have provided the impetus to investigate the utility of vWF and gylcoprotein Ib antagonists in models of platelet thrombosis. One such agent, aurin tricarboxylic acid, is a triphenylmethyl dye compound that binds to vWF and inhibits its binding to platelet glycoprotein Ib (IX) thereby inhibiting platelet adhesion and agglutination in a shear field. Aurin tricarboxylic acid abolished cyclic flow reductions in all animals in a Folt's model of platelet-dependent thrombus formation. Moreover, since stress-induced platelet aggregation proceeds independent of fibrinogen and arachidonic acid, cyclic flow reductions could not be restored following exposure to thromboxane A_2.[51] Aurin tricarboxylic acid produced no alterations in the hemodynamic or coagulation profile of any animal. Thus, the effective inhibition of glycoprotein Ib/IX-mediated platelet adhesion and agglutination by aurin tricarboxylic acid introduces a novel approach to platelet inhibition in situations of high shear.

Summary

The role of platelets in the pathophysiology of unstable coronary syndromes has been established and, until recently, aspirin has been the only antiplatelet agent with documented efficacy in reducing clinical event rates. With an ever-expanding knowledge of the pathways leading to platelet adhesion and aggregation, a multitude of new agents are becoming available that are directed at virtually every step in the cascade of platelet aggregation and thrombosis. These include: serotonin receptor antagonists, prostanoid derivatives and antagonists, fibrinogen receptor antagonists, selective thrombin inhibitors, and von Willebrand factor receptor antagonists. Further clinical trials are warranted to identify the agent or combination of selective anitplatelet and antithrombotic agents with the greatest efficacy and safety in the treatment of acute coronary syndromes.*

References

1. Davies MJ, Thomas AC, Knapman PA. Intramyocardial platelet aggregation in patients with unstable angina suffering sudden ischemic cardiac death. Circulation 1986; 73:418–427.

---

*Editor's note: Recent data give the edge to the IIb/IIIa inhibitors. However, more data are coming.

2. Davies MJ. A macro and micro view of coronary vascular insult in ischemic heart disease. Circulation 1990; (Suppl II):II-38–46.
3. Ambrose JA, Winters S, Stern A, et al. Angiographic lesion morphology and the pathogenesis of unstable angina. J Am Coll Cardiol 1985; 5: 629–638.
4. Sherman CT, Litvack F, Grundfest W, et al. Coronary angioscopy in patients with unstable angina pectoris. N Engl J Med 1986; 315:913–919.
5. Antiplatelet Trialists' Collaboration. Secondary prevention of vascular disease by prolonged antiplatelet treatment. Br Med J 1988; 296:320–331.
6. Lewis HD, Davis JW, Archibald DG, et al. Protective effects of aspirin against acute myocardial infarction and death in men with unstable angina. N Engl J Med 1983; 309:396.
7. Cairns JA, Gent M, Singer J, et al. Aspirin, sulfinpyrazone or both in unstable angina. N Engl J Med 1985; 312:1369.
8. Theroux P, Oimet H, McCans J, et al. Aspirin, heparin or both to treat acute unstable angina. N Engl J Med 1988; 319:1105–1111.
9. De Clerck F, Xhonneux B, Leysen J, et al. Evidence for functional 5-HT2 receptor sites on human blood platelets. Biochem Pharmacol 1984; 33: 2807.
10. Bevan J, Heptinstall S. Effects of combinations of 5-hydroxytryptamine receptor antagonists on 5-HT-induced human platelet aggregation. Arch Pharmacol 1986; 334:341.
11. Folts JD, Crowell EB, Rowe GG. Platelet aggregation in partially obstructed vessels and its elimination with aspirin. Circulation 1976; 54:365.
12. Folts JD, Gallagher K, Rowe GG. Blood flow reductions in stenosed canine coronary arteries: vasospasm or platelet aggregation? Circulation 1982; 65:248.
13. Golino P, Buja LM, Ashton JH, et al. Effect of thromboxane and serotonin receptor antagonists on intracoronary platelet deposition in dogs with experimentally stenosed coronary arteries. Circulation 1988; 78:701.
14. Ashton JH, Benedict CR, Fitzgerald C, et al. Serotonin as a mediator of cyclic flow variations in stenosed canine coronary arteries. Circulation 1986; 73:572.
15. Ogletree ML, Lefer AM, Smith JB, et al. Studies on the protective effect of prostacyclin in acute myocardial infarction. Eur J Pharmacol 1979; 56: 95.
16. Lefer AM, Ogletree ML, Smith JB. Prostacyclin: A potentially valuable agent for preserving myocardial tissue in acute myocardial ischemia. Science 1978; 200:52.
17. Melin JA, Becker LC. Salvage of ischemic myocardium by prostacyclin during experimental myocardial infarction. J Am Coll Cardiol 1983; 2: 279.
18. Nicolini FA, Mehta JL, Nichols WW, et al. Prostacyclin analogue iloprost decreases thrombolytic potential of tissue-type plasminogen activator in canine coronary thrombosis. Circulation 1990; 81:1115.
19. Hassan S, Pickles H. Epoprostenol (prostacyclin, PG12) increases apparent liver blood flow in man. Prostaglandins Leukot Med 1983; 10:449.
20. Swedberg K, Held P, Wadenvik H, et al. Central hemodynamic and antiplatelet effects of iloprost: a new prostacyclin analogue in acute myocardial infarction in man. Eur Heart J 1987; 8:362.

21. Sharma B, Wyeth RP, Gimenez HJ. Intracoronary prostaglandin E, plus streptokinase in acute myocardial infarction. Am J Cardiol 1986; 58:1161.
22. Fitzgerald DJ, Catella F, Fitzgerald C. Platelet activation in unstable coronary disease. N Engl J Med 1986; 315:983–989.
23. Fitzgerald DJ, Catella F, Roy F, et al. Marked platelet activation in vivo after intravenous streptokinase in patients with acute myocardial infarction. Circulation 1988; 77:142.
24. Shebuski RJ, Smith JM, Storer BL, et al. Influence of selective endoperoxide/thromboxane A_2 receptor antagonism with sulatroban on lysis time and reocclusion rate after tissue plasminogen activator-induced coronary thrombolysis in the dog. J Pharmacol Exp Ther 1988; 246:790.
25. Gan ZR, Gould RJ, Jacobs JW, et al. A potent platelet aggregation inhibitor from the venom of the viper, *Echis carinatus*. J Biol Chem 1988; 263:19–27.
26. Shebuski RJ, Ramjit DR, Bencen GH, et al. Characterization and platelet inhibitory activity of bitistatin, a potent RGD containing peptide from the viper, *Bitis arietans*. J Biol Chem 1989; 264:25–50.
27. Shebuski RJ, Stabilito IJ, Sitko GR, et al. Acceleration of recombinant tissue-type plasminogen activator-induced thrombolysis and prevention of reocclusion by the combination of heparin and the arg-gly-asp containing peptide bitistatin in a canine model of coronary thrombosis. Circulation 1990; 82:169.
28. Schulman SP, Clermont PJ, Navetta FI, et al. Integrelin in unstable angina: a double blind randomized trial. Circulation 1994: 88:32–72.
29. Huang T, Holt JC, Kirby EP, et al. Trigramin: Primary structure and its inhibition of von Willebrand factor binding to glycoprotein IIb/IIIa complex on human platelets. Biochem 1989; 28:661.
30. Coller BS, Folts JD, Scudder LE, et al. Antithrombotic effect of a monoclonal antibody to the platelet glycoprotein IIb/IIIa receptor in an experimental animal model. Blood 1986; 68:783.
31. Coller BS, Scudder LE. Inhibition of dog platelet function by in vivo infusion by F (ab')2 fragments of a monoclonal antibody to platelet glycoprotein IIb/IIIa receptor. Blood 1985; 66:1456.
32. Coller B, Folts JD, Smith SR, et al. Abolition of in vivo platelet thrombus formation in primates with monoclonal antibodies to the platelet GP IIb/IIIa receptor, correlation with bleeding time, platelet aggregation, and blockade of GP IIb/IIIa receptors. Circulation 1989; 80:1766.
33. Gold HK, Coller BS, Yasuda T, et al. Rapid and sustained coronary artery recanalization with combined bolus injection of recombinant tissue-type plasminogen activator and monoclonal antiplatelet GP IIb/IIIa antibody in a canine preparation. Circulation 1988; 77:670.
34. Yasuda T, Gold HK, Fallon JT, et al. Monoclonal antibody against the platelet glycoprotein IIb/IIIa receptor prevents coronary artery reocclusion after perfusion with recombinant tissue-type plasminogen activator in dogs. J Clin Invest 1988; 81:1284.
35. EPIC Investigators. Use of a monoclonal antibody directed against the platelet glycoprotein IIb/IIIa receptor in high risk coronary angioplasty. N Engl J Med 1994; 330:14:956–962.
36. Topol EJ, Morris DC, Smalling RW, et al. A multicenter, randomized placebo controlled trial of a new form of intravenous recombinant tissue-type

plasminogen activator in acute myocardial infarction. J Am Coll Cardiol 1987; 9:1205.
37. Verstraete M, Arnold AR, Brower RW, et al. Acute coronary thrombolysis with recombinant human tissue-type plasminogen activator: initial patency and influence of maintained infusion on reocclusion rate. Am J Cardiol 1987; 60:231.
38. Johns JA, Gold HK, Leinbach RC, et al. Prevention of coronary artery reocclusion and reduction in late coronary artery stenosis after thrombolytic therapy in patients with acute myocardial infarction. Circulation 1988; 78:546.
39. Jang IK, Gold HK, Ziskind AA, et al. Prevention of platelet rich arterial thrombosis by selective thrombin inhibition. Circulation 1990; 81:219.
40. Yasuda T, Gold HK, Yaoita H, et al. Comparative effects of aspirin, a synthetic thrombin inhibitor and a monoclonal antiplatelet glycoprotein IIb/IIIa antibody on coronary artery reperfusion, reocclusion and bleeding with recombinant tissue-type plasminogen activator in a canine preparation. J Am Coll Cardiol 1990; 16:714.
41. Greco NJ, Tenner TE, Narendra TN, et al. PPACK-thrombin inhibits thrombin-induced platelet aggregation and cytoplasmic acidification but does not inhibit platelet shape change. Blood 990; 75:1983.
42. Hanson SR, Harker LA. Interruption of acute platelet dependent thrombosis by the synthetic antithrombin D-phenylalanyl-L-prolyl-L-arginyl chloromethylketone. Proc Natl Acad Sci USA 1988; 85:3184.
43. Heras M, Chesebro JH, Penny WJ, et al. Effects of thrombin inhibition on the development of acute platelet thrombus deposition during angioplasty in pigs. Heparin versus recombinant hirudin, a specific thrombin inhibitor. Circulation 1989; 79:657.
44. Abensdshein DR, Recchia D, Meng Y, et al. Brief, profound inhibition of thrombin attenuates stenosis following balloon-induced arterial injury in hyperlipidemic miniswine. J Am Coll Cardiol 1994; 20a.
45. Meyer B, Badimon J, Fuster V, et al. Inhibition of the progression of thrombus growth on pre-existing mural thrombus: targetting optimal therapy. J Am Coll Cardiol 1994; 64a.
46. Topol EJ, Fuster V, Harrington RA, et al. Recombinant hirudin for unstable angina pectoris: A pilot multicenter randomized angiographic trial. Circulation 1994; 89:1557.
47. Lidon RM, Theroux P, Ghitescu M, et al. Anticoagulants and antithrombotic properties of hirulog in unstable angina. Circulation 1994; 88:1073.
48. Zeymer U, Jessel A, Neuhaus KL, et al. Hirudin as conjunctive therapy in patients with thrombolysis for acute myocardial infarction produced stable prolongation of ACT and APTT. Circulation 1994; 88:1072.
49. Fuchs J, McCabe CH, Antman EM, et al. Hirulog in the treatment of unstable angina: Results of the TIMI-7 trial. J Am Coll Cardiol 1994; 56a.
50. Cannon CP, McCabe CH, Henry TD. A pilot trial of recombinant desulfatohirudin compared with heparin in conjunctin with tissue-type plasminogen activator and aspirin for acute myocardial infarction: results of the thrombolysis in myocardial infarction (TIMI)-5 trial. J Am Coll Cardiol 1994; 23:993–1003.
51. Strony J, Phillips M, Brands D, et al. Aurin tricarboxylic acid in a canine model of coronary artery thrombosis. Circulation 1990; 81:1106.
52. Phillips MD, Moake JL, Nolasco L, et al. Aurin yricarboxylic acid: A novel inhibitor of the association of von Willebrand factor and platelets. Blood 1988; 72:1898.

11

Thrombolytic Therapy and the Acute Management of Unstable Angina/Complex Lesions

Srinivas Duvvuri, MD, John A. Ambrose, MD

Introduction

It was reasonable to assume that thrombolytic therapy should work in unstable angina. In most cases, unstable angina appeared to have a pathogenesis similar to acute myocardial infarction consisting of intracoronary thrombus formation on a fissured or disrupted atherosclerotic plaque.[1–9] Thrombolytic therapy by lysing intracoronary thrombus had become the "standard of care" for acute myocardial infarction presenting within 6 to 12 hours of onset of chest pain.[10–14] Furthermore, antithrombotic and anticoagulant therapies were the only classes of drugs that decreased morbidity and mortality following an episode of unstable angina.[15]

So, many angiographic and clinical trials in unstable angina evaluated various thrombolytic regimens utilizing either intravenous and/or intracoronary administration.[16–35] In general, angiographic improvement was not striking and, if present, did not correlate with clinical improvement.[17,18,25,30,32,36–40] In addition, large clinical trials such

From: Ambrose JA (ed): *Complex Coronary Lesions in Acute Coronary Syndromes.*

Table 1
Thrombolytic Trials in Unstable Angina

Trial	*Patients No.*	*Treatment*	*Angiographic Result*	*Clinical Result*
Uncontrolled				
Rentrop	5	IC SK	No change	No benefit
De Zwaan	41	IC SK, IV t-PA	Improved	No benefit
Gotoh	37	IC UK	Improved	No benefit
Ambrose	37	IC SK	No change	
Mandlekorn	17	IC SK	Improved	
Vetrovec	12	IC SK	Improved	Improved
Brochier	16	SK, t-PS, APSAC, OR UK	No change	
Controlled				
Lawrence	40	IV SK + warfarin		Improved
Ardissino	24	IV t-PA	No change	Improved
Karlson	205	IV t-PA		Improved
Gold	24	IV t-PA	Improved	Improved
Freeman	70	IV t-PA	No change	Worsened
Nicklas	40	IV t-PA	No change	No benefit
Saran	48	IV SK		Improved
Williams	67	IV t-PA	Improved	
Topol	40	IV t-PA	No change	No benefit*
Schreiber	25	IV UK	Improved	No benefit
Sansa	43	IV UK	Improved	
Neri-Serner	97	IV t-PA		No benefit
Schreiber	149	IV UK		Worsened
UNASEM	159	IV APSAC	Improved	Worsened
TIMI IIIA**	306	IV t-PA	Improved	
TIMI IIIB**	1473	IV t-PA		No change

* Pacing threshold of ischemic symptoms increased.
** Included patients with non-Q wave infarction.
Clinical end-points included recurrent angina, myocardial infarction, death, and need for coronary revascularization.

as the TIMI IIIB[36] did not find clinical benefit for these agents in combination with heparin and aspirin versus heparin and aspirin alone. Many clinical studies have even shown that thrombolytic therapy may be detrimental in unstable angina, increasing the incidence of myocardial infarction following their administration[17,18,25,30,32,36–40] (Table 1).

This chapter will discuss at length the angiographic trials of thrombolytic therapy in unstable angina and focus on the relationship between intracoronary thrombus and/or complex lesions and the response to therapy. However, as the ultimate test of a therapy is whether or not it conveys clinical benefit, the larger clinical trials will also be discussed. Finally, we will consider the potential mechanisms for these negative effects of thrombolytic therapy in unstable angina.

Thrombolytic Trials of Unstable Angina versus Acute Myocardial Infarction

Prior to discussing the results of thrombolytic therapy in unstable angina, certain methodological differences between trials of unstable angina and myocardial infarction pertaining to patient selection and timing of thrombolytic therapy should be addressed. In acute myocardial infarction, thrombolytic therapy is given within 6 to 12 hours after the onset of pain to a homogeneous group of patients presenting with ST segment elevation and chest pain whereas in unstable angina the patient population is more heterogeneous. The definition of unstable angina utilized in thrombolytic trials has been variable, and this may have accounted for some of the observed differences between the studies. This variability may have been minimized if a more uniform system was utilized, such as that of Braunwald classification[41] or the Duke angina score system.[42] Some trials have used more stringent criteria by restricting the definition of unstable angina to either new onset angina and/or rest angina only.[38] Some investigators have enrolled patients during angina and ischemic ECG changes and performed angiography during ongoing ischemic symptoms.[18] Not surprisingly, the incidence of coronary thrombus and total occlusions in these patients with more acute presentations was higher than in studies enrolling patients with a more subacute clinical presentation.

Likewise, the timing of thrombolytic therapy in unstable angina trials has been considerably more heterogeneous than in thrombolytic trials of acute myocardial infarction. Patients with unstable angina are rarely enrolled within hours of the onset of symptoms and some have been studied several hours to days after the acute presentation. However, at least angiographically in unstable angina, the presence of coronary thrombus is most apparent when patients are studied soon after the onset of symptoms or after a change in symptoms from stable to unstable angina.[18,43] As will be discussed later, this subset of patients will show some angiographic improvement following thrombolytic therapy.

Trials of Thrombolytic Therapy in Unstable Angina

Over 20 studies (published as full articles) have been reported on thrombolytic therapy in unstable angina (Table 1), and it becomes apparent that even though many of these have reported some angiographic improvement after thrombolysis, there is no consistent concordant clinical improvement. Many of the earlier studies were observational and low powered, consisting of fewer than 100 patients. Two of the largest enrollment trials, the UNASEM[37] (Unstable Angina Study Using Eminase) and the TIMI III,[36,38,39] which were reported in the last 2 years, have not been able to show that thrombolytics confer any significant angiographic or clinical benefit in unstable angina over that conveyed by heparin therapy. In fact, in the UNASEM trial, there was a higher incidence of hemorrhagic complications and recurrent angina in the thrombolytic group.

Angiographic Results

Several angiographic trials have been conducted to date, to address the issue of thrombolysis in unstable angina. Seven have been uncontrolled, observational studies[16–22] mostly employing intracoronary thrombolytics. Of the controlled prospective trials, all utilized intravenous thrombolytics.[23–37] Three parameters seem to significantly affect the angiographic outcome following thrombolytic therapy in unstable angina. These include the presence of intracoronary thrombus, the elapsed time from the last episode of ischemic symptoms to the onset of thrombolytic treatment, and the presence of total coronary occlusion prior to the treatment.

Ambrose et al.[19] studied 37 patients who presented with chest pain[29] with unstable angina and eight with non-Q-wave infarction and had lesions with >50% and <100% stenosis. Sixty-seven percent (or 24 lesions) were complex prior to an infusion of intracoronary streptokinase. They found no significant improvement in diameter stenosis from the pre- to the post-thrombolytic treatment angiograms. After streptokinase, only one lesion changed from complex to simple. Similarly, Topol et al.[31] studied 40 patients with unstable angina, and after angiography, randomized patients to intravenous rt-PA or placebo. There was no angiographic benefit in the patients treated with the thrombolytic agent compared to placebo. However, de Zwaan et al.,[17] in an uncontrolled study, evaluated 41 patients with unstable angina and performed coronary angiography 2–69 hours (mean 19 hours) after the last episode of angina. Of these, retrospective analysis was performed on 21 patients who received 250,000 units of intracoronary streptokinase, and prospective analysis was performed on 20 patients who were administered intravenous rt-PA. Both groups revealed significant improvement in percent diameter stenosis in the post-therapy angiograms. Of these, 32% had a total occlusion prior to thrombolytic therapy and 80% of lesions with total occlusion had significant improvement following treatment. The inclusion of totally occluded arteries will increase the success rate of thrombolytics whereas other investigators have selectively excluded such patients from their studies and this may have been reflected in their lower rates of angiographic success. Total occlusion in a coronary artery is intimately associated with coronary thrombosis and this may be the factor that leads to higher angiographic success with thrombolytic therapy in such lesions. It is also conceivable that some of these patients with total occlusion may have an evolving myocardial infarction rather than unstable angina. Similarly, Gotoh et al.[18] found in a subgroup of patients with ongoing "unstable angina" and ST elevation that thrombolytics were effective when there was angiographic evidence of totally or subtotally occluded coronary artery prior to therapy.

Angiographic improvement in patients with unstable angina has been strongly associated with the presence of coronary thrombus as well as total occlusion prior to thrombolytic treatment. This has been borne out in the UNASEM and TIMI IIIA trials,[37,39] the two largest randomized trials on unstable angina that have employed angiographic end-points. These trials randomized 159 and 306 patients, respectively, and the latter trial also included patients with non-Q-wave infarction.

The UNASEM trial was a large randomized placebo-controlled study designed to evaluate angiographic and clinical outcome of thrombolytic therapy in unstable angina.[37] One hundred fifty-nine patients with either crescendo and/or rest angina of less than 4 weeks' duration and electrocardiographic evidence of ischemia were enrolled. All patients received intravenous heparin infusion and were randomized within 12 hours of their last episode of angina to receive either intravenous anistreplase (Eminase) or placebo infusion. All patients underwent coronary angiography within 3 hours from the time of randomization. Thirty-three patients were excluded from the study because of angiographic evidence of either significant left main coronary stenosis (>70% lesion), normal coronaries, or nonsignificant stenosis (<50% lesion). Of the 126 eligible patients, 65 patients received Eminase and

61 received placebo infusion. Coronary angiography was repeated 12–28 hours later in all the study patients. Subsequently, all patients received aspirin (300 mg/day).

Analysis revealed that patients randomized to the Eminase group had a statistically significant decrease in the lesion severity compared to the placebo group (P = 0.002). By quantitative analysis mean diameter stenosis decreased significantly more frequently in patients receiving Eminase compared to those receiving placebo (11% vs. 3%) (P = 0.008). It was noted that 17 of 65 (26%) patients in the Eminase group and 11 of 61 (18%) patients in the placebo group had totally occluded coronary arteries at baseline angiography. In the Eminase group, 12 of the 17 occluded arteries were recanalized compared to none of the 11 in the placebo group (P = <0.05). There was no significant difference in the percent diameter stenosis reduction in patent ischemia-related arteries (i.e., significant but nontotally occluding lesions) in the two groups. Hence, the improvement noted in totally occluded coronary arteries may be responsible for the observed overall difference in the stenosis severity with thrombolytic therapy in this patient cohort (Table 2).

Table 2

Coronary Angiographic Changes of the Culprit Lesion in UNASEM

Patients with Two Angiograms	*Antistreptalase**	*Placebo*
Assessment by the angiographic Committee	64	59
I II		
● → ●	5	11
● → ○	12	0
○ → ●	1	0
○ → ○	46	48
Assessment by the CAAS system	63	57
Diameter stenosis I (%)	70	66
Diameter stenosis II (%)	59	63
Mean change in diameter stenosis I–II (%)	11†	3†
Decrease in diameter stenosis of open arteries (%)	5	3

* After antistreptalase, median degree of stenosis was significantly less severe than after placebo (p = 0.002).
† p = 0.008; I = baseline angiography; II = angiography after 12–28 hours; ● = Occluded artery; ○ = open artery.
Modified with permission from Bar et al.; Circulation 1992.

TIMI IIIA was designed to assess the angiographic effect of a moderate dose (up to 80 mg) of intravenously administered tissue plasminogen activator in patients presenting with either unstable angina or non-Q-wave infarction within 12 hours of their last ischemic episode along with ECG changes or a history of coronary artery disease.[39] The placebo arm received aspirin and intravenous heparin as well as beta blockers and calcium channel blockers. There were 391 patients who fulfilled the above criteria and were enrolled, but 314 patients were eligible for randomization after the initial catheterization.

Follow-up catheterization was available in 308 patients at 18–48 hours of which 306 film pairs were analyzed to assess the study end-points. Approximately 30% in each group had non-Q-wave infarction at presentation and the remainder had unstable angina.

The primary end-point was a measurable reduction in the percent diameter stenosis of the culprit lesion of >10% or an improvement in flow by at least two TIMI grades at follow-up compared to the baseline angiogram. A secondary end-point was the incidence of substantial improvement, defined as a reduction in the diameter stenosis of >20% or an increase by two TIMI grades at follow-up. Apparent thrombus by their definition was found in 35% of lesions at baseline. This was defined as a globular, abrupt, protruding intraluminal radiolucency that was either round or polypoid and was subclassified as small, medium, or large. Possible thrombus, defined as an intraluminal lucency with the appearance of a tightly adherent, flat, intraluminal mass was found in an additional 40% of the patients. TIMI grade 0 or 1 was found in 18% of the patients at baseline angiography. Apparent thrombus was detected in 47% of patients with non-Q-wave infarction compared to 29% of patients with unstable angina, of which recent complete occlusions were noted in 37% and 18%, respectively.

The primary end-point occurred in 25% of patients in the rt-PA group and 19% in the placebo group (P = 0.25) and was more frequent in patients with non-Q-wave infarction (35%) than in unstable angina patients (16%) (P<0.001). Substantial improvement (secondary end-point) occurred in 15% of patients in the rt-PA group versus 5% in the placebo group (P = 0.003) (Table 3). Subgroup analysis revealed that substantial improvement occurred more frequently in lesions with complete occlusion (P = 0.05), and this end-point was more frequent in patients with non-Q-wave infarction (21%) compared to those with unstable angina (5%) (P<0.001). Other features of the culprit lesion more likely to be associated with this end-point included recent occlusion and apparent thrombus (P<0.001). Overall, 15% of patients in the rt-PA group had substantial improvement and 25% had measurable im-

Table 3

Quantitative Arteriographic Analysis: Baseline Measurements and Response at 18–24 Hours of Primary Culprit Lesions to t-PA or to Placebo in TIMI-3A

	t-PA	*Placebo*	*p for Comparison*
n	150	156	—
Baseline QCA measurements* (%S, mm)	84 ± 9% S 0.43 ± 0.28 mm	84 ± 9% S 0.46 ± 0.28 mm	0.36 0.42
Percent with measureable improvement† (%)	25	19	0.25
Percent with substantial improvement (%)	15	5	0.003
Percent with measureable worsening (%)	3	1	0.16
Mean change in percent stenosis (%S)*	−6.2 ± 10.1	−4.6 ± 6.6	0.10
Mean change in minimum diameter (mm)*	+0.17 ± 0.29	+0.14 ± 0.20	0.27

QCA = Quantitative coronary arteriographic; t-PA = tissue-type plasminogen activator.
* %S is percent diameter. The lumen diameter at the point of greatest narrowing is expressed in mm.
† This is the primary end-point comparison.
Modified with permission from Brown et al.; Circulation 1993.

provement. Of lesions with apparent thrombus at baseline, measurable improvement was found in 49%, and substantial improvement in 36%. However, lesions with possible thrombus rarely showed such improvement (3%). There was no significant difference in the primary end-point using rt-PA in patients with unstable angina in the absence of an apparent thrombus or complete occlusion.

The last determinant of angiographic improvement with thrombolytic therapy in unstable angina may be the time interval between the onset of or last episode of rest pain and the thrombolytic intervention. As intracoronary thrombus appears more frequently on angiography when performed soon after rest pain,[43] this conclusion should be intuitively obvious. However, one can only suggest this is so, since no one study has evaluated the efficacy of thrombolytic therapy based on the time interval between the onset or last episode of rest pain and the thrombolytic intervention. There is angioscopic evidence to suggest a higher incidence of coronary thrombus when evaluated in the early hours after onset of ischemic pain.[44,45] In studies where thrombolytic therapy was given soon after rest pain or even during an episode of ischemia, angiographic improvement was more likely to occur than in studies where there was a longer interval between the onset of last episode of pain and the thrombolytic intervention.[18] The general trend in these studies suggests that the maximal potential angiographic benefit from thrombolytic therapy in patients with unstable angina is derived if such intervention is employed temporally as close to the index episode of angina as possible.

Clinical Outcome

The natural history data suggest that the occurrence of unstable angina portends an increased risk of cardiac events such as myocardial infarction and cardiac death in the ensuing months compared to patients with stable coronary syndromes. In patients with unstable angina treated with beta blockers and calcium blockers at 1 month, the incidence of acute myocardial infarction is 10–20% and mortality is 1–4% and the mortality rises to 10–12% at 1 year follow-up.[46,47] More recent therapeutic advances particularly with the addition of aspirin and intravenous heparin, have improved prognosis decreasing myocardial infarction and/or death by 50–70%[15] in such patients. However, since there is still a risk of death and/or myocardial infarction in spite of these agents, further therapeutic avenues need to be explored.

With this in mind, we shall evaluate the results of the various trials using thrombolytics in unstable angina where clinical end-points have been assessed either prospectively or retrospectively. The earlier observational studies of Rentrop[16] and de Zwaan[17] revealed no clinical benefit after using intracoronary streptokinase even though the latter study found a decrease in angiographic stenosis severity in the majority of the patients. In this same study, the overall incidence of myocardial infarction, persistent chest pain, and need for revascularization was very high and may have reflected a high-risk subgroup of patients with unstable angina. In the uncontrolled study of Ambrose et al.,[19] myocardial infarction was reported in two patients on follow-up after intracoronary thrombolysis even in the absence of total occlusion or impaired coronary flow at baseline. In addition, Gotoh et al.,[18] using intracoronary streptokinase, studied 37 patients with unstable angina and noted significant improvement in angiographic appearance of the lesions but this did not translate into clinical benefit. In fact, there was a high incidence (71%) of recurrent symptoms in patients with intracoronary thrombus even after successful thrombolysis compared to an incidence of 36% in those without such a thrombus on the initial angiogram. Thus, in this study, angiographic improvement did not protect against future cardiac events.

Of the randomized controlled studies, Lawrence et al.[23] noted significant clinical improvement at 6 month follow-up in 40 patients by using streptokinase 250,000 IU bolus followed by 100,000 IU/hour X 24 hours followed by warfarin for 6 months compared to warfarin alone ($P<0.02$). Similarly, Karlson et al.,[25] using intravenous rt-PA (1 mg/Kg over 4 hours) in 205 patients with unstable angina found significant improvement in clinical events such as recurrent angina, acute myocardial infarction, and exercise induced ischemia (61% in rt-PA vs. 80% in placebo, $P = 0.005$). Saran et al.,[29] using intravenous streptokinase compared to placebo in 48 patients, also found a significant decrease in recurrent angina (79% vs. 38%), acute myocardial infarction (25% vs. 12%), and mortality at 6 months (16.6% vs. 8.3%) with streptokinase. Unfortunately, coronary angiography was not performed in any of the above randomized clinical studies and this somewhat lessens their importance.

Of the angiographic studies that revealed clinical or hemodynamic improvement in patients with unstable angina, Topol et al.[31] reported a significant increase in pacing threshold to ischemia after intravenous infusion of rt-PA even in the absence of an appreciable angiographic improvement. However, this study noted that thrombolytic therapy does not protect against the need for elective or emergent revascularization. Gold et al.[26] noted clinical improvement in 23 patients after randomization to an infusion of either rt-PA or placebo and performing angiography 1–3 days later. Angiography revealed no thrombus in the rt-PA group and 79% incidence in the placebo group, even though baseline angiography was not performed in this study. Holter monitoring after the thrombolytic therapy revealed higher incidence of ischemia in the placebo group (55%) compared to the rt-PA group (8%).

Ardissino[24] studied 103 patients with unstable angina and randomized 24 of the patients who were refractory to conventional therapy that included intravenous heparin to receive either rt-PA or placebo. Baseline angiograms were performed and follow-up studies at 72 hours after the treatment revealed no significant difference in the angiographic appearance in the two groups. However, there was a significantly lower incidence of recurrent ischemia in the rt-PA group compared to placebo (0% vs. 75%) initially but ischemia recurred within a few days. The improved outcome without an apparent improvement in angiographic outcome in this study resembles the study by Topol[31] and may be related to the observation that a small increase in diameter following thrombolysis may increase distal flow and improve hemodynamics. As the pressure gradient across a coronary stenosis is directly proportional to the square of the flow and inversely to the diameter raised to the fourth power,[48] a small change in diameter by thrombolysis may cause a profound change in pressure and flow across a stenosis.

In contrast to the last two studies, in the UNASEM trial, despite angiographic improvement, there was no significant difference in the cardiac event rate between the treatment (Eminase) and the control groups. Also angiographic improvement did not correlate with clinical improvement. Thrombolytic therapy also did not seem to protect against the incidence of acute myocardial infarction. Particularly interesting was the trend towards a higher incidence of recurrent angina in the Eminase group compared to placebo although this did not attain statistical significance ($P = 0.06$). These findings persisted up to 1 year of follow-up.[39] Also, there was a statistically significant ($P = 0.001$) increase in hemorrhagic complications in the Eminase group. A similar effect was described by Schreiber et al.[35] who randomized 149 patients to three treatment arms, namely urokinase (3 million IU over 90 min) plus heparin infusion, urokinase plus aspirin, and placebo plus heparin. There was no statistical difference in the clinical end-points of recurrent angina, need for revascularization, or death in the three groups. In the interim analysis there was a trend towards a higher incidence of myocardial infarction in the urokinase group (10.2% vs 6.4%) and the initially projected enrollment size of 600 patients was reduced to 149 patients.

The TIMI IIIB trial[36] was designed to assess the effect on clinical outcome of patients treated with rt-PA compared to placebo since the TIMI IIIA study was only an angiographic study. In addition, however, in the former study, patients were also randomized to either an early invasive arm or to conservative therapy. Enrollment included 1,473 patients with unstable angina or non-Q-wave infarction of which 740 patients were randomized to early invasive therapy (and intervention if deemed suitable after the 18–48 hour angiogram). A similar number of patients (733) were randomized to the conservative arm of the study and were treated with conventional medical therapy which included intravenous heparin, beta blockers, calcium blockers, and aspirin. This latter group underwent angiography only for recalcitrant angina or recurrent or provocable ischemia, and revascularization was performed in these patients if indicated. Clinical end-points included death, myocardial infarction, stroke, and failure of medical therapy. The incidence of death or myocardial infarction was not significantly different between rt-PA and the placebo groups at 42 days and at 1 year. There was a significantly higher incidence of stroke and fatal and nonfatal myocardial infarction in the rt-PA group compared to placebo. There were also no significant differences in death, myocardial infarction, or unsatisfactory symptom limited exercise stress test at 6 weeks for invasive and conservative strategies.

The results of most of the earlier smaller trials and the recently published larger trials such as UNASEM and TIMI IIIA or B demonstrate that there is no identifiable clinical benefit even in the presence of angiographic benefit for thrombolytic therapy in patients with unstable angina. In fact, the data on clinical outcome suggest that such therapy may in fact be deleterious. From the results of nine randomized placebo-controlled studies, Waters and Lam[49] suggested that in patients with unstable angina, the relative risk for myocardial infarction is increased with thrombolytic therapy compared to conventional therapy.

Reasons for the Variable Response to Thrombolytic Therapy in Unstable Angina

The beneficial effects of thrombolytic therapy in acute myocardial infarction are potentially overwhelming both from angiographic as well as from clinical end-points in several different trials.[10–14] In spite of the apparent pathogenetic similarities between unstable angina and transmural myocardial infarction,[1–9,50–57] there must be major differences that are contributing to the dissimilar effects that thrombolytics exert in these two syndromes. These may include differences between syndromes in the design of thrombolytic trials, as well as differences in the coronary substrate and hence the therapeutic response to such therapy (Table 4).

Patient Selection and Clinical End-Points

The efficacy of thrombolytic therapy in myocardial infarction has been assessed by assigning major end-points of improvement in mortality and left ventricular function in studies employing thousands of patients. End-points such as recurrent angina, myocardial infarction, need for revascularization, and cardiac death have been studied in un-

Table 4
Reasons for Variable Response of Thrombolytic Therapy in Unstable Angina

Group I
Studies not powered to show an effect due to small sample size and low incidence of hard end-points in unstable angina trials.
Group II
Differences in the anatomy and pathology of the thrombus between acute myocardial infarction (fibrin-rich totally occlusive thrombus) and unstable angina (platelet-rich mural thrombus).
Group III
Absence of thrombus in some patients with unstable angina.
Group IV
Platelet stimulating or procoagulant effects of thrombolytic agents.

stable angina. The mortality at 7 days in unstable angina treated with beta blockers, calcium blockers, aspirin, and intravenous heparin infusion is about 2% and of refractory angina is about 10%.[15] With such a low mortality in this group, a reduction of 25% in the mortality rate would require a very large sample size of several thousands of patients. Most trials, with the exception of TIMI III, have been conducted with under 200 patients. Additionally, in unstable angina most patients have a patent but stenosed artery, and to demonstrate a change in the diameter stenosis or minimal luminal diameter, quantitative techniques must be employed. While these techniques eliminate the problem of subjective variability, even the most sophisticated of quantitative techniques are not without potential theoretical flaws. Also, the end-points chosen (such as 10% vs. 20% reduction in diameter stenosis) in unstable angina have varied and may not be expected to have the same impact on clinical outcome as establishing patency from a recent totally occluded vessel (the usual angiographic end-point of thrombolytic trials in acute myocardial infarction).

Coronary Substrate

From necropsy and angiographic studies, the plaque in acute myocardial infarction is often of moderate severity and the terminal event that occludes the artery is a freshly formed thrombus[1,2] composed of red cells and fibrin. The plaque in most patients with unstable angina leads to a luminal stenosis of 70–99% with a superimposed thrombus that is usually small and nonocclusive.[24,43,58] In the minority of patients with unstable angina who have total occlusion of the culprit artery, there may be more extensive thrombus similar to that in myocardial infarction. Such lesions may be more responsive to thrombolytic therapy and angiographic improvement may be readily detected.

As the thrombus is mural and nonocclusive in unstable angina, we have suggested that these differences in the thrombus between unstable angina and acute myocardial infarction can be explained by the fact that the thrombus is platelet-rich in unstable angina while platelets and fibrin are present in acute myocardial infarction.[50] Pathologically, the head of a coronary thrombus is platelet-rich while the intraluminal component is composed of red cells and fibrin. It is this trailing thrombus that is missing in most cases of unstable angina. The angioscopic findings of Mizuno et al.[44] are consistent with this hypothesis. The thrombus in unstable angina was white or whitish-red while in acute myocardial infarction Mizuno et al found that it was predominantly red. It is the fibrin-rich thrombus that is responsive to thrombolytic agents. The platelet-rich thrombus may not only be resistant to thrombolytics but it may also exert effects that limit the ability of thrombolytic agents to lyse thrombus.[59] It has been shown by some investigators that platelet incorporation into the thrombus leads to decreased binding of rt-PA and hence decreased fibrinolytic activity.[60] Platelets undergo a change in shape upon activation and this facilitates their binding to the fibrin in the thrombus via their GP IIb/IIIa complex, a process that leads to clot retraction. Inhibition of this clot retraction has been shown to abolish the antifibrinolytic effect of platelets described above. Thus, inhibition of fibrin-bound thrombin as well as of platelet activation is important in thrombolysis. Recently, several studies have been conducted with novel antiplatelet agents some of which have shown promise in animal studies. Using the anti-GP IIb/IIIa antibody 7E3, Coller[61,62] and Yasuda et al.[63] have shown that inhibiting platelet and fibrin interaction may decrease the resistance of the platelet-rich thrombus to thrombolytic therapy. Subsequently, other studies using platelet IIb/IIIa inhibitors have shown a similar effect. A similar effect was also seen with the thrombin inhibitor Argatroban[64] in "red-thrombi" (which are erythrocyte- and fibrin-rich).

Procoagulant Effects of Thrombolytic Agents

There is evidence that thrombolytic agents in addition to their primary role in fibrinolysis, exert procoagulant actions[67–69] and this is in part related to the exposure of fibrin-bound thrombin which is a potent stimulus for rethrombosis. This action is mediated by fibrinogen, platelet activation,[70] and an increase in PA-I (plasminogen activator inhibitor). The breakdown products of fibrinogen, fibrinopeptide-A, and thrombin-antithrombin complexes, which are markers of thrombin activity, have been demonstrated after thrombolytic treatment.[71,72] Thrombolytic agents may also directly activate platelets, particularly in the initial hours after their administration. The platelet-rich thrombus in unstable angina may thus be adversely affected by thrombolytic agents. Heparin may not effectively inhibit the increased thrombin activity during thrombolysis and novel antithrombins such as hirudin may more specifically inhibit clot-bound thrombin.[73] In a multicenter trial, recombinant hirudin (a potent specific inhibitor of thrombin) was used for the treatment of unstable angina[65] and resulted in a significantly greater improvement in coronary luminal cross sectional area and minimal luminal diameter compared with heparin treatment. There was also a tendency towards a reduction in the incidence of myocardial infarction from 8% in the heparin group to 2.6% in the hirudin group ($P = 0.11$). Similarly, hirulog (a direct inhibitor of free and clot-bound thrombin) in low and high doses was used in the TIMI 7 trial[66] in unstable angina patients, and at the higher dose revealed a significant decrease in death and nonfatal myocardial infarction at hospital discharge and at 6 weeks' follow-up when compared to the lower dose. All patients received aspirin but heparin was not used in this study. The encouraging results from this have led to the TIMI 8 trial (in progress) which is an international, randomized, double blind, placebo-controlled trial of heparin versus hirulog in patients with unstable angina and non-Q-wave infarction.*

Conclusion

In spite of unequivocal clinical benefit of thrombolytic therapy in patients with acute Q-wave infarction and the similarities in pathogenesis between unstable angina and myocardial infarction, the data suggest that angiographic benefit of thrombolytic therapy in unstable angina may be realized only in lesions that have a significant thrombus burden, particularly if there was a recent onset total occlusion of the vessel. The majority of lesions with complex morphology do not change significantly with thrombolytic therapy. Clinical benefit with thrombo-

* Editor's note: Taps for TIMI-8—it was canceled!

lytics is also limited and the therapy may even prove harmful. Preliminary results with the thrombin inhibitors have been encouraging. The results of large trials with these newer agents should become available in the future and it is hopeful that these agents may prove to be more beneficial than thrombolytic therapy in unstable angina (see Chapters 10 and 12).

References

1. DeWood MA, Spores J, Notske R, et al. Prevalence of total coronary occlusion during the early hours of transmural myocardial infarction. N Engl J Med 1980; 303:897–902.
2. Falk E. Plaque rupture with severe preexisting stenosis precipitating coronary thrombosis: Characteristics of coronary plaques underlying fatal occlusive thrombi. Br Heart J 1983; 50:127–134.
3. Davies MJ, Thomas AC. Plaque fissuring: The cause of acute myocardial infarction, sudden ischemic death, and crescendo angina. Br Heart J 1985; 53:363–373.
4. Fuster V, Steele PM, Chesebro JH. Role of platelets and thrombosis in coronary disease and sudden death. J Am Coll Cardiol 1985; 5:175B-184B.
5. Falk E. Unstable angina with fatal outcome: Dynamic coronary thrombosis leading to infarction and/sudden death. Circulation 1985; 71:699–708.
6. Fuster V, Badimon L, Cohen M. Insights into the pathogenesis of acute coronary syndromes. Circulation 1988; 77(6):1213–1220.
7. Bugiardini R, Pozzati A, Borghi A, et al. Angiographic morphology in unstable angina and its relation to transient myocardial ischemia and hospital outcome. Am J Cardiol 1991; 67:460–464.
8. Badimon L, Chesebro JH, Badimon JJ, et al. Thrombus formation on ruptured atherosclerotic plaques and rethrombosis on evolving thrombi. Circulation 1992; 86(6):(Suppl)III-74.
9. Davies MJ. Thrombosis and coronary atherosclerosis. In: Julian DG, Kubier W, Norris RM, Swan HJ, Collen D, Verstraete M, eds: Thrombolysis in Cardiovascular Disease. New York, Marcel Dekkar, 1989, pp. 25–43.
10. Gruppo Italiano per lo studio della streptokinase nel infarcto miocardico. Effectiveness of intravenous thrombolytic therapy in acute myocardial infarction. Lancet; 1:397–402.
11. The TIMI study group: 1985. The thrombolysis in myocardial infarction trial: Phase I findings. N Engl J Med 1986; 312:932–936.
12. Williams DO, Borer J, Braunwald E, Chesebro J, et al. Intravenous recombinant t-PA in patients with acute myocardial infarction. A report from NHLBI thrombolytics in myocardial infarction trial. Circulation 1986; 73: 338–346.
13. Verstraete M, Bernard R. Randomized trial of intravenous recombinant t-PA versus intravenous streptokinase in acute myocardial infarction: Report from European Cardiovascular Society Group. Lancet 1985; 1: 842–847.

14. ISIS-2 (Second International Study of Infarct Survival) Collaborative Group. Randomized trial of intravenous streptokinase, oral aspirin, both or neither among 17,187 cases of suspected acute myocardial infarction. Lancet 1988; 2:349–360.
15. Theroux P, Quimet H, McCans J, et al. Aspirin, heparin, or both to treat acute unstable angina. N Engl J Med 1988; 319:1105–1111.
16. Rentrop KP, Blanke H, Karsh KR, et al. Selective intracoronary thrombolysis in acute myocardial infarction and unstable angina pectoris. Circulation 1981; 63:307–317.
17. De Zwaan C, Bar FW, Janssen JHA, et al. Effects of thrombolytic therapy in unstable angina: Clinical and angiographic results. J Am Coll Cardiol 1988; 12:301–309.
18. Gotoh K, Minamino T, Katoh O, et al. The role of intracoronary thrombus in unstable angina: Angiographic assessment and thrombolytic therapy during ongoing angina attacks. Circulation 1988; 77:526–534.
19. Ambrose JA, Hjemdahl-Monsen C, Borico S, et al. Quantitative and qualitative effects of intracoronary streptokinase in unstable angina and non-Q wave infarction. J Am Coll Cardiol 1987; 9:1156–1165.
20. Mandlekorn JB, Wolf NR, Sing S, et al. Intracoronary thrombus in nontransmural myocardial infarction and unstable angina pectoris. Am J Cardiol 1983; 52:1–6.
21. Vetrovec GE, Leinbach RC, Gold HK, et al. Intracoronary thrombolysis in syndromes of unstable ischemia: Angiographic and clinical results. Am Heart J 1982; 104:946–952.
22. Brochier ML, Raynaud P, Rioux P, et al. Thrombosis and thrombolysis in unstable angina. Am J Coll Cardiol 1991; 68:105B-109B.
23. Lawrence JR, Shepher JT, Bone I, et al. Fibrinolytic therapy in unstable angina pectoris: A placebo-controlled clinical trial. Thromb Res 1980; 17: 767–777.
24. Ardissino D, Barberis P, DeServi S, et al. Recombinant tissue-type plasminogen activator followed by heparin compared with heparin alone for refractory unstable angina pectoris. Am J Cardiol 1990; 66:910–914.
25. Karlsson JE, Berglund U, Hamberger A, et al. Thrombolysis with recombinant human plasminogen activator during instability in coronary artery disease: Effect on myocardial ischemia and need for coronary revascularization. Am Heart J 1992; 12:1419–1426.
26. Gold HK, Johns JA, Leinbach RC, et al. A randomized, blinded, placebo-controlled trial of recombinant human tissue-type plasminogen activator in patients with unstable angina pectoris. Circulation 1987; 75:1192–1199.
27. Freeman MR, Langer A, Wilson RF, et al. Thrombolysis in unstable angina: A randomized double-blind trial of t-PA and placebo. Circulation 1992; 85:150–157.
28. Nicklas J, Topol EJ, Kander N, et al. A randomized double-blind, placebo-controlled trial of tissue plasminogen activator in unstable angina. J Am Coll Cardiol 1989; 13:434–441.
29. Saran RK, Bhandari VS, Narain RC, et al. Intravenous streptokinase in the management of a subset of patients with unstable angina. A randomized-controlled trial. Int J Cardiol 1990; 28:840–844.
30. Williams DO, Topol EJ, Califf RM, et al. Intravenous recombinant tissue-

type plasminogen activator in patients with unstable angina pectoris. Circulation 1990; 82:376–383.
31. Topol EJ, Nicklas JM, Kander NH, et al. Coronary revascularization after intravenous tissue plasminogen activator for unstable angina pectoris: Results of a randomized, double-blinded, placebo-controlled trial. Am J Cardiol 1988; 62:368–371.
32. Schreiber T, Macina G, McNulty A, et al. Thrombolytic therapy in unstable angina and non-Q wave myocardial infarction: A randomized trial of urokinase vs aspirin. Am J Cardiol 1989; 64:840–844.
33. Sansa M, Cernigliaro C, Campi A, et al. Effects of urokinase and heparin on minimal cross-sectional area of the culprit narrowing in unstable angina pectoris. Am J Cardiol 1991; 68:451–456.
34. Neri-Serneri GGN, Gensini GF, Poggesi L, et al. Effect of heparin, aspirin, or alteplase in reduction of myocardial ischemia in refractory unstable angina. Lancet 1990; 335:615–618.
35. Schreiber T, Rizik D, White C, et al. Randomized trial of thrombolysis versus heparin in unstable angina. Circulation 1992; 86(5):1407–1414.
36. TIMI IIIB Investigators. Effects of tissue plasminogen activator and a comparison of early invasive and conservative strategies in unstable angina and non-Q-wave myocardial infarction: Results of the TIMI IIIB Trial. Circulation 1994; 89:1545–1556.
37. Bar FW, Verheugt FW, Col J, et al. Thrombolysis in patients with unstable angina improves the angiographic but not the clinical outcome. Results of UNASEM. Circulation 1992; 86:131–137.
38. TIMI III Investigators. Early effects of tissue-type plasminogen activator added to conventional therapy on the culprit coronary lesion in patients presenting with ischemic cardiac pain at rest. Circulation 1993; 87:38–52.
39. TIMI IIIA Investigators. Early effects of tissue-type plasminogen activator added to conventional therapy on the culprit coronary lesion in patients presenting with ischemic cardiac pain at rest: results of the Thrombolysis in Myocardial Ischemia (TIMI IIIA) Trial. Circulation 1993; 87:38–52.
40. Moliterno DJ, Sapp SK, Topol E. The paradoxical effect of thrombolytic therapy for unstable angina: Meta-analysis. J Am Coll Cardiol 1994; 288A: No.774–3.
41. Braunwald E. Unstable angina: A classification. Circulation 1991; 80: 410–414.
42. Califf RM, Mark DB, Harrel FE, Hlatky MA, Lee KL, Rosati RA, Pryor DB. Importance of clinical measures of ischemia in the prognosis of patients with documented coronary artery disease. J Am Coll Cardiol 1988; 11:20–26.
43. Freeman MR, Williams AE, Chisholm RJ, et al. Intracoronary thrombus and complex morphology in unstable angina: Relation to timing of angiography and in-hospital cardiac events. Circulation 1989; 80:17–23.
44. Mizuno K, Satomura K, Miyamoto A, et al. Angioscopic evaluation of the character of coronary thrombi in acute coronary syndromes. N Engl J Med 1992; 326:287–291.
45. Sherman CT, Litvack F, Grundfest W, et al. Coronary angioscopy in patients with unstable angina pectoris. N Engl J Med 1986; 315:913–919.

46. Mulcahy R, Al Awdahi AH, de Buitleor M, et al. Natural history and prognosis of unstable angina. Am Heart J 1985; 109:753–758.
47. Wallace WA, Richeson JF, Yu PN, et al. Unstable angina pectoris. Clin Cardiol 1990; 13(10):679–686.
48. Gould KL. Dynamic coronary stenosis. Am J Cardiol 1980; 45:286–292.
49. Waters D, Lam JYT. Is thrombolytic therapy striking out in unstable angina? Circulation 1992; 86:(5)1642–1643.
50. Ambrose JA. Plaque disruption and the acute coronary syndromes of unstable angina and myocardial infarction: If the substrate is similar, why is the clinical presentation different? J Am Coll Cardiol 1992; 19:1653–1658.
51. Ambrose JA, Winters SL, Stern A, et al. Angiographic morphology and the pathogenesis of unstable angina. J Am Coll Cardiol 1985; 5:609–616.
52. Ambrose JA. Coronary angiography in the acute coronary syndromes. In: Bliefeld W, Hamm CW, Braunwald E, eds: Unstable angina. New York, Springer-Verlag, 1990, pp. 112–128.
53. Haft JI, Goldstein JE, Niemiera ML, et al. Coronary arteriographic lesion of unstable angina. Chest 1987; 92:609–612.
54. Williams AE, Freeman MR, Chisholm RJ, et al. Angiographic morphology in unstable angina pectoris. Am J Cardiol 1988; 62:1024–1027.
55. Ambrose JA, Israel DH. Angiography in unstable angina. Am J Cardiol 1991; 68(7):78B-84B.
56. Ambrose JA, Winters SL, Arora RR, et al. Angiographic evaluation of coronary morphology in unstable angina. J Am Coll Cardiol 1986; 7: 472–478.
57. Ambrose JA, Hjemdahl-Monsen CE. Acute ischemic syndromes: Coronary pathophysiology and angiographic correlations. In: Gersh BJ, Rahimtoola SH, eds. Acute Myocardial Infarction. New York, Elsevier, 1991, pp. 64–77.
58. Chesebro JH, Fuster V. Thrombosis in unstable angina. N Engl J Med 1992; 327(3):192–194.
59. Jang IK, Gold HK, Zisking AA, et al. Differential sensitivity of erythrocyte-rich and platelet-rich arterial thrombi to lysis with recombinant tissue-type plasminogen activator: A possible explanation for resistance to coronary thrombolysis. Circulation 1989; 79:920–928.
60. Kunitada S, Fitzgerald GA, Fitzgerald DJ, et al. Inhibition of clot lysis and decreased binding of tissue-type plasminogen activator as a consequence of clot retraction. Blood 1992; 79(6):1420–1427.
61. Coller B. Platelets and thrombolytic therapy. N Engl J Med 1990; 322(1): 33–40.
62. Coller BS. The role of platelets in thrombolytic therapy. In: Haber E, Braunwald E, eds. Thrombolysis: Basic Contributions and Clinical Progress. St. Louis, Mosby Year Book, 1991, pp. 155–178.
63. Yasuda T, Gold HK, Fallon JT, et al. Monoclonal antibody against the platelet glycoprotein IIb/IIIa receptor prevents coronary artery reocclusion following reperfusion with recombinant tissue-type plasminogen activator in dogs. J Clin Invest 1988; 81:1284–1291.
64. Jang IK, Gold HK, Ziskind AA, Leinbach RC, Fallon JT, Collen D. Prevention of platelet rich arterial thrombus by selective thrombin inhibitor. Circulation 1990; 81:219–215.

65. Topol EJ, Fuster V, Harrington RA, Califf R, Kleiman NS, et al. Recombinant hirudin for unstable angina pectoris: A multicenter, randomized angiographic trial. Circulation 1994; 89:1557–1566.
66. Hirulog in the treatment of unstable angina. J Am Coll Cardiol 1994; Abstract No.712–1.
67. Fitzgerald DJ, Wright F, Fitzgerald FA. Increased thromboxane biosynthesis during coronary thrombolysis. Circ Res 1989; 65(1):83–94.
68. Owen J, Friendman K, Grossman BA, et al. Thrombolytic therapy with tissue plasminogen activator or streptokinase induces transient thrombin activity. Blood 1988; 72(2):616–620.
69. Seitz R, Blanke H, Pratorius G, et al. Increased thrombin activity during thrombolysis. Thromb Haemost 1988; 59:541–542.
70. Aronson DL, Chang P, Kessler CM. Platelet-dependent thrombin generation after in vitro fibrinolytic treatment. Circulation 1992; 85:1706–1712.
71. Eisenberg PR, Sherman LA, Jaffe AS. Paradoxic elevation of fibrinopeptide A after streptokinase: Evidence of continued thrombosis despite intense fibrinolysis. J Am Coll Cardiol 1987; 10(3):527–529.
72. Eisenberg PR, Miletich JP. Induction of marked thrombin activity by pharmacologic concentrations of plasminogen activators in nonanticoagulated whole blood. Thrombosis Res 1989; 55:635–643.
73. Rudd MA, George D, Johnstone MT, et al. Effect of thrombin inhibition on the dynamics of thrombolysis and on platelet function during thrombolytic therapy. Circ Res 1992; 71(4):829–834.

12

Angioplasty in Unstable Angina/Complex Lesions

John A. Ambrose, MD, Sabino Torre, MD

Introduction

When percutaneous transluminal coronary angioplasty (PTCA) was first introduced into clinical cardiology practice in 1978,[1] its application was limited to patients with stable angina pectoris who had single-vessel disease. The target lesion was generally a single, discrete, concentric, subtotal stenosis situated in the proximal portion of the coronary vessel. Eligible patients also generally had normal left ventricular function. However, as operator experience developed, technology improved and success rates increased patient selection broadened to include higher-risk patients with more complicated lesions.

One important group of patients that were difficult to manage in clinical practice were those with medically refractory unstable angina in whom the only available treatment option had been coronary artery bypass surgery. These patients were generally considered at higher risk than those treated in the early period of PTCA because of the presence of multivessel coronary disease, eccentric or ulcerated lesions often associated with the presence of intracoronary thrombus, and the presence of impaired left ventricular function. Nevertheless, reports of the efficacy of PTCA as an alternative to surgical revascularization in these patients first appeared in 1981. Today, PTCA has gained wide-

From: Ambrose JA (ed): *Complex Coronary Lesions in Acute Coronary Syndromes.*

spread acceptance in the treatment of patients with refractory unstable angina; however, acute complications tend to be higher.

This chapter will first discuss the safety and efficacy of PTCA in the management of patients with unstable angina from a historical perspective. Procedural factors such as the timing of PTCA, the presence of complex lesions, and the presence of single or multivessel disease will be discussed as they relate to the differences in outcome and complications following PTCA. Finally, the use of adjunctive pharmacological agents such as thrombolytics and preliminary data with the newer antithrombin and antiplatelet agents will also be reviewed.

Safety and Efficacy

All patients with unstable angina should initially be managed with bed rest and pharmacological treatment, including aspirin, heparin, nitrates, beta blockers, and often calcium channel blockers. In general, the heart rate should be slowed to about 60 beats/minute and, if elevated, the systolic blood pressure lowered to between 100 and 140 mm Hg. In the majority of patients, clinical symptoms can be stabilized.

The first published reports of the use of PTCA in patients with unstable angina appeared in 1981, one from North America and the other from Europe. The first of these described 17 patients with unstable angina who underwent PTCA, with successful dilation achieved in 13 patients (76%).[2] All of these patients had disabling angina, including angina at rest, with 10 experiencing medically refractory angina during hospitalization. Although all four failures underwent coronary bypass surgery only one of these was performed as an emergency. The only death occurred in a patient undergoing elective coronary surgery after the lesion could not be crossed with the guidewire. No myocardial infarctions occurred in this early series. At a mean follow-up of approximately 11 months, all patients were alive, with all but one patient asymptomatic, and none had a myocardial infarction.

Similiar results were also reported from Germany.[3] Forty patients who underwent PTCA in the setting of unstable angina with rest pain and transient ST or T-wave changes had a success rate of 63%. One patient required emergency bypass surgery after abrupt occlusion with the subsequent development of a myocardial infarction. Of the 14 failures, 11 underwent elective bypass surgery. No other complications or deaths were observed in this series.

These early series clearly demonstrated the feasibility of PTCA in selected patients with unstable angina, including patients with rest

Table 1
Angioplasty in Unstable Angina

	N	*Success*	*Death (%)*	*MI (%)*	*CABG (%)*
• Initially stabilized (1986–1992)	1,036	89%	0.3	5.1	5.8
• Refractory (1987–1990)	1,438	85%	1.3	6.3	6.8
• Post-MI (1986–1990)	634	88%	1.1	6.3	6.5
• Stable Angina (1985–1992)	10,129	92%	0.7	1.6	2.5

Modified from de Feyter and Serruys: PTCA for unstable angina. In Textbook of Interventional Cardiology, edited by Topol EJ, WB Saunders, 1994 (with permission). MI = myocardial infarction.

angina, demonstrating at least modest success rates with minimal complication rates and mortality. Since then, a number of other publications[4–14] have reported their experiences with PTCA in the setting of unstable angina, with larger numbers of patients and overall success rates approaching 90% (Table 1). Thus, PTCA has been demonstrated to be safe and effective in patients with unstable angina who have been initially stabilized with medical therapy and has also proved to be safe and effective in those patients refractory to intensive medical therapy. In the former patients, PTCA success rates have averaged 89%, and in the latter group have averaged 85%.

The immediate mortality rates in these studies has ranged from 0% to 5.4% and acute myocardial infarction complicating the procedure has been reported to occur in 0% to 12% of attempted procedures.[2–14] Although emergency coronary bypass surgery has been necessary in 2–13% of cases, most of the larger series have reported rates of about 6%.[10,12–14] With the introduction of better percutaneous revascularization equipment such as more steerable guidewires, smaller profile balloons, and "bail-out" devices such as perfusion balloons, directional atherectomy, and stents, acute procedural success rates have increased while acute complications have decreased significantly.[15–17] At the present time, most institutions with experience in acute coronary syndrome percutaneous revascularization are reporting angiographic success rates approaching 95% with fewer than 5% of patients experiencing a major ischemic complication such as Q-wave myocardial infarction, coronary bypass surgery, or death. In our experience with the Thrombolysis and Angioplasty in Unstable Angina (TAUSA) trial, angiographic success was about 95% in the 233 patients in the placebo arm of the trial undergoing PTCA for unstable angina with an emergency bypass rate of only 2%.[18]

Procedural Factors

Importance of Complex Lesions

Serial angiography has demonstrated that many patients with unstable angina will have rapidly progressive lesions[19,20] that have complex features, including lesions that may be irregular, ulcerated, or contain intraluminal thrombus, as well as lesions that have led to total occlusion.[21] These factors help to explain the relatively high acute occlusion rates during or after PTCA with subsequent procedural-related myocardial infarction, since more complex lesions are dilated in unstable angina patients[7,13] compared to patients with stable angina, in whom lower rates of myocardial infarction are generally anticipated. Concerning specifically the presence of intracoronary thrombus and the risk of acute complications, most studies demonstrate a higher incidence of procedural complications when intracoronary thrombus is present prior to PTCA.[12,22,23]

Timing of PTCA

The high procedural major complication rate of PTCA in patients with unstable angina may be less if one would allow initial "stabilization" of the unstable lesion and then perform PTCA. The exact time period required for stabilization of an unstable lesion is unknown and the reported data are conflicting. In our experience reported preliminarily, PTCA within 48 hours from the last episode of rest pain was associated with the highest risk of major complications.[24] de Feyter et al. found a high complication rate of PTCA in patients initially stabilized but scheduled for PTCA within a week of stabilization.[7] Data from Myler et al.[25] and Stammen et al.[26] suggest that a stabilization period of as much as 2 weeks may be necessary. Myler et al.[25] demonstrated that patients with angina of less than 2 weeks' duration at the time of angioplasty suffered significantly higher major complication rates than did patients with angina of greater than 2 weeks' duration. The results of several nonrandomized studies indicate that stabiliza-

Table 2
Relation of Timing of PTCA for Unstable Angina and Major Complications

Author	Stabilization Period	Major Complications Death %	MI %	CABG %
de Feyter	<1 week	0	10	12
Myler	<1 week	0.3	6.5	9.4
Myler	1–2 weeks	0	6.6	6.1
Stammen	>2 weeks	0.3	3.6	4.7
Myler	>2 weeks	0.3	1.6	4.8

Adapted from de Feyter and Serruys: PTCA For Unstable Angina. In Textbook of Interventional Cardiology, edited by Topol EJ, WB Saunders, 1994 (with permission).

tion and pretreatment with heparin for one to several days does reduce the procedure-related complication rate[7–12,24–32] (Table 2). Patients treated with intravenous heparin for at least 24 hours prior to PTCA have been shown in noncontrolled studies to have a lower incidence of acute closure (0–5.7%) than patients in whom heparin was not given (8–33%).[29–32]

Based on these incomplete data, de Feyter and Serruys have suggested the practical policy of "cooling off" the unstable patient for 3 days with heparin, aspirin, and a combination of beta blockers, and then proceeding to angioplasty. The impact of introducing a stabilization period on the logistics of patient management and costs is substantial and more studies are needed to substantiate this policy.[33]

While the above approach is a safe and conservative approach to coronary intervention in unstable angina, it is often impossible and/or impractical to delay intervention. Furthermore, not all the data suggest that a "cooling off" period is necessary. In a retrospective analysis of unstable patients undergoing PTCA from the TAUSA trial, there was no additional protective effect of heparin administration prior to intervention on the incidence of acute closure or in-hospital ischemic events.[34] It has been our policy over the past few years not to delay angiography more than 24 hours once a patient is admitted to the hospital with rest angina. In most cases, if a coronary intervention is required it is performed in the same setting. One exception is when filling defects are present (usually distal to the culprit lesion). In this case, the intervention is delayed until the defects can be adequately resolved usually with an intracoronary infusion of a thrombolytic drug.

PTCA of the "Culprit" Lesion with Multivessel Disease

Overall, the majority of patients with unstable angina have multivessel disease; however, a substantial number of patients who are either young or have new onset angina or both may have single-vessel disease. Thus, the issue in multivessel disease patients of single versus multilesion angioplasty is very relevant since many of those undergoing single-lesion PTCA remain incompletely revascularized. Dilating only the ischemia-causing vessel (the "culprit" lesion) has been recommended as an initial approach to stabilize the patient's condition.[35,36] Identification of the culprit lesion is often possible using the combined evidence of either transient electrocardiographic changes during ischemia or angiographic findings (irregular lesions, ulcerated lesions, intracoronary thrombus, and severity of the lesion) or both. The primary success rates with this approach are generally excellent with subsequent resolution of symptoms in most patients.

While long-term follow-up of successfully treated patients using this strategy reveals that many patients will remain clinically improved,[35,36] the results of exercise testing and radionuclide scintigraphy suggest that a significant number of patients will have residual ischemia. This is presumably because of incomplete revascularization in most and restenosis of the dilated lesion in others. In addition, there is a higher recurrence rate of angina in the multivessel disease patients following "culprit" lesion PTCA (incompletely revascularized).[36] Careful clinical follow-up of patients with multivessel disease should be maintained as those with incomplete revascularization may potentially continue to have myocardial ischemia as documented by either recurrent symptoms or "positive" electrocardiography and perfusion scintigraphy during exercise.[7] Prospective studies, preferably randomized, will be required to confirm the overall efficacy and safety of culprit lesion angioplasty versus multilesion angioplasty in patients with unstable angina and multivessel disease. Meanwhile, it does appear that in selected patients, PTCA remains a worthwhile alternative to surgery.

Restenosis and Unstable Angina/Complex Lesions

There are conflicting data on the importance of complex lesions and/or unstable angina as a risk factor for restenosis. In some studies, eccentricity, lesion length, and the presence of thrombus were positively associated with restenosis.[37,38] Ellis et al. found morphology to be less important.[39] Recently, de Groote et al. found a greater loss in minimal lumen diameter and a higher rate of restenosis in culprit compared to nonculprit lesions in unstable angina.[40]

The data are likewise conflicting as to the importance of unstable angina as a risk factor for restenosis. Some studies have found higher rates while others have not.[33]

Thrombolytic Therapy as an Adjunct to Angioplasty

As mentioned previously, acute coronary occlusion following coronary angioplasty is increased in patients presenting with unstable angina and thrombus formation at the site of balloon dilatation has been suggested as a possible mechanism for the increase in acute closure. Angiographically, the presence of a complex lesion or an intracoronary thrombus on angiography prior to angioplasty is associated with a higher incidence of adverse events. Thrombolytic therapy infused intravenously or directly into the coronary artery has been advocated either before, during, or immediately after angioplasty to prevent complications associated with the procedure.

Thrombolytic Therapy Prior to Angioplasty

Even in the New Approaches to Coronary Intervention (NACI) Registry, in which devices other than angioplasty balloons were primarily used, the presence of intracoronary thrombus was associated with a lower success rate (85% vs. 93% for procedures without intracoronary thrombus) and an increased complication rate of either death, Q-wave myocardial infarction, or coronary bypass surgery (9% vs. 3%, respectively).[41] Because of this association between intracoronary thrombus and complications of angioplasty, thrombolytic therapy and/or prolonged infusions of heparin have been advocated prior to angioplasty as a means of improving success. Several studies have reported the results of thrombolytics in small numbers of patients in whom large filling defects were lysed by intracoronary infusions prior to angioplasty[42–45] (Table 3). Infusions of intravenous or intracoronary thrombolytics, in general, reduced thrombus burden and allowed angioplasty to proceed with few or no complications. Even when thrombus was not present prior to angioplasty, Topol et al. noted that intravenous t-PA given prior to angioplasty may facilitate the safety of angioplasty in unstable angina.[46]

Table 3
Intravenous or Intracoronary Thrombolytic Therapy in Native Vessels or SV Grafts to Decrease Intracoronary Thrombus Prior to Angioplasty

Name	*No.*	*Agent*	*Delay in PTCA*	*Decrease in T*	*Results of PTCA*
Hurley	3	IV t-PA × 6 hr	24–72 hr	Yes	No complications
Goudreau	8	IC UK × ~30–60 min	—	Yes in 7/8	7 of 8 without complications
Grill	12	IC SK/IV t-PA × 60 min–3 hr	.3 to 4 d	Yes in 8/12	All 8 without complications
Chapekis	21	IC UK × 24 hr	24 hr	Yes	19 to 20 without complications

t-PA = tissue plasminogen activator; UK = urokinase; SK = streptokinase.

Anecdotally, we have infused intracoronary thrombolytic therapy (usually urokinase) for a period of one to several hours prior to angioplasty in patients with obvious abundant intracoronary thrombus. In these instances, the thrombus was usually a large filling defect (>2 mm in length) located proximal or in most cases distal to a significant lesion. It has been our policy to infuse the drug through a diagnostic catheter located in the ostium of the coronary artery. However, it is possible to infuse medication through infusion catheters that can be advanced up to the lesion. We have been reluctant, however, to use these types of catheters in the left coronary artery but have used them often in the right coronary artery or in saphenous vein grafts, particularly when the coronary thrombus was located in a distal segment. In general, this approach has been very satisfactory with excellent results both in dissolving thrombus and allowing angioplasty to proceed safely (Figures 1 and 2).

The Mechanism of Acute Closure during Angioplasty in Unstable Angina

Can one be sure of the mechanism of acute closure during angioplasty? This is, of course, an important question. If the mechanism of acute closure is coronary dissection, it is possible that a thrombolytic agent could conceivably worsen the results (see the results of the TAUSA Trial). If one or multiple filling defects are noted in the artery

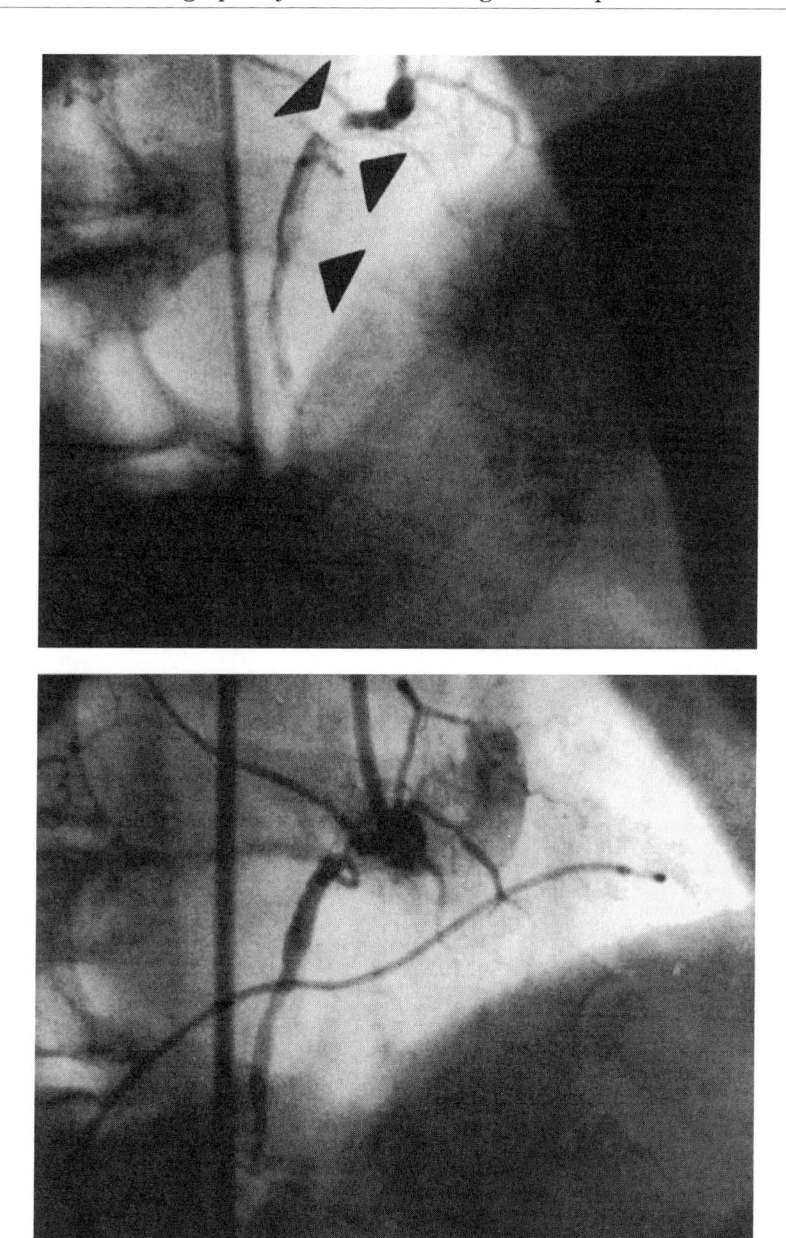

Figure 1: RCA in the RAO projection. The patient had a recent inferior wall myocardial infarction. In the top panel, the two lower arrows point to the extensive thrombus that was dissolved (lower panel) by a 6-hour infusion of urokinase (800,000 units) through a 6 French diagnostic catheter.

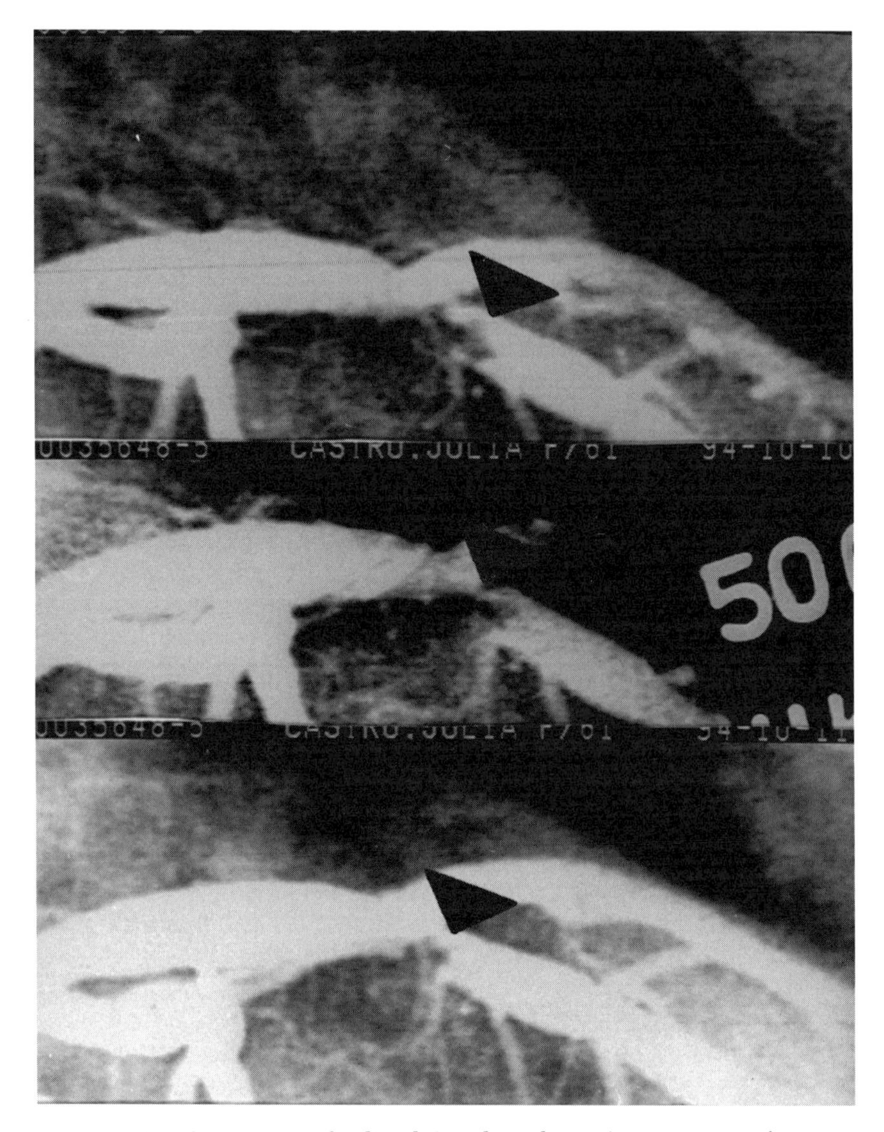

Figure 2: Another strategy for dissolving thrombus prior to coronary intervention. This patient had an anterior wall myocardial infarction 2 days prior to angiography. Serial angiograms of the left anterior descending artery are seen in the RAO projection. The top panel shows a significant lesion with a filling defect distal to the narrowing. In the middle panel, the patient had received a 45-minute infusion of 500,000 units of urokinase through a diagnostic catheter positioned in the proximal LAD. The patient was brought back to the catheterization laboratories after 18 additional hours of IV heparin (heparin had been given continuously for 2 days prior to angiography) and the lower angiogram was recorded. This shows further resolution of thrombus. PTCA was performed uneventfully.

just prior to or immediately after opening the artery or if the patient was known to have had thrombus in the artery prior to angioplasty, one can assume in the absence of a significant angiographic dissection that the mechanism is probably thrombotic. If an angiographic dissection is seen, it is likely the cause of closure and it is prudent not to use thrombolytic agents. One further point must be stressed. Thrombus formation develops over about 10 to 15 minutes following angioplasty. Therefore, delayed views at 15 minutes may be necessary to exclude thrombus formation post angioplasty in unstable patients.

Two recent observations offer conflicting data concerning the importance of thrombotic occlusion as the mechanism of acute closure following angioplasty in unstable angina. In a preliminary investigation utilizing the technique of percutaneous angioscopy, Jain et al. reported that while intravascular thrombi were usually seen at the site of acute closure, thrombus was rarely its cause.[47] In 8 of 10 abrupt closures undergoing angioscopy, an occlusive dissection was present. On the other hand, indirect evidence for the importance of thrombus in acute closure comes from the EPIC trial (The Evaluation of $7E_3$ for the Prevention of Ischemic Complications). In the treatment group assigned to a bolus and 12-hour infusion of $c7E_3$, there was a significantly lower incidence ($<1\%$) and a marked reduction in the need for urgent PTCA during the first 48 hours after angioplasty in comparison to placebo (heparin group).[48]

Thrombolytic Therapy for Acute Closure

Several other noncontrolled studies have also suggested a possible role for intracoronary thrombolytic therapy in the setting of acute closure during angioplasty[43,49–53] (Table 4). In these studies, once acute closure had occurred, repeat dilatation alone was usually ineffective in reopening the artery. The use of intracoronary streptokinase, urokinase, or t-PA in addition to redilatation improved angiographic results and avoided ischemic complications.

The analyses of the data from the studies contained in Table 4 were usually retrospective. There was also no standardization in the methods for giving the thrombolytic agents and/or repeating angioplasty. Furthermore, Gulba et al. found re-occlusion in over 50% in 24 to 36 hours following opening.[52] Therefore, while initially appearing beneficial, the importance of thrombolytics versus prolonged and repeated balloon inflations versus stenting in this situation is difficult to understand. In addition, not all studies have shown positive results

Table 4
Intracoronary Thrombolysis for Acute Closure after Transluminal Coronary Angioplasty*

Study	*n*	*Drug*	*Dose*	*Angiographic Success (%)*
Suryapranata	12	IC SK	2.5×10^5	75
de Feyter	34	IC SK	$2.5–15 \times 10^5$	65
Verna	23	IC UK	$1–3.6 \times 10^5$	65
Goudreau	14	IC UK	$1.5–5 \times 10^5$	72
Gulba	27	IC/IV t-PA	20 mgs IC & 50 mgs IV	82
Scheiman	48	IC UK	$1–2.5 \times 10^5$	90

SK = streptokinase; UK = urokinase; t-PA = tissue plasminogen activtor; IC = intracoronary.
* In all studies except that of Scheiman, thrombolytic agent given after repeated dilation failed to reopen the acute closure.

with thrombolytic agents. In a retrospective analysis of patients from two large referral centers, Lincoff et al. were unable to show any benefits from intracoronary thrombolytic therapy in the treatment of abrupt vessel closure complicating angioplasty.[54] A prospective trial that unfortunately was not placebo-controlled has been carried out to better assess the role of intracoronary urokinase at the time of acute closure. Schieman et al. followed a standardized protocol in 75 patients in whom acute or threatened closure occurred following angioplasty.[53] Small doses of intracoronary urokinase infused over about 30 to 40 minutes through a guiding catheter along with redilitation resulted in an angiographic success rate of 90% without ischemic events or procedure-related myocardial infarction. This study, although not randomizing thrombolytic agents once acute closure was suspected, provides additional data for the beneficial effects of urokinase.

Based on all the above data, we think it is reasonable to adopt the following approach. In a patient with acute closure that is presumed to be secondary to thrombotic causes and refractory to at least one long repeat dilatation, it is reasonable to infuse urokinase directly into the artery in a dose of about 250,000 to 750,000 units over a period of 20 minutes to 1 hour along with careful redilatation of the artery. We believe the strategy should be carried out prior to assuming that this represents an angioplasty failure and the patient should be sent for another intervention. Since the newer methods of nonsurgical intervention except for perhaps the transluminal extraction catheter are relatively useless in patients with large amounts of intracoronary thrombus, the thrombolytic/redilatation approach may be the best chance for maintaining patency. Whether newer antithrombin agents like hirudin may prove to be more beneficial remains to be determined. Anecdotally, an infusion of a monoclonal antibody to the glycoprotein IIb/IIIa receptor on the platelet (c7E_3) has also been shown to improve coronary flow following angioplasty in a small number of patients with "threatened" acute closure.[55] Preliminary observations with the local delivery of a thrombolytic agent by the Dispatch catheter (Scimed Life Systems) indicates that this catheter may be able to rapidly dissolve intracoronary thrombi using substantially less drug than standard thrombolytic techniques.[56] In other cases, particularly when the mechanism of acute closure is not clearly thrombus, stenting may be the appropriate strategy for acute closure.

Prophylactic Thrombolytic Therapy during Angioplasty in Unstable Angina

Studies without a matching control group have suggested that in certain patients who are at high risk for acute closure during angioplasty, small doses of intracoronary urokinase infused immediately before angioplasty will increase the success rate of the procedure and decrease complications.[57,58] While intracoronary thrombus defined as filling defects proximal or distal to a stenosis appear to benefit from long infusions of thrombolytic therapy prior to angioplasty, do the above data suggest that thrombolytic therapy should be used prophylacticly during angioplasty in unstable angina even when apparent thrombus is not present? While there could be some benefit as suggested by the data of Anwar et al.[56] there is also a potential detrimental effect for this type of therapy. Thrombin-bound fibrin is active and its release by thrombolytic therapy could result in further thrombosis.[59] Furthermore, hemorrhage into the wall of an artery has been demonstrated pathologically by Waller et al. when angioplasty was performed after thrombolysis for acute infarction.[60] Because the major mechanism of angioplasty involves splitting and dissection of the plaque, thrombolytic therapy in unstable angina could be detrimental by either extending the dissection or preventing the dissection from sealing with further inflations of the balloon. Finally, since the thrombus in unstable angina is presumed to be platelet-rich and thrombolytic therapy activates platelets, such therapy may lead to further thrombus formation or increased vasomotor tone.[61]

The TAUSA Trial

To ascertain whether or not there was a role for prophylactic thrombolytic therapy during angioplasty in unstable angina, a randomized, multicenter, double-blind trial was instituted. The hypothesis of the Thrombolysis and Angioplasty in Unstable Angina (TAUSA) Trial was that prophylactic thrombolytic therapy could decrease the incidence of intraluminal thrombus formation and acute closure after angioplasty as well as decrease adverse in-hospital ischemic events. For inclusion into this study, patients had to have ischemic rest pain (unstable angina) with angioplasty performed within 1 week of an episode of rest pain. Patients with non-Q or Q-wave infarction and recurrent pain were also included if the last episode of rest pain was within 7 days of angioplasty. In a small randomized double-blind pilot study of 92 patients, 150,000 units of intracoronary urokinase was shown to decrease angiographic filling defects after angioplasty. However, acute closure and in-hospital ischemic events were not prevented by this dose.[62]

In the larger TAUSA Trial, 469 patients were randomized in double-blind fashion to receive either intracoronary urokinase or placebo during angioplasty.[18] All patients were pretreated with aspirin; heparin was given to maintain an ACT >300 seconds and heparin therapy was continued overnight after angioplasty. In phase I, 257 patients received 250,000 units of urokinase or placebo in divided dosages given immediately before wire placement and immediately after the 1 minute post PTCA angiogram. In phase II, 212 patients received a 500,000 unit infusion of urokinase or placebo in divided doses before and immediately after PTCA. Angiograms were performed at 1 and 15 minutes following PTCA and read by a core laboratory. This analysis was done for the presence of filling defects, acute closure, and dissection. In-hospital events (ischemic chest pain with or without electrocardiographic changes, myocardial infarction, emergency bypass surgery, and death) served as clinical end-points. The results are summarized in Table 5.

The major results of the TAUSA Trial indicated that while there was a decrease in filling defects post PTCA with urokinase, the harder end-points of acute closure and early ischemic events were increased particularly during phase II in which the higher dose of urokinase was infused. The results with urokinase appeared worse in unstable angina without recent infarction than in the group undergoing angioplasty after recent infarction. This was opposite to what we found in the pilot study in which only patients with unstable angina and no recent infarc-

Table 5
TAUSA Trial: Angiographic and In-hospital Outcome

	Urokinase n (%) *n = 232*	*Placebo n (%)* *n = 237*
Filling Defect (15 min)	30 (13.8)	41 (18.0)
Major Dissection	22 (9.5)	19 (8.0)
Acute Closure	23 (10.2)	10 (4.3)*
Ischemia	23 (9.9)	8 (3.4)**
CABG	12 (5.2)	5 (2.1)†
MI	9 (3.9)	5 (2.1)
Any clinical end-point	30 (12.9)	15 (6.3)‡

* P <0.02; ** P <0.005; † P = 0.009; ‡ P = 0.018.

tion seemed to improve following the small dose of intracoronary urokinase. The reason for this difference is unknown but may relate to patient selection or to differences in the urokinase dose between studies.

Based on this trial, thrombolytic therapy should be avoided as prophylactic therapy in patients undergoing angioplasty in unstable angina or recent infarction. It is likely that these negative results are related to one of two mechanisms. Urokinase given in the fashion as infused in the TAUSA Trial will increase intimal disruption or prevent intimal sealing. The second mechanism may relate to the possibility that urokinase and other thrombolytic agents may at least, early after infusion, activate platelets. If there is very little fibrin thrombus present at the time of angioplasty, the effects of a thrombolytic agent would be negligible and the potential detrimental effects of the thrombolytic agent on activating platelets may be more important.

Angioplasty in Complex Lesions

The large number of patients undergoing angioplasty in the TAUSA Trial afforded us an opportunity to study the effects of complex lesion morphology on the results of angioplasty. Of the 469 patients randomized into the trial, 459 ultimately underwent angioplasty and of these a morphology of the culprit lesion was available in 458. In the following discussion, *complex* is defined as lesions with overhanging edges, irregular borders or ulcerations, or filling defects proximal or distal to a significant stenosis. In addition, total coronary occlusion with angiographic features of thrombus were also included in the diagnosis of complex although total occlusion was present in only 9% prior to angioplasty. Of the 458 patients with data available, 245 (53.5%) had complex lesions while the remaining 213 had simple lesions. Baseline characteristics were similar including the percentage of patients in whom heparin therapy was given prior to angioplasty. The overall success rate for complex lesions was 94.7% versus 97.2% in the simple group P = NS. *Success* was defined as a residual stenosis <50%. Angiographic and clinical end-points are contained in Table 6. Complex lesion angioplasty was associated with a significantly higher incidence of definite thrombus and acute closure as well as a higher incidence of recurrent angina and emergency bypass surgery.[63]

In the group with complex culprit lesions, 127 (51.8%) had received urokinase while 118 were in the placebo group. Again, baseline characteristics were similiar between urokinase and placebo. The results of angioplasty are contained in Table 7. The success of angioplasty was lower (91.3%) in the urokinase group versus 97.5% in the placebo group. Filling defects post angioplasty were slightly decreased by urokinase. However, acute closure was significantly increased with urokinase being 15% in this group versus 6% in the placebo group. Clinical endpoints were also worse with urokinase than with placebo with the biggest difference being in the incidence of post angioplasty ischemia. When we analyzed separately the 56 with pre-PTCA filling defects proximal or distal to a stenosis, there were also no differences between urokinase and placebo.

Table 6
TAUSA Trial: Angiographic and Clinical Results Based on Lesion Morphology

	Simple *N = 213*	*Complex* *N = 245*	*P*
Angiographic			
• Definite thrombus (%)	5.6	22.0	<0.001
• Acute closure (%)	3.3	10.6	<0.003
Clinical			
• Recurrent angina (%)	3.3	9.0	<0.02
• MI (%)	1.9	3.3	NS
• CABG (%)	0.9	5.2	<0.02
• Death (%)	0	0	NS
• Composite (%)	5.2	12.2	<0.01

MI = myocardial infarction; CABG = coronary artery bypass graft.

Table 7
TAUSA Trial: End-points in Complex Lesions

	Urokinase *n = 127*	*Placebo* *n = 118*
Definite filling defects	18.9%	25.4%
Acute closure	15.0%	5.9%*
Major dissection	11.0%	5.9%
Ischemia	14.2%	4.2%**
MI	3.9%	3.4%
CABG	7.1%	2.5%
Any clinical end-point	17.3%	6.8%§

** P <.007; * P <.03; § P <0.02.
MI = myocardial infarction; CABG = coronary artery bypass graft.

In the 213 simple, "culprit" lesions, there were no significant differences in clinical end-points with angioplasty between urokinase and placebo. However, as for the entire group, there was a trend to a significant reduction in filling defects following angioplasty in the group given urokinase (P<0.06). When we analyzed separately the placebo group, which included 233 culprit lesions undergoing angioplasty, 118 had complex lesions and 115 had simple lesions. The incidence of definite filling defects following angioplasty was increased threefold in the complex group and this difference was highly significant. Acute closure was also increased over twofold from 2.6% in the simple group to 5.9% in the complex group but this difference was not significant.

We can therefore draw the following conclusions about angioplasty for complex lesions based on the results of TAUSA:

1. Complex lesions are associated with a higher incidence of complications than simple lesions.

2. Urokinase as administered in this trial had an adverse effect on the angioplasty results of complex lesions and there was no benefit even in the group with pre-PTCA filling defects. The results of angioplasty in the placebo group were quite good even in the group with complex lesions, suggesting that unless other interventional techniques prove better (e.g., directional atherectomy or stents), angioplasty is a good technique for at the acute management of complex lesions. However, the incidence of acute closure was nearly 6% for complex lesions with aspirin and heparin alone. It is likely that newer adjunctive therapies e.g., antiplatelet or antithrombin agents, should improve on these results with intervention.

In analyzing these results, one may be puzzled by the fact that filling defects proximal or distal to a stenosis were not beneficially treated by urokinase. As mentioned earlier in this section, urokinase seemed to improve the results of angioplasty when thrombus was present proximal or distal to a lesion. We suspect that the difference between these prior studies and the results of the TAUSA Trial are probably in the way the urokinase was administered. If used, urokinase should be infused slowly prior to angioplasty as outlined previously. In addition, the "prophylactic" infusion of urokinase as done in the TAUSA Trial immediately after angioplasty might possibly create or increase the amount of intimal dissection is not recommended.

Newer Adjunctive Agents and Angioplasty

The beneficial response of thrombolytic agents in acute myocardial infarction and the lack of efficacy of these agents in unstable angina along with a better understanding of the importance of platelets and thrombin in acute syndromes has spurred further development of different classes of agents to modify thrombus formation. Newer, direct thrombin inhibitors such as hirudin and hirulog and antiplatelet agents that specifically block the glycoprotein IIb/IIIa receptor have been used during PTCA to decrease acute complications and possibly prevent restenosis.

Preliminary results with both hirudin or hirulog during PTCA have been reported recently.[64,65] Periprocedural infarction or bypass surgery were significantly reduced with a hirudin infusion of 24 hours in comparison to heparin. The Hirulog Angioplasty Study, a large multicenter randomized trial of hirulog versus heparin during intervention in unstable angina, showed no decrease in the combined end-points of death, infarction, or the need for emergent bypass with hirulog in comparison to heparin, 4.6% versus 5.2% respectively, P = NS. However, a significant reduction in these adverse end-points occurred in a subgroup with postinfarction angina receiving hirulog (6.6% with heparin vs. 2.5% with hirulog, $P<0.01$). Overall, hirulog was also associated with a significant reduction in bleeding complications in comparison to heparin. A monoclonal antibody known as $7E_3$ against the platelet receptor IIb/IIIa was developed and has been shown to be an effective antiplatelet agent in both animals and humans. A chimeric form of the drug ($c7E_3$) has been used during angioplasty. The EPIC Trial randomized over 2,000 patients to either $c7E_3$ given as a bolus, a bolus of $c7E_3$ plus a 12-hour infusion, or placebo during PTCA.[48] All received heparin. In comparison to placebo, the bolus plus infusion resulted in a 35% reduction (12.8 vs. 8.3%, P = 0.008) in ischemic events over a 30–day period. The results in unstable angina were even more striking with a 71% reduction in comparison to placebo (13.0 vs. 3.8%, P = 0.004). At 6-month follow-up, late death and infarction were also significantly reduced with the bolus and infusion in comparison to placebo.[66] Similiar results have been reported with other IIb/IIIa receptor blockers. This improvement in short-term ischemic complications was associated with an increased risk of bleeding and the need for transfusions. Recent data suggest that the bleeding may be more related to the heparin dose than to the $c7E_3$.[67] Current studies during PTCA are evaluating the use of $c7E_3$ with lower doses of heparin to achieve similar results to EPIC in reducing ischemic complications without increasing bleeding. Integrelin, a reversible cyclic heptapeptide blocker with a short half-life, reduced ischemic complications in comparison to heparin in a small randomized trial.[68] In the near future, large trials with these or newer agents will be published. These agents will likely improve on the results of PTCA and/or other interventions in these high-risk populations with unstable angina, acute myocardial infarction, or complex lesions. Large trials with integrelin, $c7E_3$, and MK-383, a nonpeptide IIb/IIIa inhibitor, are presently ongoing. Orally active IIb/IIIa inhibitors have also been developed and trials are planned.

References

1. Gruntzig A. Transluminal dilatation of coronary artery stenosis (letter). Lancet 1978; 1:263.
2. Williams DO, Riley RS, Singh AK, Gewirtz H, Most AS. Evaluation of the role of coronary angioplasty in patients with unstable angina pectoris. Am Heart J 1981; 102:1–9.
3. Meyer J, Schmitz H, Erbel R, et al. Treatment of unstable angina pectoris with percutaneous transluminal coronary angioplasty (PTCA). Cathet Cardiovasc Diagn 1981; 7:361–371.
4. Meyer J, Schmitz HJ, Kiesslich T, et al. Percutaneous transluminal coronary angioplasty in patients with stable and unstable angina pectoris: Analysis of early and late results. Am Heart J 1983; 106:973–980.
5. de Feyter PI, Serruys PW, van den Brand M, et al. Emergency coronary angioplasty in refractory unstable angina. N Engl J Med 1985; 313:3426.
6. Quigley PJ, Erwin J, Maurer BJ, Walsh MJ, Gearty GF. Percutaneous transluminal coronary angioplasty in unstable angina: comparison with stable angina. Br Heart J 1986; 55:227–230,
7. de Feyter PJ, Serruys PW, Suryapranata H, Beatt K, van den Brand M. Coronary angioplasty early after diagnosis of unstable angina. Am Heart J 1987; 114:48–54.

8. Steffenino G, Meier B, Finci L, Rutishauser W. Follow-up results of treatment of unstable angina by coronary angioplasty. Br Heart J 1987; 57: 416–419.
9. Timmis AD, Griffin B, Crick IC, Sowton E. Early percutaneous transluminal coronary angioplasty in the management of unstable angina. Int J Cardiol 1987; 14:25–31.
10. Plokker TWH, Ernst SM, Bal ET, et al. Percutaneous transluminal coronary angioplasty in patients with unstable angina pectoris refractory to medical therapy: long-term clinical and angiographic results. Cathet Cardiovasc Diagn 1988; 14:15–18.
11. Sharma B, Wyeth RP, Kolath GS, Gimenez HI, Franciosa IA. Percutaneous transluminal coronary angioplasty of one vessel for refractory unstable angina pectoris: Efficacy in single and multivessel disease. Br Heart J 1988; 59:280–286.
12. de Feyter PI, Suryapranata H, Serruys PW, et al. Coronary angioplasty for unstable angina: Immediate and late results in 200 consecutive patients with identification of risk factors for unfavorable early and late outcome. J Am Coll Cardiol 1988; 12:324–333.
13. Perry RA, Seth A, Hunt A, Shiu MF. Coronary angioplasty in unstable angina and stable angina: A comparison of success and complications. Br Heart J 1988; 60:367–372.
14. Kamp O, Beatt KI, de Feyter PI, et al. Short, medium and long term follow-up after percutaneous transluminal coronary angioplasty for stable and unstable angina pectoris. Am Heart J 1989; 117:991–996.
15. Stack RS, Quigley PJ, Collins G, Philips HR. Perfusion balloon catheter. Am J Cardiol 1988; 61:77G-88G.
16. Simpson JB, Johnson DE, Braden LJ, Gifford HS, Thapliyal HV, Selmon MR. Transluminal coronary atherectomy: Results in 21 human cadaver vascular segments. Circulation 1986; 74:II-202A.
17. Roubin GS, Douglas JS Jr, Lembo NJ, Black AJ, King SB. Intracoronary stenting for acute closure following PTCA. Circulation 1988; 78:II-407A.
18. Ambrose JA, Almeida OD, Sharma S, Torre S, Marmur J, Israel D, Ratner D, Weiss M, et al., for the TAUSA investigators. Adjunctive thrombolytic therapy during angioplasty for ischemic rest angina: Results of the TAUSA Trial. Circulation 1994; 90:69–77.
19. Kimbiris D, Iskandrian A, Saras H, et al. Rapid progression of coronary stenosis in patients with unstable angina pectoris selected for coronary angioplasty. Cathet Cardiovasc Diagn 1984; 10:101–114.
20. Ambrose JA, Winters SL, Arora RR, Riccio A, Gorlin R, Fuster V. Angiographic evolution of coronary morphology in unstable angina. J Am Coll Cardiol 1986; 7:472–478.
21. Ambrose JA, Winters SL, Arora RR, Haft JI, Goldstein J, Rentrop KP, Gorlin R, Fuster V. Coronary angiographic morphology in myocardial infarction: A link between the pathogenesis of unstable angina and myocardial infarction. J Am Coll Cardiol 1985; 6:1233–1238.
22. Mabin TA, Holmes DR, Smith HC, et al. Intracoronary thrombus: role in coronary occlusion complicating percutaneous transluminal coronary angioplasty. J Am Coll Cardiol 1985; 5:198–202.
23. Arora RR, Platko WP, Bhadwar K, Simfendorfer C. Role of intracoronary

thrombus in acute complications during percutaneous transluminal coronary angioplasty. Cathet Cardiovasc Diagn 1989; 16:226–229.
24. Torre SR, Ambrose JA, Sharma SK, Untereker WJ, Weiss WB, Monsen C, Marshall J, Grunwald A, Moses J, Israel D. Relationship between recent rest pain and acute complications of PTCA in unstable angina. J Am Coll Cardiol 1992; 19:230A
25. Myler RK, Shaw RE, Stertzer SH, et al. Unstable angina and coronary angioplasty. Circulation 1990; 82(Suppl II)II:88–95.
26. Stammen F, De Scheerder I, Glazier JI, et al. Immediate and follow-up results of the conservative coronary angioplasty strategy of unstable angina pectoris. Am J Cardiol 1992; 69:1533.
27. Morrison DA. Percutaneous transluminal coronary angioplasty for rest angina pectoris requiring intravenous nitroglycerin and intra-aortic balloon counterpulsation. Am J Cardiol 1990; 66:168.
28. Rupprecht MJ, Brennecke R, Kottmeyer M, Bernhard G, Erbel R, Pop T, Meyer R. Short- and long-term outcome after PTCA inpatients with stable and unstable angina. Eur Heart J 1990; 11:1964.
29. Hettleman BD, Aplin RA, Sullivan PR, et al. Three days of heparin pretreatment reduces major complications of coronary angioplasty in patients with unstable angina (abstr). J Am Coll Cardiol 1990; 25:154.
30. Laskey MAL, Deutsch E, Barnathan E, et al. Influence of heparin therapy on percutaneous transluminal coronary angioplasty outcome in unstable angina pectoris. Am J Cardiol 1990; 65:1425.
31. Pow TK, Varrichione TR, Jacobs AK, et al. Does pretreatment with heparin prevent abrupt closure following PTCA? J Am Coll Cardiol 1988; 11: 238A.
32. Lukas MA, Deutsch E, Hirschfeld JW, et al. Influence of heparin on percutaneous transluminal coronary angioplasty outcome in patients with coronary arterial thrombus. Am J Cardiol 1990; 65:179.
33. de Feyter PJ, Serruys PW. PTCA for unstable angina. In Topol EJ (ed): Textbook of Interventional Cardiology, 2nd edition, Philadelphia, WB Saunders Company, 1994.
34. Ambrose JA, Almeida OD, Ratner D, Torre S, Sharma SK, Marmur JD, Israel D, for the TAUSA trial. Heparin administered prior to angioplasty does not decrease angioplasty complications: TAUSA trial results. Circulation 1994; 90:I-374A.
35. Wohlgelertner D, Cleman M, Mighinan HA, et al. Percutaneous transluminal coronary angioplasty of the "culprit lesion" for management of unstable angina pectoris in patients with multivessel coronary artery disease . Am J Cardiol 1986; 58:460.
36. de Feyter PJ, Serruys PW, Arnold A, et al. Coronary angioplasty of the unstable angina related vessel in patients with multivessel disease. Eur Heart J 1986; 7:460.
37. Hirshfeld JW, Schwartz SJ, Jugo R, et al., and the M-Heart Investigators. Restenosis after coronary angioplasty: a multivariate statistical model to relate lesion and procedural variables to restenosis. J Am Coll Cardiol 1991; 18:647–656.
38. Bourassa MG, Lesperance J, Eastwood C, Schwartz L, Cote G, Kazim F,

Hudon G. Clinical, physiologic, anatomic, and procedural factors predictive of restenosis after PTCA. J Am Coll Cardiol 1991; 18:368–376.
39. Ellis SG, Roubin GS, King SB, Douglas JS Jr, Cox WR. Importance of stenosis morphology in the estimation of restenosis risk after elective PTCA. Am J Cardiol 1989; 63:30–34.
40. de Groote P, Bauters C, Mc Fadden EP, Lablanche JM, Leroy F, Bertrand ME. Local lesion-related factors and restenosis after coronary angioplasty: Evidence from a quantitative angiographic study in patients with unstable angina undergoing double-vessel angioplasty. Circulation 1995; 91: 968–972.
41. O'Neill WW, Sketch MH Jr, Steenkiste A, Detre K, for the NACI Registry Investigators. New Device Intervention in the treatment of intracoronary thrombus. Report of the NACI Registry. Circulation 1993; 88(no. 4, part 2):I-595A.
42. Hurley DV, Bresnahan DR, Holmes DR Jr. Staged thrombolysis and percutaneous transluminal coronary angioplasty for unstable and postinfarction angina. Cathet Cardiovasc Diagn 1989; 18:67–72.
43. Goudreau E, DiSciascio G, Vetrovec GW, Chami Y, Kohli R, Warner M, Sabri N, Cowley MJ. Intracoronary urokinase as an adjunct to percutaneous transluminal angioplasty in patients with complex coronary narrowings or angioplasty-induced complications. Am J Cardiol 1992; 69:57–62.
44. Grill HP, Brinker JA. Nonacute thrombolytic therapy: An adjunct to coronary angioplasty in patients with large intravascular thrombi. Am Heart J 1989; 118:662.
45. Chapekis AT, George BS, Candela RJ. Rapid thrombus dissolution by continuous infusion of urokinase through an intracoronary perfusion wire prior to and following PTCA: results in native coronaries and patent saphenous vein grafts. Cathet Cardiovas Diagn 1991; 23:89–92.
46. Topol EJ, Nicklas JM, Kander NH, Walton JA, Ellis SG, Gorman L, Pitt B. Coronary revascularization after intravenous tissue plasminogen activator for unstable angina pectoris: Results of a randomized, double-blind, placebo-controlled trial. Am J Cardiol 1988; 62:368–371.
47. Jain SP, White CJ, Collins TJ, Escobar A, Ramee SR. Etiologies of abrupt occlusion after PTCA: Angioscopic morphology. J Am Coll Cardiol 1993; 21:484A.
48. EPIC investigators. Use of a monoclonal antibody directed against the platelet glycoprotein IIb/IIIa receptor in high risk coronary angioplasty. N Engl J Med 1994; 330:956–961.
49. Suryapranata H, de Feyter PJ, Serruys PW. Coronary angioplasty in patients with unstable angina pectoris: is there a role for thrombolysis? J Am Coll Cardiol 1988; 12:69A-77A.
50. de Feyter PJ, van den Brand M, Laarman GJ, van Domburg R, Serruys PW, Suryapranata H, Jaarman G. Acute coronary artery occlusion during and after percutaneous coronary angioplasty: frequency, prediction, clinical course, management, and follow-up. Circulation 1991; 83:927–936.
51. Verna E, Repetto S, Boscarini M, Onofri M, Qing LG, Binaghi G. Management of complicated coronary angioplasty by intracoronary urokinase and immediate re-angioplasty. Cathet Cardiovasc Diagn 1990; 19:116–122.
52. Gulba DC, Daniel WG, Simon R, Jost S, Barthels M, Amende I, Rafflenbeul

W, Lichtlen PR. Role of thrombolysis and thrombin in patients with acute coronary occlusion during percutaneous transluminal coronary angioplasty. J Am Coll Cardiol 1990; 16:563–568.
53. Schieman G, Cohen BM, Kozina J, Erickson JS, Podolin RA, Peterson KL, Ross J Jr, Buchbinder M. Intracoronary urokinase for intracoronary thrombus accumulation complicating percutaneous transluminal coronary angioplasty in acute ischemic syndromes. Circulation 1990; 82:2052–2060.
54. Lincoff AM, Popma JJ, Ellis SG, Hacker JA, Topol EJ. Abrupt vessel closure complicating coronary angioplasty: clinical, angiographic and therapeutic profile. J Am Coll Cardiol 1992; 19:926–935.
55. Anderson VH, Kirkeeide RL, Krishnaswami A, Weigelt LA, Revana M, Weisman HF, Willerson JT. Cyclic flow variations after coronary angioplasty in humans: clinical and angiographic characteristics and elimination with $7E_3$ monoclonal antiplatelet antibody. J Am Coll Cardiol 1994; 23:1031–1037.
56. Mitchel JF, Azrin MA, Fram DB, Hong MK, Wong SC, Barry JJ, Bow LM, Curley TM, Kiernan FJ, et al. Inhibition of platelet deposition and lysis of intracoronary thrombus during balloon angioplasty using urokinase-coated hydrogel balloons. Circulation 1994; 90:1979–1988.
57. Anwar A, Myler RK, Nguyen K, Shaw RE, Webb J, Anwar LB, Murphy MC, Cumberland DC, Stertzer SH. Combined coronary angioplasty, urokinase and heparin in the treatment of acute ischemic syndromes. J Invasive Cardiol 1991; 3:41–48.
58. Pavlides GS, Schreiber TL, Gangadharan V, Puchrowicz S, O'Neill WW. Safety and efficacy of urokinase during elective coronary angioplasty. Am Heart J 1991; 121:731–737.
59. Chesebro JH, Goldhelyi P, Fuster V. Pathogenesis of thrombosis in unstable angina. Am J Cardiol 1991; 68:2B-10B.
60. Waller BF, Rothbaum DA, Pinkerton CA, Cowley MJ, Linnemeier TJ, Orr C, Irons M, Helmuth RA, Wills ER, Aust C. Status of the myocardium and infarct-related coronary artery in 19 necropsy patients with acute recanalization using pharmacological (streptokinase, r-tissue plasminogen activator), mechanical (percutaneous transluminal coronary angioplasty) or combined types of reperfusion therapy. J Am Coll Cardiol 1987; 9: 785–801.
61. Coller BS. Role of platelets in thrombolytic therapy. In: Haber E, Braunwald E (eds): Thrombolysis: Basic Contributions and Clinical Progress. St. Louis, Mosby Year Book, 1991, pp 155–178.
62. Ambrose JA, Torre SR, Sharma SK, Israel DH, Monsen CE, Weiss M, Untereker W, Grunwald A, Moses J, Marshall J, Bunnell P, Sobolski J. Adjunctive thrombolytic therapy for angioplasty in ischemic rest angina: Results of a double-blinded randomized pilot study. J Am Coll Cardiol 1992; 20:1197–1204.
63. Mehran R, Ambrose JA, Bongu RM, Almeida OA, Israel DH, Torre S, Sharma SK, Ratner DE. Angioplasty of complex lesions in Ischemic Rest Angina- Results of the TAUSA Trial. J Am Coll Cardiol (submitted for publication).
64. van den Bos AA, Deckers JW, Heyndrickx GR, Laarman GJ, Rijnierse J,

et al. PTCA with hirudin associated with less acute cardiac complications than with heparin. Circulation 1992;(Suppl) 86:1482A.
65. John Bittl. Personal communication.
66. Lincoff AM, Califf RM, Anderson K, Weisman HF, Topol EJ for the EPIC investigators. Striking clinical benefit with platelet GP IIb/IIIa inhibition by $c7E_3$ among patients with unstable angina pectoris: Outcome in the EPIC trial. Circulation 1994; 90(No.4, Part 2):I-21A.
67. Lincoff AM, Tcheng JE, Bass TA, Popma JJ, Teirstein PS, Kleiman NS, Weisman HF, Musco MH, Catherine FC, Berdan LG, Califf RM, Topol EJ , Prolog Investigators. A multicenter, randomized, double-blind pilot trial of standard versus low dose weight-adjusted heparin in patients treated with the platelet GP IIb/IIIa receptor antibody $c7E_3$ during percutaneous coronary revascularization. J Am Coll Cardiol 1995; 80A (abstract).
68. Tcheng JE, Ellis SG, Kleiman NS, Harrinton RA, Mick MJ, Navetta FI, et al. Outcome of patients treated with the GPIIb/IIIa inhibitor Integrelin during coronary angioplasty: Results of the IMPACT Study. Circulation 1993; 88 (no. 4, part 2):I-595 (abstract).

13

Complex Lesions and Newer Interventional Techniques

Samin Sharma, MD

Coronary lesions with a complex morphology, as mentioned previously, are in most studies associated with a relatively high risk of abrupt closure or suboptimal angiographic results after balloon angioplasty.[1] This is, in part, caused by failure of balloon inflation to exert uniform radial force due to mechanical elasticity and recoil in the eccentric, ulcerated, and disrupted lesions or thrombus propagation or embolization in the lesions with filling defects. In addition, balloon dilatation creates an uncontrolled tear or dissection in the plaque or at times even in the normal vessel wall. One or more of these factors can lead to abrupt occlusion and perhaps higher restenosis. A number of new interventional techniques have been introduced in an attempt to overcome these limitations of balloon angioplasty. These newer interventional techniques can be grouped in broad categories: (1) directional coronary atherectomy, (2) devices to treat lesions with a large thrombus burden, (3) other interventional devices.

Directional Coronary Atherectomy

Directional coronary atherectomy (DCA) may be well suited for complex lesion subtypes because of its ability to directly excise an ulcerated or irregular lesion or intimal flap and to remove atherosclerotic

From: Ambrose JA (ed): *Complex Coronary Lesions in Acute Coronary Syndromes.* © Futura Publishing Co., Inc., Armonk, NY, 1996.

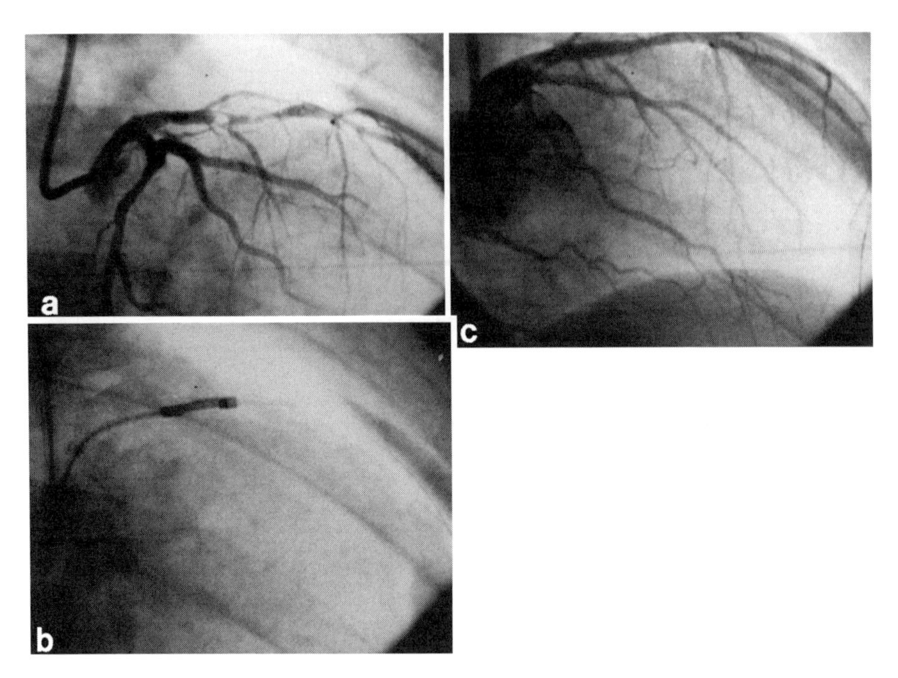

Figure 1: Directional coronary atherectomy of a complex lesion. **(a)** 90% complex—eccentric stenosis in proximal LAD. **(b)** 7 Fr atherocath in LAD. **(c)** Post-DCA smooth large lumen without any dissection.

plaque and intraluminal thrombus (Figures 1A-C). Also, coronary atherectomy by directionally excising the plaque in these complex lesions potentially reduces trauma to the normal vessel segment (Figures 2A-E). In these cases, DCA results in a widely patent vessel lumen without dissection with a resultant decrease in turbulent blood flow. It is to be noted that although DCA effectively excises the plaque, it is not the sole mechanism for all the angiographic improvement as balloon dilatation after initial cuts ("facilitated balloon angioplasty"), contributes equally.[2]

The first published report of the success of DCA in complex lesion morphology was by Hinohara et al. in 1990.[3,4] Immediate success and complication rates of coronary atherectomy were evaluated in three different types of complex lesion subsets, namely ulceration, intimal flaps, and spontaneous or angioplasty (PTCA)-induced coronary dissection. The initial procedural success was 97% for ulcerated lesions (n = 38), 88% for intimal flaps lesions (n = 8), and 77% for lesions with dissection (n = 13). The need for emergency coronary artery bypass

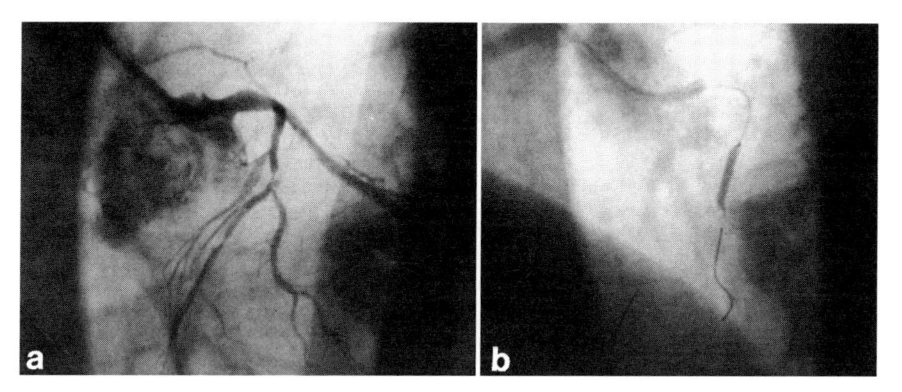

Figure 2: Directional coronary atherectomy of an angiographically suboptimal TCA result. **(a)** Complex lesion with ulcer crater in proximal LAD involving the ostium of first diagonal branch. **(b)** Kissing balloon technique in LAD and diagonal. Continued.

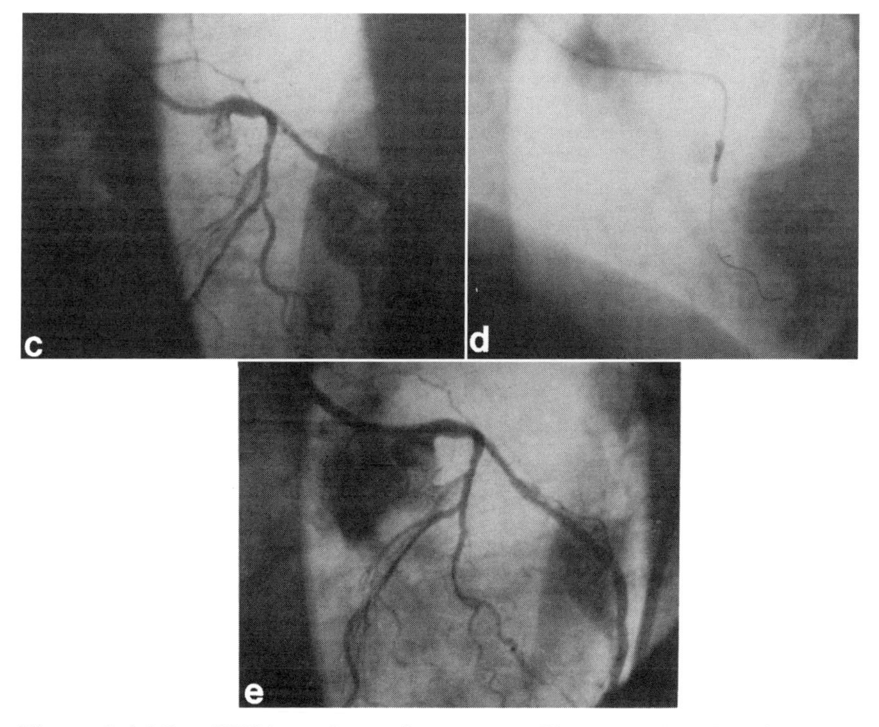

Figure 2: **(c)** Post-PTCA results—ulcer crater still present. **(d)** 6 Fr atherocath with the guidewire in diagonal. **(e)** Post-DCA results—smooth lumen without ulcer crater.

graft (CABG) was highest in the latter subgroup (23% compared to 3% in ulcerated lesion and 0% in the intimal flap). Therefore, in this uncontrolled study, DCA was beneficial in most of these lesions.

Ellis et al. published an in-depth systematic analysis of the relation of stenosis morphology to the procedural results of directional coronary atherectomy for 400 lesions from 378 patients consecutively treated at six major institutions.[5] Lesion success and complications were closely correlated with modified American College of Cardiology/American Heart Association Task force lesion morphology: for type A lesions, 93% success and 3% complications; for type B1 lesions, 88% success and 6% complications; and for type B2 lesions, 75% success and 13% complications. There were too few type C lesions treated for analysis. Multivariate analysis revealed complex probably thrombus associated lesions to have a favorable outcome ($P = 0.05$) while stenosis angulations ($P<0.001$), proximal tortuosity ($P<0.001$), decreased pre-DCA minimal luminal dimension ($P = 0.03$), and calcification ($P = 0.04$) correlated independently with an adverse outcome. These authors concluded that specific lesion subsets such as complex lesions may have a relatively better outcome with DCA compared to PTCA. In this study, lesions associated with large (>2 mm) thrombi were generally avoided.

A similar observation of the effectiveness of DCA in complex lesions was reported in 447 lesions of which 12% had abnormal contour and 2% had an associated thrombus.[6] In this series of primary lesions with abnormal contour, the primary success rate of DCA was 97% with 3.2% major complications, and for lesions with thrombus, primary success was 100% with 0% major complications. In the balloon restenotic lesions, the corresponding rates of primary success was slightly lower and complication rates were higher.

A report by Umans et al. of DCA for treating coronary artery stenoses with complex lesion morphology revealed success rates of 95% and major complications (death, myocardial infarction (MI), urgent CABG) of 5% in 113 lesions from two European centers.[7] Quantitative coronary analysis revealed a residual minimal luminal diameter of 2.42 mm ± 0.52 mm and a diameter stenosis of 26 ± 12% after DCA.

Holmes et al., in a preliminary publication, also reported the results of DCA in 30 thrombus-containing lesions (defined as discrete intraluminal filling defects or gross luminal irregularity) compared to 370 lesions without thrombus.[8] Baseline clinical characteristics revealed a higher incidence of myocardial infarction and unstable angina in patients with thrombus-containing lesions while the baseline diameter stenosis was similar in the two groups. Procedural success was 100% in lesions with thrombus compared to 87% in lesions without thrombus.

Also, procedural complications were 0% in lesions with thrombus compared to 9% in lesions without thrombus. The authors hypothesized that this observed benefit was related to removal of the unstable, lesion-associated thrombus by DCA rather than remodeling of these lesions which usually takes place after PTCA.

Limitations of Directional Coronary Atherectomy

The most important limitation of the DCA technique is the rigid housing and relatively large profile. A tortuous vessel, angulated lesions, and diffusely diseased vessels or diffusely diseased saphenous vein grafts (SVG) are usually considered to be a contraindication for directional atherectomy. Heavy lesion or vessel calcification is also a major obstacle to atherectomy because of the difficulty in crossing the lesion and the inability of the cutter to shave off the calcified plaque. There also appears to be a greater risk of coronary perforation in this setting. Finally, when there is a large thrombus burden, defined as filling defects >2 mm in length, the risk of distal embolization may be excessive.

Devices to Treat Lesions with a Large Thrombus Burden

Complex lesions with an associated large thrombus are at a high risk of distal embolization with the high-profile Simpson atherocath.[9] This is especially true for lesions in degenarated saphenous vein grafts which usually contain soft friable atheromata as well as thrombus. Pretreatment with short-term or prolonged urokinase infusions in the presence of thrombus in native vessels or SVGs has resulted in the increased success of interventional procedures in this setting.[10] In addition to thrombolytic therapy, a number of interventional modalities are available to treat these thrombus-containing complex lesions.

Transluminal Extraction Catheter (TEC)

The TEC device consists of a rotating hollow torque tube with two cutting blades at its cone-shaped distal end. Rotation of the catheter excises soft thrombus and atheromatous material from the lesion and suction applied through the center of the torque tube aspirates the resulting debris into a vacuum system. The TEC device has a unique advantage in removing the excised tissue by vacuum extraction without having to cross the lesion and thereby reducing the propensity of distal embolization. In a preliminary report from the TEC registry, procedural success was reported to be 93% for both native coronary arteries and saphenous vein grafts.[11] Major complications were noted in 5.8% of cases (death 2.8%, Q-wave MI 0.9%, and emergency CABG 2.1%. Mortality was noted to be higher in patients with SVG treatment compared to native coronary arteries (3.2% vs. 1.6%; P = 0.09) but the need for emergency CABG was lower in the SVG patients (0.4% vs. 3.6%; P<0.01). The complication rates were also lower when the TEC procedure was performed in the absence of acute myocardial infarction (Figure 3).

Popma et al. presented procedural results after coronary angioplasty using the TEC catheter in 51 patients with complex lesion anatomy, defined as ostial location, intraluminal thrombus, lesion irregularity, ulceration, or length >10 mm and SVG lesions with extensive degeneration. The procedural success (<50% final diameter obstruction and the absence of major complications) was obtained in 42 patients (84%) with major complications occurring in 14%.[12] Only lesion thrombus correlated with an unsuccessful outcome. This same group also reported preliminarily the results of TEC in SVG lesions.[13] The incidence of distal embolization in SVG lesions with thrombi was noted in 10 of the 76 lesions (14%) treated with TEC, and was associated in most cases with adjunctive balloon dilatation. Also, distal embolization was associated with lower procedural and higher complication rates including mortality after the procedure.

A recent report from the NACI registry evaluating the incidence and angiographic determinants of risks and outcome of coronary embolus and myocardial infarction in 239 lesions (210 patients) with TEC revealed an overall incidence of 5.2% for coronary embolus and myocardial infarction (11 patients) each. Ten of these 11 patients had both coronary embolus and myocardial infarction.[14] Predictors of coronary embolus were thrombus in the lesion, total occlusion, SVG lesions, and left ventricular ejection fraction <50%. Predictors of myocardial infarction were family history of coronary artery disease, thrombus, and target vessel tortuosity. There was higher incidence of CABG in patients with myocardial infarction (27% vs. 1% without infarction; P<0.001) and higher mortality in patient with coronary embolus (36.4% vs. 3.5% without embolus; P<001). Thus, while the presence of large thrombus may be adequately managed with TEC, the complication rate is not small.

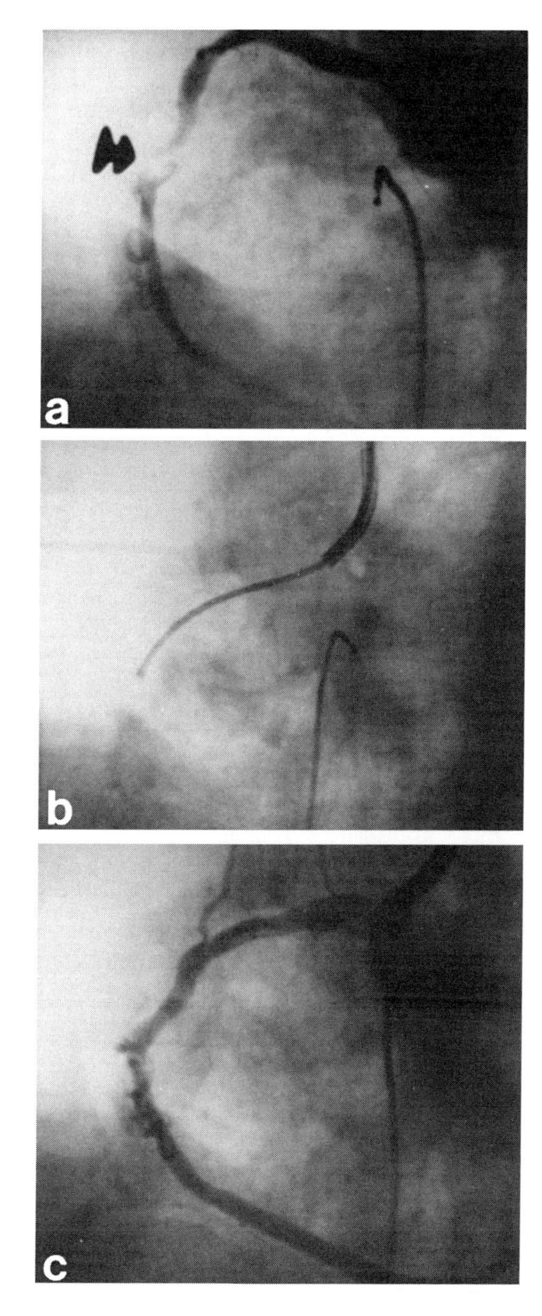

Figure 3: TEC atherectomy of a mid-RCA lesion with a large distal thrombus (arrow). (**a**) Mid-RCA lesion. (**b**) TEC device. (**c**) final result after adjunctive balloon therapy.

Currently a "no-touch policy" has been recommended for elective patients with large amounts of thrombus consisting of the TEC procedure followed by oral anticoagulation and performing the definitive intervention 6–8 weeks later. This method in anecdotal reports has shown to be highly successful with very low complication rates. Another potential scenario would be to use adjunctive thrombolytic therapy as a continuous infusion for several hours prior to the use of TEC or some other interventions.

Percutaneous Thrombectomy Device

The percutaneous thrombectomy catheter (hydrolyser catheter) consists of a 7 French double lumen drainage catheter based on the Venturi effect created by a high-pressure jet. A recent report described the preliminary results of thrombectomy catheters in seven SVG lesions associated with filling defects.[15] All procedures were successful, requiring adjunctive balloon dilatation in six. There were no complications including distal embolization in this small series. The thrombectomy catheter may be a potential treatment for extensively degenerated vein grafts.

Laser Thrombolysis

Lasers have the potential for rapid and safe removal of intravascular thrombus as all types of thrombi avidly absorb a wide range of laser wavelengths that can produce an efficient vaporization or plaque ablation. Lasers may prove to be useful as the sole therapy for acute or chronic thrombosis, as a rescue therapy for failed pharmacological thrombolysis, or as an adjunctive therapy along with other catheter-based devices. The promise of laser thrombolysis is based on the fact that removal of thrombi without significantly damaging the underlying vessel may be preferred to the current techniques and if adjunctive mechanical recanalization is needed, results may be superior with less intimal disruption than with standard techniques. Various lasers are suitable for thrombolysis but most promising are the holmium: YAG laser, fluid-core laser catheter and excimer laser.

Holmium: YAG Laser Coronary Angioplasty

A fresh thrombus is known to have a high water content which results in a large thermal sink and consequently dissipation of laser energy . Since absorption of laser radiation is a function not only of the pigmented component of blood but also of the aqueous component, the holmium laser, whose wavelength coincides with strong water absorption peak, appears to be ideal for thrombolysis.[16] Topaz et al. reported their experience with holmium: YAG laser angioplasty in 13 patients each with a contraindication to thrombolysis and an occlusive thrombus in the infarct-related artery. All lesions were successfully crossed by a wire followed by slow advancement of the holmium: YAG laser catheter across the lesion and subsequent balloon dilatation to achieve the optimal angiographic results.[16] There was no distal embolization or intimal dissection and residual stenosis was minimal in all lesions (<20%). This initial, small clinical experience demonstrated that the holmium: YAG laser was safe in lesions with thrombus, even in those associated with acute infarction.

Fluid-Core Laser Catheter

Delivery of laser energy for thrombolysis is accomplished with a fluid-core light guide causing a low index of refraction and transmission of laser energy distally into the vessel via free-flowing fluid through the open distal end. Fluid-core laser thrombolysis has been used successfully during acute myocardial infarction and may have promise in lesions with large amounts of thrombus.[17]

Excimer Laser Catheter (ELCA)

The excimer laser has been extensively used in the treatment of coronary stenoses unfavorable for balloon angioplasty.[18,19] Rosenfield et al. in a preliminary investigation, described the successful results of excimer laser thrombolysis in lesions with either a high risk for embolization or failed conventional thrombolysis.[20]

Laser-Balloon Angioplasty (LBA)

The laser-balloon angioplasty device pioneered by Spears et al. had shown to be highly effective (>90%) in the treatment of acute thrombotic occlusion de novo or post-PTCA.[21] Unfortunately, because of the high expense, limited potential market, and high restenosis rates when used as a bail-out, this device has been withdrawn from clinical trials.

Other Interventional Devices

Ultrasound Angioplasty

High-intensity, low-frequency ultrasonic energy, if delivered via a catheter, can cause atherosclerotic plaque ablation and clot lysis both in vivo and in vitro by causing direct mechanical trauma to the plaque and cavitation of thrombi. Siegel et al. have described the safety and feasibility of ultrasonic angioplasty in 51 patients with unstable angina of which seven lesions had angiographic evidence of thrombus.[22] Procedural success (<50% diameter stenosis) was achieved by ultrasonic catheter alone in 39 lesions and with adjunctive PTCA in 48 lesions. There were no major complications in this small series. The post-procedure residual lumen was free of haziness or dissection.

Coronary Stent

Stents are available in various design configurations with two important potential indications: preventing early abrupt closure and reducing restenosis. The Cook stent (Gianturco-Roubin) has been approved as a bail-out device after PTCA for abrupt closure or threatened closure caused by intimal dissections. The multicenter registry data suggest that intracoronary stenting can be achieved in the setting of acute and threatened closure with a high degree of technical success. Furthermore, the incidence of major complications (MI, CABG, death) appears acceptably low.[23] Because of the thrombogenic nature of the stent, it should be clearly avoided in thrombotic occlusions.

The Palmaz-Schatz stent (Johnson and Johnson) has been shown to be effective in comparison to routine PTCA in reducing restenosis.[24,25] Recently, the Palmaz-Schatz stent has been approved for lesions in native vessels of >3.0 mm to decrease restenosis. This stent will be favored particularly in eccentric or complex lesions, without large amounts of angiographically visible thrombus (filling defects), to obtain optimal angiographic results (Figure 4A-B). The stents have also been shown to prevent elastic recoil.

It should be remembered that the deployment of an intracoronary stent is not a benign procedure, with stent thrombosis and complications at the vascular access site being its two major limitations. Hopefully, with continued improvements in stent design, e.g., coating the stents with anticoagulants or less aggressive use of anticoagulation in

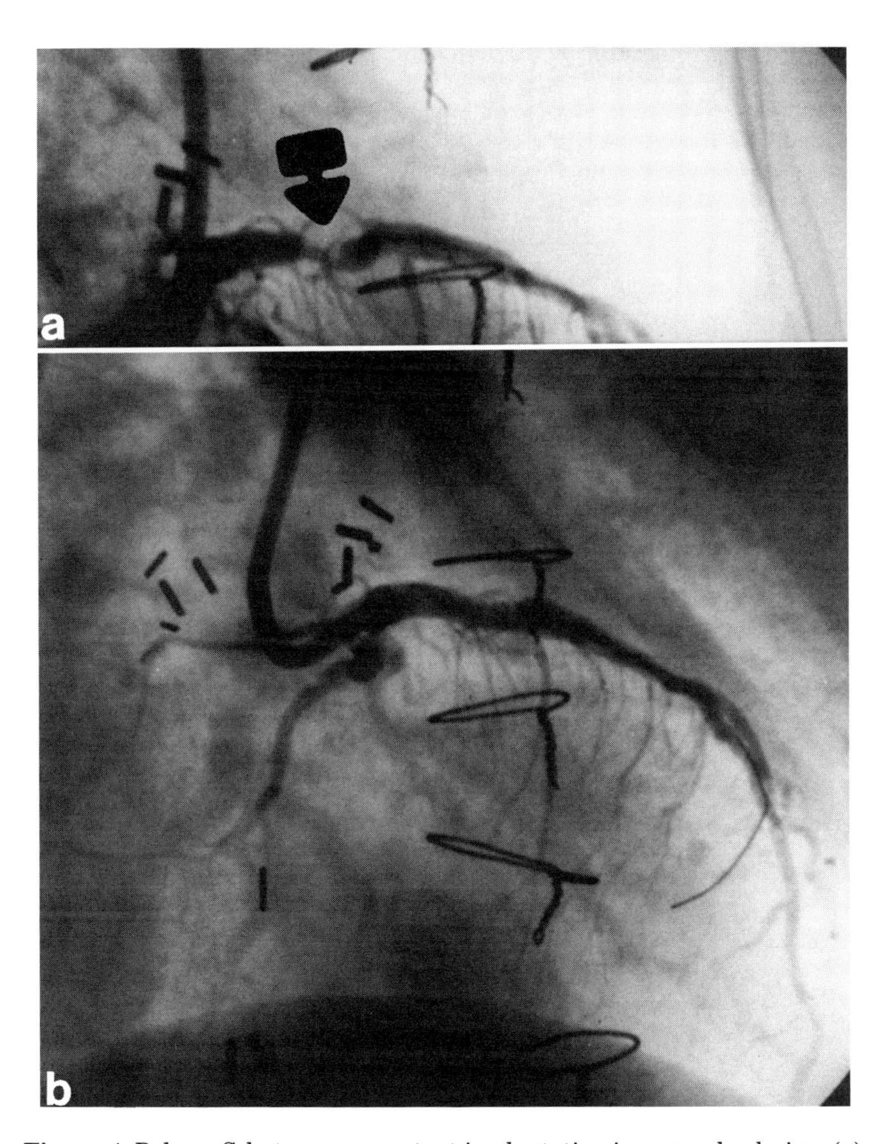

Figure 4: Palmaz-Schatz coronary stent implantation in a complex lesion. **(a)** 80% complex-eccentric stenosis in proximal LAD (arrow). **(b)** Post-stent results with smooth borders.

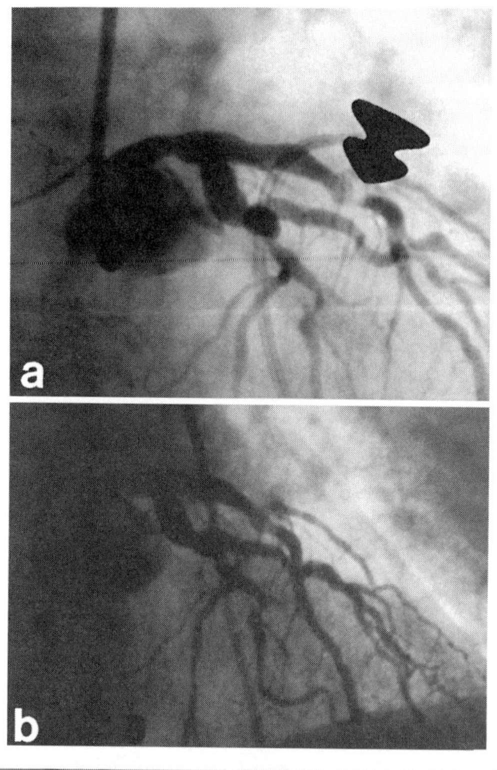

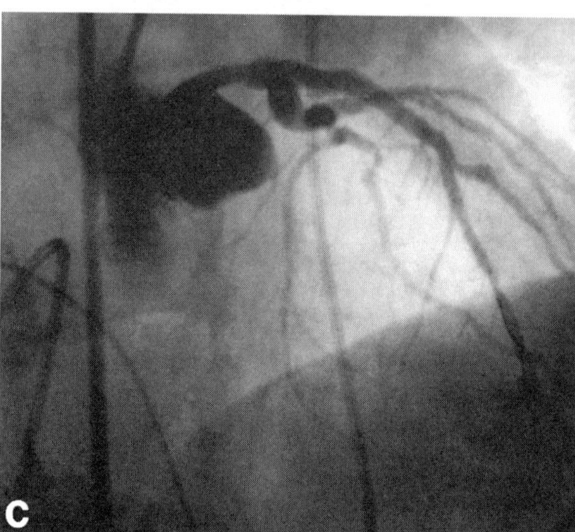

Figure 5: Rotablator atherectomy of a complex lesion in the mid-LAD. **(a)** Complex lesion in the mid-LAD. **(b)** After rotablator (1.5 ± 2.0 mm burrs), the lesion had a good lumen but was a little hazy. **(c)** Following Palmaz-Schatz stent and high-pressure balloon, the artery was widely patent.

the presence of a fully expanded stent confirmed by the use of intravascular ultrasound,[26,27] these limitation will be overcome.

Rotablator

Rotational atherectomy does not appear to have a direct role in complex lesions as use of this device is associated with distal embolization and no-reflow phenomena even in lesions without complex features. However, patients who have been stabilized on medical therapy and have lesions with some complex features but without filling defects, can probably safely undergo rotablator. (Figure 5A-C).

Conclusions

Complex lesions in acute coronary syndromes present a difficult problem for the interventionalist. Conventional balloon angioplasty has been associated with a relatively high incidence of acute thrombotic closure, dissection, elastic recoil, and distal embolization. It appears that improved results may be obtained employing lesion-specific interventional devices such as directional atherectomy or primary stenting for complex/irregular lesions in a large vessel (>3 mm) and the TEC device for native or vein graft thrombotic lesions. However, even in the NACI registry, new interventions are associated with lower success rates and higher complications when thrombus is present.[28] Adjunctive pharmacotherapy consisting of aspirin, prolonged heparinization preprocedure, and perhaps newer antithrombotic or antiplatelet drugs and thrombolytic agents, especially urokinase pre- and intraprocedure, may result in a lower incidence of preprocedural ischemic and clinical complications. However, more studies will need to be reported before deciding what is the optimal interventional therapy for these angiographic complex lesions.

References

1. Ellis SG, Roubin GS, King SB, et al. Angiographic and clinical predictors of acute closure after native vessel coronary angioplasty. Circulation 1988; 77:372–379.
2. Penny W, Schmidt D, Safian R, et al. Insight into the mechanism of luminal improvement after directional coronary atherectomy. Am J Cardiol 1991; 67:435–447.

3. Robertson GC, Rowe M, Selmon M, et al. Directional coronary atherectomy for lesions with complex morphology. Circulation 1990; 82:III-312.
4. Hinohara T, Rowe M, Robertson G, et al. Directional coronary atherectomy for the treatment of coronary lesion with abnormal contour. J Interven Cardiol 1990; 2:57–63.
5. Ellis SG, DeCesare NB, Pinkerton CA, et al. Relation of stenosis morphology and clinical presentation to the procedural results of directional coronary atherectomy. Circulation 1991; 84:644–653.
6. Hinohara T, Rowe M, Robertson G, et al. Effect of lesion characteristics on outcome of directional coronary atherectomy. J Am Coll Cardiol 1991; 17:1112–1120.
7. Umans V, Haine E, Raskin J, et al. One hundred and thirteen attempts at directional coronary atherectomy: the early and combined experience of two European Centers using quantitative angiography to assess their results. Eur Heart J 1992; 139:918–924.
8. Holmes D, Ellis S, Garratt K. Directional coronary atherectomy for thrombus containing lesions: Improved outcome. Circulation 1991; 84:II-26.
9. Holmes D, et al., for the CAVEAT II investigators. The Coronary Angioplasty versus Excisional Atherectomy Trial (CAVEAT II: Preliminary results. Circulation 1993; 88:I-594.
10. Sabri M, Johnson D, Waren M, Cowly M, et al. Intracoronary thrombolysis followed by directional atherectomy. Cathet Cardiovasc Diagn 1992; 26: 15–18.
11. O'Neill W, Kramer B, Sketch M, et al. Mechanical extraction atherectomy: Report of the US Transluminal Extraction Catheter Investigation. Circulation 1992; 86:I-779.
12. Popma J, Leon M, Mintz G, et al. Results of coronary angioplasty using the transluminal extraction catheter. Am J Cardiol 1992; 70:1526–1532.
13. Hong M, Popma J, Leon M, et al. Distal embolization after transluminal extraction catheter treatment of saphenous vein graft lesions. J Am Coll Cardiol 1993; 21:228A.
14. Moses J, Tierstein P, Sketch M, et al. Angiographic determinants of risk and outcome of coronary embolism and myocardial infarction (MI) with the transluminal extraction catheter (TEC): A report from the new approaches to coronary intervention (NACI) registry. J Am Coll Cardiol 1994; 23:218A.
15. Fajadet J, Bar O, Jordan C, et al. Human percutaneous thrombectomy using the new hydrolyser catheter: Preliminary results in saphenous vein graft. J Am Coll Cardiol 1994; 23:220A.
16. Topaz O, Rozenbaum TA, Battista S, et al. Laser facilitated angioplasty and thrombolysis for acute myocardial infarction complicated by prolonged or recurrent chest pain. Cathet Cardiovasc Diagn 1993; 28:7.
17. Gregory KW, Block PC, Knopf WA, et al. Laser thrombolysis in acute myocardial infarction. J Am Coll Cardiol 1993; 21:289A.
18. Bittl JA, Sanborn TA. Excimer laser coronary angioplasty. Circulation 1992; 86:71–78.
19. Cook SL, Eigler NL, Shefer, et al. Percutaneous excimer laser coronary angioplasty for lesions not ideal for balloon angioplasty. Circulation 1991; 84:632–643.

20. Rosenfield K, Pieczek A, Losordo D, et al. Excimer laser thrombolysis for rapid clot dissolution in lesion at high risk for embolization: A potentially useful new application for excimer laser. J Am Coll Cardiol 1992; 19:104A.
21. Spears JR, Safian RD, Douglas R, et al., and LBA study group. Multicenter acute and chronic results of laser balloon angioplasty for refractory abrupt closure after PTCA. Circulation 1991; 84:II-517.
22. Siegel R, Gum J, Ashan A, et al. Percutaneous therapeutic coronary ultrasound angioplasty: Initial clinical experience. European Heart J 1994; (Suppl)15:337.
23. Roubin GS, Cannon AD, Agarwal SK, et al. Intracoronary stenting for acute and threatened closure complicating percutaneous transluminal coronary angioplasty. Circulation 1992; 85:916–927.
24. Serruys PW, Jaegere P, Kiemenij F, et al. A comparison of balloon-expandable-stent implantation with balloon angioplasty in patients with coronary artery disease. N Engl J Med 1994; 33:489–495.
25. Fischman DL, Leon MB, Baim DS, et al. A randomized comparison of coronary-stent placement and balloon angioplasty in the treatment of coronary artery disease. N Engl J Med 1994; 33:496–501.
26. Goldberg SL, Colombo A, Nakamura S, Almagor Y, Maiello L, Tobias J. Benefit of intracoronary ultrasound in the deployment of Palmaz-Schatz stents. J Am Coll Cardiol 1994; 24:996–1003.
27. Mudra H, Klauss V, Blasini R, et al. Ultrasound guidance of Palmaz-Schatz intracoronary stenting with a combined intravascular ultrasound balloon catheter. Circulation 1994; 90:1252–1261.
28. O'Neill W, Sketch M, Steinkiste A, Detre M, for the NACI registry investigators. New device intervention in the treatment of intracoronary thrombus: Report of the NACI registry. Circulation 1993; 88:I-595.

14

Conclusions

John A. Ambrose, MD

Like most medical texts, some sections of this book may not be up to date due to the obligatory delay in publication. As there have been several recent articles of interest on the subject matter contained in this book, I have waited as long as I could to write this last chapter (much to the chagrin of the publishers). This provides the reader with some of the most recent data through the middle of 1995. I have divided this chapter into sections on pathogenetic mechanisms, invasive diagnosis, and medical and interventional therapy.

Pathogenetic Mechanisms

Both postmortem analysis of the coronary arteries and directional atherectomy tissue analysis of culprit lesions in acute syndromes have provided us with some new insights into the mechanisms and factors predisposing to plaque disruption. Computer analysis of plaques indicates that plaque rupture occurs at the point of maximal wall stress in about 60% of cases.[1] The lipid content of the plaque contributes significantly to its propensity of plaque disruption with a lipid volume greater than 40% showing the greatest likelihood.[2] Several angiographic trials of lipid-lowering therapy have been recently published and there is a discrepancy between the degree of plaque regression (which is very small) and the reduction in clinical events on therapy (which is very large).[3,4] It has been suggested that removal of lipid

From: Ambrose JA (ed): *Complex Coronary Lesions in Acute Coronary Syndromes*.

from the plaque may stabilize the plaque and make it less susceptible to plaque disruption.[5] In particular, it has been hypothesized that the ratio of liquid to cholesterol monohydrate crystals may be an important determinant of plaque rupture.[6] The concentration of monohydrate crystalline cholesterol is related to stiffness of the plaque liquid pool and an increase in stiffness reduces stress on the fibrous cap. If the ratio is increased (more liquid or less crystalline cholesterol), the chances of plaque disruption are increased while a decrease in this ratio makes plaque rupture less likely. Lowering plasma LDL and/or increasing HDL by diet, exercise, or drugs may selectively decrease the amount of liquid cholesterol in the plaque and thus stabilize the plaque.

Additional studies have been reported on the role of inflammation in acute coronary syndromes. As has been previously reviewed in Chapters 1, 3, and 7, inflammation is an important component of cap stability with macrophage infiltration common to sites of plaque disruption and thrombus formation. Recent data indicate the importance of cytokines elaborated by T-lymphocytes and metalloproteinases produced by activated macrophages in the genesis of plaque disruption.[7,8] Inflammation can also be demonstrated with directional atherectomy tissue analysis of culprit lesions in unstable angina and non-Q-wave infarction.[9] Plaques showing inflammation also usually contain thrombus.[10] In fact, inflammation and thrombus are undoubtedly interrelated such that inflammation promotes thrombosis and visa versa.

Are there other roles for inflammation in acute syndromes and what is the site of activation? The presence of inflammation as detected by an increase in C-reactive protein and serum amyloid protein on hospital admission has been shown to worsen in-hospital prognosis in patients with unstable angina and prolonged rest pain even when there is no enzymatic evidence of myocardial necrosis.[11] C-reactive protein is a cytokine-mediated acute phase reactant produced in the liver. What activates this protein in unstable angina is at present unclear. However, it appears that the microcirculation and myocardium may also be a site of inflammatory activation in unstable angina as well as in myocardial infarction. In a preliminary investigation of patients with unstable angina, de Servi et al. found that an increase in white cell markers of inflammation were present across the microcirculation (between the distal coronary artery and the coronary sinus) rather than across the culprit lesion in the epicardial coronary artery (between the systemic artery and the coronary artery just distal to the lesion).[12] Thus, in certain situations, ischemia might lead to myocardial effects provoking an inflammatory reaction.

Invasive Diagnosis Angioscopy

Angioscopy

More data have been published concerning the comparison of angiography and angioscopy. While angiography underestimates intracoronary thrombus, its specificity is very high while sensitivity is low.[13,14] For a diagnosis of intracoronary thrombus, angioscopy is thus the image tool of choice. In patients with postinfarction angina, Tabata et al. identified intracoronary thrombus by angioscopy in all 17 patients while in postinfarction patients without recurrent angina pectoris, intracoronary thrombus was identified in only 15%. ($P<0.01$).[15]

Intravascular Ultrasound

This technique has gained increased popularity over the past few years for assessing the extent of atherosclerosis and the results of percutaneous coronary intervention. With intracoronary ultrasound (ICUS), two-dimensional, tomographic views of the coronary arteries provide accurate information on lumen diameter and wall structures including the extent of atherosclerotic plaque formation and calcification.[16,17] Compared to contrast angiography, it is a more sensitive technique for defining these characteristics. ICUS has also been used to assess lesional morphology and thus can be related to the clinical presentation of the patient and compared to angiographic morphology. The use of ICUS involves over-the-wire techniques similar to angioplasty. It is associated with a minor risk, particularly of transient vascular spasm. The complication rate of ICUS (but not necessarily the direct cause of) was increased in patients with acute coronary syndromes in comparison to stable angina or asymptomatic patients.[18]

Plaque Morphology and Angiography

With ICUS, one can divide atherosclerotic plaques into soft, fibrous, calcified, and mixed (Figure 1). Soft plaques have homogeneous intimal echoes less than that of the adventitia and calcification is not present. At least 80% of the plaque area had this composition. Fibrous plaques had at least 80% of the plaque with an echodensity greater than or equal to that seen for the adventitia without the presence of calcium. The other plaque classifications are combinations of the above.

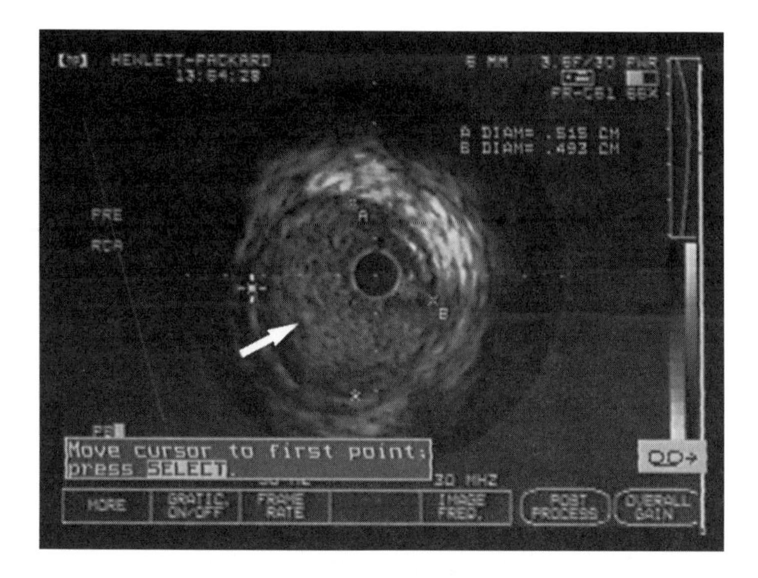

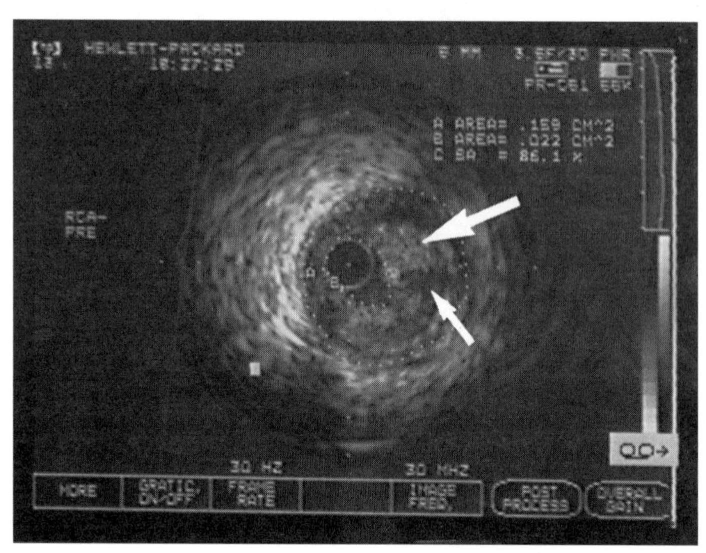

Figure 1: Top: ICUS of a lesion in the right coronary artery showing soft plaque (small arrow). **Bottom:** ICUS of a different lesion also in the right coronary artery with mixed soft (small arrow) and fibrotic (larger arrow) plaque.

Soft plaques are noted to have a high content of lipid and thrombi and would be more common in acute syndromes. Unfortunately, the ability of ICUS to specifically detect thrombus is limited. Patients with unstable angina had a significantly increased incidence of soft plaque with fewer calcified and mixed plaques and less intralesional calcium deposits than lesions from patients with stable angina.[19,20] It was also reported that the ICUS demonstration of soft plaque was more sensitive though less specific (74% and 59%, respectively) than the sensitivity and specificity of a complex lesion as assessed by angiography (40% and 82%, respectively) for a clinical diagnosis of unstable angina.[19,20]

Medical Management

New Antithrombin and Antiplatelet Agents

The results of several large trials with the use of new antithrombin and antiplatelet agents have yet to be reported. Preliminary data are available (Table 1). Hirudin has been evaluated in GUSTO II and several different intravenous IIb/IIIa blockers have been or are being evaluated in clinical trials in unstable angina.[21–23] The results of the large trials should be available in 1996. Hirulog was evaluated in the TIMI-

Table 1
New Antithrombotics for Acute Coronary Disease: Clinical Trials

	Trial		
New Agents	*Unstable Angina*	*Myocardial Infarction*	*PTCA Occlusion*
Hirudin	GUSTO Pilot GUSTO-II OASIS	TIMI-5 Pilot (rt-PA) TIMI-6 Pilot (SK) TIMI-9 GUSTO-II OASIS	Rotterdam Pilot GUSTO II HELVETICA
Hirulog	Montreal Pilot TIMI-7 Pilot TIMI-8	Montreal Pilot (SK) ISIS-5 HERO(SK)	Topol et al.
IIb/IIIa Receptor blocker	ECSG Pilot Hopkins Pilot CAPTURE	TAMI-8 IMPACT (MI)	EPIC IMPACT (PTCA)

With permission of V. Fuster and Circulation 1994; 90:2140.

7 trial comparing four different doses of hirulog and aspirin in over 400 patients with unstable angina in a randomized, double-blind study.[24] Death and myocardial infarctions were significantly reduced at hospital discharge and after 6 weeks with the three higher doses of hirulog compared to the lowest dose of hirulog which was essentially homeopathic (12–50 times lower than the other three doses). Unfortunately, no comparison to heparin was done. These results were supposed to be tested in the larger TIMI-8 trial, but the trial has been canceled.

Prolonged Infusions of Thrombolytic Therapy in Unstable Angina

While the results of most trials of thrombolytic therapy in unstable angina have either been negative or even detrimental, (increased clinical events in thrombolytic-treated patients), nearly all trials have infused thrombolytic therapy for no more than 12 hours. Prolonged infusions have rarely been performed. Recently, Romeo et al. reported the results of a randomized trial of 3 days of low dose t-PA plus heparin versus heparin alone in 67 patients with refractory unstable angina.[25] In patients treated with t-PA, there was a significant reduction in acute myocardial infarction in hospital as well as a significant decrease in chest pain and myocardial ischemia on follow-up. However, in contrast to the above, in a preliminary investigation, Oltrona et al. found no benefit to a 48-hour infusion of streptokinase in new-onset angina pectoris versus either standard therapy or a 90-minute streptokinase infusion.[26] As reviewed in Chapter 11, I doubt that thrombolytic therapy, even given as a prolonged infusion, will be beneficial in unstable angina.

Interventional Therapy

Perfusion Balloon Angioplasty

In the randomized perfusion balloon catheter trial, patients undergoing PTCA were randomized to one of two primary balloon strategies.[27] The standard strategy included one to four dilatations of up to 60 seconds while the prolonged strategy required an inflation of up to 15 minutes which could be repeated. In both strategies, the lesion was crossed with a perfusion balloon. In patients with irregular, ulcereous, thrombus-laden lesions (complex lesions), the success rate was higher for the prolonged versus the standard strategy (98% versus 87%, respectively) and major dissections were less (3% versus 14%, respectively). However, there was no difference in the 6–month restenosis rate (52% versus 43%, respectively).[28]

Coronary Stenting

Stenting has become very popular in the treatment of complex lesions in acute syndromes as long as one or more large filling defects (the definition of intracoronary thrombus used by some investigators) are not present. Of course, in this situation, thrombus can be lysed prior to deployment of the stent (see Chapter 12). As most of these lesions are highly eccentric, the Palmaz-Shatz stent has been the stent of choice as it is more likely to prevent prolapse of intima into the lumen than the looser coil stents. However, no randomized trial has prospectively addressed this group of lesions. In the STRESS trial, a subgroup of 82 lesions were complex and ulcerated and could be compared retrospectively.[29] Lesion morphology did not influence the acute procedural results between stenting and angioplasty but the relative benefits of stents over balloon angioplasty alone on late follow-up were greater for concentric lesions in comparison to complex, ulcerated lesions.

Cardiac Surgery

To the noninterventionalist, this book may appear skewed since we did not consider bypass surgery as therapy. However, as the subject of the book was the complex lesion, management was focused on the treatment of this lesion. Nevertheless, all interventionalists realize that for the treatment of the patient, bypass surgery is, in some cases, the only option. In unprotected left main artery disease, three-vessel disease particularly with left ventricular dysfunction, or patients with less than suitable lesions for percutaneous intervention, surgery may be either absolutely indicated or preferable, depending on the situation.

In conclusion, the treatment of a complex lesion in some cases is neither simple nor uncomplicated. Therapy is evolving so we must remain open-minded and receptive to new approaches. We should, however, not forget that the therapy of lesions is secondary to the well-being of our patients. Whatever our approach, patient safety and benefit must always be foremost in our minds.

References

1. Cheng GC, Loree HM, Kamm RD, Fishbein MC, Lee RT. Distribution of circumferential stress in ruptured and stable atherosclerotic lesions. Circulation 1993; 87:1179–1187.
2. Davies MJ, Richardson PD, Woolf N, et al. Risk of thrombosis in human atherosclerotic plaque: Role of extracellular lipid, macrophage and smooth muscle content. Br Heart J 1993; 69:377–381.
3. Brown G, Albers JJ, Fisher LD, et al. Regression of coronary artery disease as a result of intensive lipid-lowering therapy in men with high levels of apolipo-protein B. N Engl J Med 1990; 323:1289–1298.
4. Watts GF, Lewis B, Brunt JNH, et al. Effects on coronary artery disease of lipid lowering diet, or diet plus cholestryramine, in the St. Thomas Atherosclerosis Regression Study (STARS). Lancet 1992; 339:563–569.
5. Brown BG, Zhao XQ, Sacco DE, Albers JJ. Lipid-lowering and plaque regression: New insights into prevention of plaque disruption and clinical events in coronary disease. Circulation 1993; 87:1781–1791.
6. Loree HM, Tobias BJ, Gibson LJ, et al. Mechanical properties of model atherosclerotic lesion lipid pools. Athero Thromb 1994; 14:230–234.
7. Libby P, Lee RT. Role of Activated macrophages and T-lymphocytes in rupture of coronary plaques. In Braunwald WE: Heart Disease. Update 2: 1–9, Philadelphia, W.B. Saunders Co., 1995.
8. Galis Z, Sukhova G, Lark M, Libby P. Increased expression of matrix metalloproteinases and matrix degrading activity in vulnerable regions of human atherosclerotic plaques. J Clin Invest 1994; 94:2493–2503.
9. Moreno PR, Falk E, Palacios FI, et al. Macrophage infiltration in acute coronary syndromes. Circulation 1994; 90:775–778.
10. Ambrose JA, Fyfe BS, Sharma SK, et al. Clinical-pathologic observations of rest angina from atherectomy tissue analysis: Role of lipids, inflammation, and thrombus. J Am Cell Cardiol, submitted for publication.
11. Liuzzo A, Biasucci LM, Gallimore JR, et al. The prognostic value of C-reactive protein and serum amyloid 'a' protein in severe unstable angina. N Engl J Med 1994; 331(7):417–424.
12. de Servi S, Mazzone A, Ricevuti G, et al. Site of leukocyte activation in unstable angina. J Am Coll Cardiol 1995; 312A (abstract).
13. Heijer PD, Foley DP, Escaned J, et al. Angioscopic versus angiographic detection of intimal dissection and intracoronary thrombus. J Am Coll Cardiol 1994; 24:649–654.
14. Manzo K, Nesto R, Sassower M, et al. Coronary lesion morphology by angioscopy vs. angiography: The ability of angiography to detect thrombi. J Am Coll Cardiol 1994; I-484A (abstract).
15. Tabata H, Mizuno K, Arakawa K, et al. Angioscopic identification of coronary thrombus in patients with postinfarction angina. J Am Coll Cardiol 1995; 25:1282–1285.
16. Nissen SE, Grines CL, Gurley JC, et al. Application of a new phased-array ultrasound imaging catheter in the assessment of vascular dimensions. In vivo comparison to cineangiography. Circulation 1990; 119:1392–1400.
17. Barzilai B, Saffitz JE, Miller JG, Sobel BE. Quantitative ultrasonic charac-

terization of the nature of atherosclerotic plaques in human aorta. Circ Res 1987; 60:459–63.
18. Hausmann D, Erbel R, Marie J, et al. The safety of intracoronary ultrasound. Circulation 1995; 91:623–630.
19. Hodgson J McB, Reddy KG, Suneja R, et al. Intracoronary ultrasound imaging: Correlation of plaque morphology with angiography, clinical syndrome and procedural results in patients undergoing coronary angioplasty. J Am Coll Cardiol 1993; 21:35–44.
20. Rasheed Q, Nair R, Sheehan H, et al. Correlation of ultrasound plaque characteristics in atherosclerotic coronary artery disease patients with clinical variables. Am J Cardiol 1994; 73:753–758.
21. Schulman SP, Pascal JGC, Clermont G. Integrelin in unstable angina: A double-blind randomized trial. Circulation 1993; 88(no. 4, part 2):I-608A (abstract).
22. Simoons ML, de Boer MJ, van den Brand, et al. Randomized trial of a GPIIB/IIIA platelet receptor blocker in refractory unstable angina. Circulation 1994; 89:596–603.
23. Theroux P, White H, David D, et al. A heparin-controlled study of MK-383 in unstable angina. Circulation 1994; 90(no. 4, part 2):I231 (abstract).
24. Fuchs J, Mc Cabe CH, Antman EM, et al., for the TIMI-7 Investigators. Hirulog in the treatment of unstable angina: Results of the TIMI-7 trial. J Am Coll Cardiol 1994; 56A (abstract).
25. Romeo F, Rosano GMC, Martuscelli E, et al. Effectiveness of prolonged low dose recombinant tissue-type plasminogen activator for refractory unstable angina. J Am Coll Cardiol 1995; 25:1295–1299.
26. Oltrona L, Merlini PA, Spinola, et al. A randomized trial on prolonged streptokinase infusion with concomitant heparin administration in unstable angina pectoris. Circulation 1993; 88(no. 4, Part 2):I-608A (abstract).
27. Ohman EM, Marquis JF, Ricci DR, et al. A randomized comparison of the effects of gradual prolonged versus standard primary balloon inflation on early and late outcome: Results of a multicenter clinical trial. Circulation 1994; 89:1118–1125.
28. Kereiakes DJ, Sketch MH Jr., Ohman EM. Perfusion balloon angioplasty in patients with complex coronary lesion morphology. J Interven Cardiol 1995; 7:4B—8B(Suppl B).
29. Savage M, Fischman D, Hirshfeld J, et al. Effect of lesion morphology on angiographic outcome after balloon angioplasty and coronary stenting: Result from the STRESS trial. Circulation 1994; 90:I-324.

Index